Current Topics in Microbiology
154 and Immunology

Cytomegaloviruses

Edited by J. K. McDougall

With 58 Figures

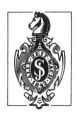

Springer-Verlag
Berlin Heidelberg NewYork
London Paris Tokyo HongKong

JAMES K. MCDOUGALL PhD.
Research Professor of Pathology
University of Washington,
Member, Fred Hutchinson Cancer Research Center,
1124, Columbia Street, Seattle, WA 98104 , USA

ISBN 3-540-51514-3 Springer-Verlag Berlin Heidelberg NewYork
ISBN 0-387-51514-3 Springer-Verlag NewYork Berlin Heidelberg

© Springer-Verlag Berlin Heidelberg 1990
Library of Congress Catalog Card Number 15-12910
Printed in Germany

The use of registered names, trademarks, etc. in this publication does not imply, even in the
absence of a specific statement, that such names are exempt from the relevant protective
laws and regulations and therefore free for general use.

Product Liability: The publisher can give no guarantee for information about drug dosage
and application thereof contained in this book. In every individual case the respective user
must check its accuracy by consulting other pharmaceutical literature.

Typesetting: Thomson Press (India) Ltd., New Delhi
Offsetprinting: Saladruck, Berlin; Bookbinding: B. Helm, Berlin
2123/3020-543210 — Printed on acid-free paper.

Preface

Named for the enlarged, inclusion-bearing cells characteristic of infection by these viruses, cytomegaloviruses present a significant challenge to both microbiologist and immunologist. Although most primary infections in humans are subclinical, cytomegalovirus can be associated with a wide spectrum of disease, particularly when infection occurs in the immuno-compromised individual or as a result of congenital or perinatal infection. Although reinfection with cytomegalovirus has been demonstrated, most recurrent and persistent infections result from the reactivation of latent virus. Cytomegaloviruses, like other members of the Herpesviridae family, have the capacity to establish latency after a primary infection but the mechanisms for establishing the nonreplicating but reactivatable state have not been defined. The factors responsible for the spectrum of manifestations of cytomegalovirus infection are largely undetermined but host immunological function, route of infection, and size of inoculum all contribute to the extent and severity of disease.

Cytomegaloviruses have the largest genomes in the herpes-virus family, approximately 240 kilobase pairs, providing a potential coding capacity for more than 200 proteins of which less than one-fourth have been mapped and described. There are many similarities to other herpesviruses in genome structure and gene expression; for example, three temporal classes of genes can be identified as α (immediate-early), β (early), and γ (late) products. The first five chapters of this volume review and describe recent developments in understanding the transcription and regulation of these gene classes. Analysis of the molecular biology of cytomegaloviruses has progressed more slowly than that of herpes simplex virus or Epstein-Barr virus but has now received a significant boost from the progress made by Barrell's group in sequencing the complete genome of human cytomegalovirus strain AD 169. Their analysis of the open reading frames in the AD 169 sequence is in the sixth chapter. A knowledge of proteins involved in the sequential steps of virus replication and assembly can provide the basis for antiviral strategies as well as for an understanding of the host's immune response, a subject dealt with in the last section of this book. Efforts to establish a basis upon which effective prevention or modulation of cytomegalovirus infection can be developed are making good progress.

We hope that the reviews and the new results presented herein will provide encouragement to researchers in this field and to those dealing with often insidious consequences of infection by cytomegalovirus.

James K. McDougall
Seattle, Spring 1989

List of Contents

Gene Expression

T. STAMMINGER and B. FLECKENSTEIN: Immediate-Early
Transcription Regulation of Human
Cytomegalovirus   3

D. H. SPECTOR, K. M. KLUCHER, D. K. RABERT, and
D. A. WRIGHT: Human Cytomegalovirus Early
Gene Expression   21

E. S. MOCARSKI, Jr., G. B. ABENES, W. C. MANNING,
L. C. SAMBUCETTI, and J. M. CHERRINGTON:
Molecular Genetic Analysis of Cytomegalovirus and
Gene Regulation in Growth, Persistence and Latency   47

J. A. NELSON, J. W. GNANN, JR., and P. GHAZAL:
Regulation and Tissue-Specific Expression of Human
Cytomegalovirus   75

H. C. ISOM and C. Y. YIN: Guinea Pig Cytomegalovirus
Gene Expression   101

Protein Coding

M. S. CHEE, A. T. BANKIER, S. BECK, R. BOHNI, C. M.
BROWN, R. CERNY, T. HORSNELL, C. A. HUTCHISON, III,
T. KOUZARIDES, J. A. MARTIGNETTI, E. PREDDIE,
S. C. SATCHWELL, P. TOMLINSON, K. M. WESTON, and
B. G. BARRELL: Analysis of the Protein-Coding
Content of the Sequence of Human Cytomegalovirus
Strain AD 169   125

G. JAHN and M. MACH: Human Cytomegalovirus
Phosphoproteins and Glycoproteins and Their
Coding Regions.   171

Immune Response

U. H. KOSZINOWSKI, M. DEL VAL, and M. J. REDDEHASE:
Cellular and Molecular Basis of the Protective
Immune Response to Cytomegalovirus Infection . .   189

L. RASMUSSEN: Immune Response to Human
Cytomegalovirus Infection   221

E. GÖNCZÖL and S. PLOTKIN: Progress in Vaccine
Development for Prevention of Human CMV
Infection   255

Subject Index   275

List of Contributors

(Their addresses can be found at the beginning of the respective chapters)

ABENES, G. B.
BARRELL, B. G.
BANKIER, A. T.
BECK, S.
BOHNI, R.
BROWN, C. M.
CERNY, R.
CHEE, M. S.
CHERRINGTON, J. M.
DEL VAL, M.
FLECKENSTEIN, B.
GHAZAL, P.
GNANN, Jr., J. W.
GÖNCZÖL, E.
HORSNELL, T.
HUTCHISON, III, C. A.
ISOM, H. C.
JAHN, G.
KLUCHER, K. M.
KOSZINOWSKI, U. H.

KOVZARIDES, T.
MACH, M.
MANNING, W. C.
MARTIGNETTI, J. A.
MOCARSKI, E.
NELSON, J. A.
PLOTKIN, S.
PREDDIE, E.
RABERT, D. K.
RASMUSSEN, L.
REDDEHASE, M. J.
SAMBUCETTI, L. C.
SATCHWELL, S. C.
SPECTOR, D. H.
STAMMINGER, T.
TOMLINSON, P.
WESTON, K. M.
WRIGHT, D. A.
YIN, C. Y.

Gene Expression

Immediate-Early Transcription Regulation of Human Cytomegalovirus

T. Stamminger and B. Fleckenstein

1 Genomic Localization of Immediate-Early Genes   3
2 Pattern of Immediate-Early Gene Transcription   4
3 Functional Organization of the Immediate-Early-1-Upstream Region   6
4 Structural and Functional Organization of the Enhancer Region   8
References   16

1 Genomic Localization of Immediate-Early Genes

Herpesvirus genomes are expressed in three temporally regulated phases during productive infection. The first period of transcription, commonly termed "immediate early" (IE), follows entry of the virus into the host cell. It is independent of de novo synthesis of viral proteins. In general, a second ("early") phase follows, when a number of regulatory proteins and viral enzymes are synthesized. During the third phase ("late"), which begins with onset of virion DNA replication, viral structural proteins are synthesized (Honess and Roizman 1974, 1975). Immediate-early proteins are thought to exert important regulatory functions in the switch from the IE to the early phase. If permissive cells are infected in the presence of cycloheximide or anisomycin, both potent inhibitors of protein synthesis, viral IE RNA is accumulated. This approach was applied to investigate IE transcription in various strains of human cytomegalovirus (HCMV) (Wathen and Stinski 1982; McDonough and Spector 1983; Wilkinson et al. 1984; DeMarchi 1981). The IE RNA of HCMV arises from a few distinct regions of the viral genome. The region of highest transcriptional activity is localized between map units 0.66 and 0.77 in the genomes of all HCMV strains that have been investigated (Fig. 1). This region is part of the large unique compartment of the viral genome, for instance corresponding to the HindIII-E fragment of HCMV strain AD169 and the XbaI-E and -N fragments of strain Towne. It comprises approximately 20 kb.·

The four transcription units with most abundant IE expression have been termed IE-1 to IE-4 (Jahn et al. 1984; Stinski et al. 1983) (Fig. 1). The major transcript from the IE-1 gene was found to be a polyadenylated mRNA of 1.9 kb (Jahn et al. 1984; Stinski et al. 1983). The IE-2 gene is expressed into mRNA of

Institut für Klinische und Molekulare Virologie der Universität Erlangen-Nürnberg, Loschgestraße 7, D-8520 Erlangen, FRG

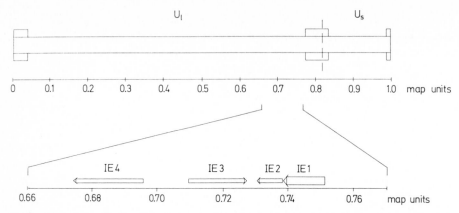

Fig. 1. Genomic localization of the four major IE transcription units within the HCMV genome. The four major IE transcription units (IE-1 to IE-4) are located between map units 0.66 and 0.77 of the HCMV genome. The entire genome has about 230 kb. U_l, long unique segment; U_s, short unique segment of the viral genome

approximately 2 kb (JAHN et al. 1984; STINSKI et al. 1983; WILKINSON et al. 1984). Some controversy remained about the IE-3 region (map units 0.709–0.728) which codes for a 2.2-kb transcript in strain AD169 and for a 1.95-kb message in the strain Towne of HCMV. While JAHN et al. (1984), WILKINSON et al. (1984), and STINSKI et al. (1983) classified this transcript as immediate early, STAPRANS and SPECTOR (1986) reported early transcription from this region of the viral genome. The IE-4 gene appeared highly unusual in structure and expression pattern. It is transcribed into a 5-kb RNA. While part of this RNA is polyadenylated, the majority of the transcripts were found in nonpolyadenylated fractions. In contrast to other IE genes of HCMV, the DNA coding for the 5-kb RNA is also expressed during late virus replication in high quantities. No compelling evidence could be found for a protein to be encoded (PLACHTER et al. 1988) within the entire nucleotide sequence of the IE-4 gene. This genomic region is devoid of translational reading frames greater than 200 nucleotides in the direction of transcription; part of it was shown to be capable of transforming primary embryonic rat fibroblasts and NIH3T3 cells in vitro (NELSON et al. 1982, 1984).

Low-abundance IE transcription was also reported from a number of other genomic regions (DEMARCHI 1981; MCDONOUGH and SPECTOR 1983; WATHEN and STINSKI 1982). At least four additional IE-mRNAs that are differentially spliced could be assigned to the unique short HCMV genome region (WESTON 1988).

2 Pattern of Immediate Early Gene Transcription

The IE-1 region, also referred to as the major IE gene, codes for the most abundant type of IE RNA with a size of about 1.9 kb under the experimental conditions of cycloheximide block (STINSKI et al. 1983; WILKINSON et al. 1984; JAHN et al. 1984). The predominant RNA is transcribed from right to left in the prototype

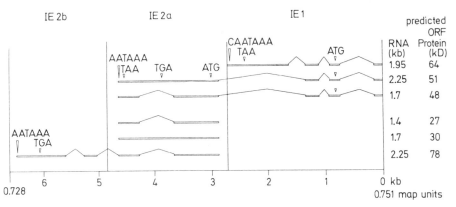

Fig. 2. Splicing pattern of IE-1 and IE-2-specific transcripts. Direction of transcription is *from right to left*. The exons of the six known mRNAs originating from this region are given in *double lines*. Start and stop codons for reading frames and polyadenylation sites are indicated by *triangles*. (Data taken from HERMISTON et al. 1987). After submission of this manuscript STENBERG et al. (1989) reported that HCMV strain Towne does not have a stop codon at nt. 1092 within the IE-2 sequence. Thus the unspliced 1.7 kb message derived from IE-2 is capable of coding for a protein of 40 kd whereas the spliced messages of 1.7 and 2.25 kb code for proteins of 55 and 86 kd, respectively

arrangement of the HCMV genome (0.739–0.751 map units) (Fig. 2). The gene has been determined in nucleotide sequence, and the transcripts were analyzed by nuclease mapping (STENBERG et al. 1984; AKRIGG et al. 1985). The major 1.9-kb IE transcript is made up of three small (121, 88, and 185 nt) and one large exon (1342 nt). The three introns (827, 114, and 70 nt) are located near the 5' end of the gene. The single open reading frame starts in the second exon and has the coding capacity for a polypeptide of 491 amino acids; the molecular weight was calculated to be 63.8 kDa (AKRIGG et al. 1985). If the mRNA was selected by hybridization to immobilized DNA of the IE-1 region and translated in vitro, it could be shown that it encodes the predominant protein found in infected cells within the first hour after infection (STENBERG et al. 1984). The protein is quickly accumulated in the nucleus of infected cells (MICHELSON-FISKE et al. 1977). The molecular weight of this IE protein was estimated by polyacrylamide gel electrophoresis to be approximately 75 kDa (BLANTON and TEVETHIA 1981; CAMERON and PRESTON 1981; GIBSON 1981; WILKINSON et al. 1984). A proline-rich region near the N terminus of the predominant IE protein might explain anomalous mobility in SDS polyacrylamide gels due to disruption of the helical protein structure (AKRIGG et al. 1985). Since it could be shown that the major IE protein is phosphorylated (GIBSON 1981), it was suggested that posttranslational modification may contribute to the unexpected migration pattern (STINSKI et al. 1983).

The IE-2 region lies immediately downstream to region 1 (Fig. 2). Northern blot analyses detected at least four classes of mRNA in the size range from 1.1 to 2.25 kb (STENBERG et al. 1985; AKRIGG et al. 1985). This suggested that the various mRNAs are formed through differential splicing from a rather small part of the genome. The IE-2 gene is transcribed in the same direction as the major IE-1 gene. A functional promoter with the CAAT and TATA sequence elements was found located between the 3' terminus of the IE-1 gene and the transcription initiation site of IE-2. A polyadenylation signal is located about 1.6 kb downstream. The single open reading frame starts with nucleotide 252, ending with nucleotide 1092. It forms the reading frame for a polypeptide of 280 amino acids (30 kDa) in the unspliced transcript. By splicing nucleotide 836 onto nucleotide 1301, the first stop codon is eliminated and the reading frame extends to a second stop at nucleotide 1481. Thus, the spliced RNA has a reading frame for 252 amino acids (27 kDa). A less abundant spliced RNA was detected that uses a splice donor site upstream of the second stop codon and is spliced onto sequences about 2 kb downstream (STENBERG et al. 1985) (Fig. 2). This led to the subdivision of the IE-2 region into IE-2a and IE-2b (Fig. 2). The IE-2b gene contains one additional intron. The resulting IE-2b transcript has 2.25 kb and is able to code for a protein of 78 kDa (HERMISTON et al. 1987). Two additional types of mRNA were detected in which the RNA from the first three exons of the IE-1 gene are differentially spliced to region 2 transcripts, extending the number of IE-2 proteins (Fig. 2). Remarkably, the relative abundancy of the various IE-2 transcripts varies with the time course of HCMV infection; the spliced IE-2 transcripts were preferentially found during the initial IE phase, while, later on in the replication cycle, unspliced transcripts from this genomic region dominated (STENBERG et al. 1985). The predominant IE-2 protein had a molecular weight of 56 kDa, whereas several other proteins in the molecular weight range from 16.5 to 42 kDa could also be detected (STINSKI et al. 1983).

Immediate-early proteins are assumed to exert regulatory functions by acting in *trans* on *cis* elements such as promoters or enhancers. EVERETT and DUNLOP (1984) could show that cotransfection of the herpes simplex virus type 1 glycoprotein D or the rabbit β-globin gene with the entire major IE gene region (*Xba*I-E fragment of strain Towne, *Hind*III-E fragment of strain AD169) resulted in activation of the heterologous promoters by the HCMV IE gene products. HERMISTON et al. (1987) found that a plasmid expressing the IE-1 and IE-2 genes activated the adenovirus E-2 promoter. In this experiment, the IE-1 protein did not function independently as gene activator, while the IE-2 proteins did. Transactivation by IE-2 proteins was augmented in the presence of IE-1 polypeptide. It suggested that IE-2 gene products might exert maximal stimulatory effects only if combined with the IE-1 protein. Since transactivator and inhibitor effects in various cell lines depend on numerous factors (such as concentration of transactivating proteins, their relative abundancy, differentiation of cells), far more work will be required to define the regulatory effect of each single IE-1/2 protein at various stages of replication and persistence in different cell types.

3 Functional Organization of the Immediate Early-1-Upstream Region

The IE-1 gene is efficiently expressed immediately following entry of virions into permissive cells (MICHELSON-FISKE et al. 1977). This could be taken as a hint that strong *cis*-regulatory elements may govern the IE-1 promoter. TATA and CAAT sequence elements are found within 65 bp upstream of the transcription initiation site. These sequences form the IE-1 promoter and are required for a low level of gene expression in intact cells and in cell-free transcription systems (STINSKI and ROEHR 1985; GHAZAL et al. 1987, 1988b). A strong enhancer was found upstream of the IE-1 promoter by the "enhancer trap" CI (WEBER et al. 1984; BOSHART et al. 1985). Linearized SV40 genomes with deletion of the two major functional enhancer domains were cotransfected with randomly fragmented DNA of the HCMV IE region. Spontaneous intracellular ligation resulted in replication-competent SV40-type recombinant viruses with HCMV DNA sequences replacing the genuine enhancer. The respective HCMV DNA fragments, representing the upstream region between nucleotides -528 and -118, fulfilled the essential criteria of a eukaryotic enhancer element (BOSHART et al. 1985). It strongly activates transcription in a wide variety of cells, including *Xenopus laevis* and *Drosophila melanogaster* cells (BOSHART et al. 1985; FÖCKING and HOFSTETTER 1986; SINCLAIR 1987). It is able to stimulate transcription from its cognate promoter and from heterologous promoters (STINSKI and ROEHR 1985; BOSHART et al. 1985). The transcription-enhancing effect could also be demonstrated in a cell-free transcription system (THOMSEN et al. 1984; GHAZAL et al. 1987). The nucleotide sequences between -120 and -65 were also able to stimulate transcription at least by a factor of 10 (GHAZAL et al. 1988b), suggesting that the transcription-enhancing domain extends beyond the enhancer sequence described by BOSHART et al. (1985). Thus, HCMV enhancer activity is localized at least between nucleotides -520 and -65. Enhancer sequences of comparable strength were also found upstream of the IE genes of the mouse cytomegalovirus (MCMV) (DORSCH-HÄSLER et al. 1985) and the simian cytomegalovirus (SCMV) (JEANG et al. 1987). No comparable enhancer could be found within all other herpesvirus genomes investigated so far. Thus, strong constitutive enhancers seem to be characteristic of cytomegalotype herpesviruses.

Although the functional relevance of the enhancer in human cytomegalovirus is obvious, the mechanisms by which these sequences mediate the enhancing effect remain to be elucidated. While most proteins binding the HCMV enhancer have not been identified so far, four high-affinity binding sites for nuclear factor 1 (NF-1) have been mapped between nucleotides -780 and -610 in the upstream region of the IE-1 enhancer/promoter (HENNIGHAUSEN and FLECKENSTEIN 1986; JEANG et al. 1987) (Fig. 3). One additional strong NF-1-binding position appeared in the first intron of the IE-1 gene (HENNIGHAUSEN and FLECKENSTEIN 1986). The NF-1-binding sites of the HCMV IE upstream sequences fall into regions that have been shown to be

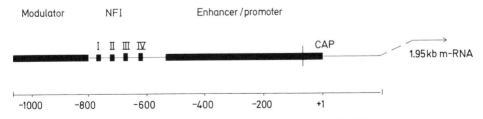

Fig. 3. The four functional domains in the upstream sequence of the major IE gene

sensitive to DNAase I in the active gene, but are not sensitive in the silent gene (NELSON and GROUDINE 1987). A cluster of at least 20 NF-1-binding sites has been observed upstream of the IE regulatory region of SCMV (JEANG et al. 1987). As the dominant IE gene of SCMV is expressed in a broad spectrum of cell types (LaFEMINA and HAYWARD 1988), it has been speculated that NF-1 may influence cell-type-specific expression of the linked IE-1 gene (JEANG et al. 1987; HENNIGHAUSEN and FLECKENSTEIN 1986).

Additional DNAase I hypersensitive sites were mapped in the region further upstream of the HCMV IE-1 promoter between nucleotides -1185 and -750, suggesting that this region also acts as target for *trans*-regulating factors (NELSON and GROUDINE 1987). To investigate the role of these elements, the corresponding fragments were placed in front of homologous and heterologous promoters linked to the CAT reporter gene. Transient expression assays showed that the element was able to modulate gene expression in nonpermissive cells in a negative manner, whereas it positively influenced expression in permissive cells (NELSON et al. 1987). This was confirmed by transcription in vitro; nuclear extracts of various cell lines were tested for the ability to mediate transcription in the presence or absence of the IE-1 upstream region between nucleotides -1145 and -524 (LUBON et al. 1989). This region, termed modulator region, mediates transcriptional repression in certain cell lines, whereas it augments transcription in other cells. It suggests a cell-specific regulatory mechanism of IE-1 gene expression.

In summary, the complex IE-1 upstream region of HCMV can be divided into at least four domains. The promoter (nucleotides -65 to $+3$) appears sufficient for a low level of transcription. The enhancer (-520 to -65) stimulates downstream gene expression from cognate and foreign promoters to a high level in a wide variety of cell types. The modulator segment (nucleotides -1145 to -750) which acts on gene expression in a differentiation-dependent fashion is located upstream of the cluster of NF-1-binding sites (-780 to -610) (Fig. 3).

4 Structural and Functional Organization of the Enhancer Region

The nucleotide sequence of the IE-1 enhancer of HCMV revealed four characteristic types of repeat elements with 17, 18, 19, and 21 bp, respectively, each represented three to five times (AKRIGG et al. 1985; BOSHART et al. 1985; STINSKI and ROEHR 1985; THOMSEN et al. 1984) (Fig. 4). The repeats are partially arranged in a nonabutting manner and are interspersed between various stretches of unique DNA. Some repeats are adjacent or overlapping (Fig. 4). DNAase I footprinting experiments with HeLa cell nuclear extracts revealed at least 13 sites of protein/DNA interaction scattered over the entire length of the promoter/enhancer region (GHAZAL et al. 1987, 1988b). This was consistent with the demonstration of DNAase I hypersensitive sites that were mapped to the HCMV enhancer region (NELSON and GROUDINE 1986). Sites of DNA-protein interaction correlated well with repeat

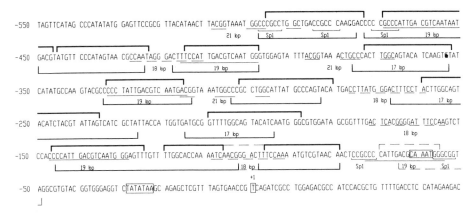

Fig. 4. Nucleotide sequence of the major HCMV enhancer/promoter. Four characteristic repeat elements of 17 bp (......), 18 bp (-----), 19 bp (———), and 21 bp (-.-.-.-.) are arranged in a nonabutting manner between -520 and -50. CAAT and TATA motifs and the transcription initiation site are *boxed*. Sequences which are protected in DNase I footprinting experiments are indicated by *solid* and *thin brackets* for each DNA strand

sequences, suggesting that each of the repeat motifs acts as target sequence for specific transcription factors (GHAZAL et al. 1987, 1988a). Additional sites of protein-DNA interaction were found in unique sequences. The intensity of DNAase I protection was different for the various classes of repeats, and each single repeat within one class appeared to bind proteins with different affinity (GHAZAL et al. 1987). These features are consistent with the model of a large nucleoprotein complex forming on the enhancer sequence and allowing for extensive protein-protein interactions.

The palindromic repeat element of 19 bp is represented four times within the HCMV enhancer sequence. Contransfection of CAT-fusion genes containing the HCMV enhancer/promoter with cloned synthetic 19 bp repeats strongly reduced CAT activity upon transient expression, indicating that the 19-bp palindrome contributes to the constitutive activity of the enhancer (FICKENSCHER et al. 1989). This was confirmed by competition assays with synthetic oligonucleotides in transcription assays with cell-free nuclear extracts (GHAZAL et al. 1988a). To investigate the action of a single 19-bp repeat in the enhancer, deletion variants of HCMV enhancer/SV40 recombinants were constructed that contained only one intact 19-bp palindrome (BOSHART et al. 1985; FICKENSCHER et al. 1989). All of those recombinant SV40-type viruses strongly expressed T-antigen and were replication competent. If one or two nucleotides were inserted into the center of the single palindromic 19-bp repeat, enhancing activity appeared not to be reduced. Removing four nucleotides, however, from the center of the palindrome diminished transcription as much as deleting the entire repeat. This was taken as evidence that the 19-bp repeat is a functional important element of the HCMV enhancer. Protein binding of the 19-bp palindrome could also be demonstrated by gel retardation assays using synthetic oligonucleotides (Fig. 5). There was a good correlation between protein-binding activity of the 19-bp sequence and the mutated derivatives with their

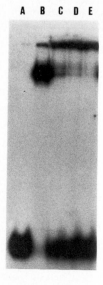

Fig. 5. Gel retardation of a synthetic double-stranded oligonucleotide representing the 19-bp repeat of the HCMV enhancer. *Lane A*, labeled oligonucleotide without addition of protein; *lane B*, gel shift of the oligonucleotide after addition of 5 μg HeLa cell nuclear extract in the presence of 1 μg polydIdC as unspecific competitor; *lane C*, same as in *B* with the addition of 5 ng unlabeled homologous oligonucleotide, *lane D*, same as in *B* with the addition of 10 ng unlabeled homologous oligonucleotide; *lane E*, same as in *B* with the addition of 20 ng unlabeled homologous oligonucleotide

function as an enhancer component (FICKENSCHER et al. 1989). If 1 or 2 bp were inserted into the 19-bp palindromic oligonucleotide (corresponding to a functional element), protein was strongly bound from cell extracts. If the core was deleted to a nonfunctional sequence, protein binding was weak. The residual binding, however, was to the same protein(s) as it could be competed by oligonucleotides with the entire palindrome.

DNA sequence motifs with dyad symmetry related to transcription control were identified in prokaryotic and, in a few cases, in eukaryotic genes. They may be imperfect palindromes that are symmetrical around a central nucleotide, such as the binding site for *cro* and repressor proteins of phage lambda (TAKEDA et al. 1983) or GCN-4 protein in yeast (HILL et al. 1986; STRUHL 1987). Alternatively, the two domains can form an ideal palindrome. This was found in the *ocs* element of the plant octopine synthase enhancer (ELLIS et al. 1987), in a 14-bp consensus from *Drosophila* heat shock genes (PARKER and TOPOL 1984), and in a regulatory response element of a human glycoprotein hormone gene (DELEGEANE et al. 1987; SILVER et al. 1987) and of the rat somatostatin gene (MONTMINY et al. 1986). As far as investigated, each half side of the dyad symmetries in yeast and in the prokaryots was found to be a binding site for a monomer of the respective dimeric proteins (TAKEDA et al. 1983; PTASHNE 1986; HOPE and STRUHL 1987). Computer searches indicated that a 12-nucleotide core sequence of the HCMV 19-bp repeat is conserved in the IE upstream sequence of other cytomegalo type herpesviruses (β-herpesviruses), but not within the entire sequence of herpes simplex virus (McGEOCH, personal communication) and varicella zoster virus (DAVISON and SCOTT 1986) (α-herpesviruses) and within DNA of Epstein-Barr virus (γ-herpesviruses) (BAER et al. 1984). The palindromic 19-bp repeat is largely conserved in the MCMV enhancer (DORSCH-HÄSLER et al. 1985) and in the SCMV IE upstream regulatory sequence, where it occurs 11 times between nucleotides −500

Table 1. Sequence homologies to the 19-bp palindrome

				Localization	Gene	Reference
g CCC	ATTGAC	GTCAAT	a a t	−469/−451	HCMV major IE enhancer	BOSHART et al. 1985
t t CC	ATTGAC	GTCAAT	GGG	−416/−398		
CCCt	ATTGAC	GTCAAT	Ga C	−333/−315		
CCCC	ATTGAC	GTCAAT	GGG	−147/−129		
CCCC	ATTGAC	Gc a AAT	GGG	−73/−55		
CCCC	ATTGAC	GTCAAT	GGt	−488/−470	SCMV IE enhancer	JEANG et al. 1987
t CCt	ATTGAC	GTCAt a	t GG	−453/−435		
t CCt	ATTGAC	GTa t AT	GGc	−430/−412		
CCCC	ATTGAC	GTCAAT	t a c	−406/−388		
g CCC	ATTGAC	GTCAAT	a GG	−363/−345		
Ca CC	ATTGAC	GTCAAT	GGG	−338/−320		
CCCt	ATTGAC	GTCAAT	Ga c	−284/−266		
TCCC	ATTGAC	GTCAAT	GGc	−167/−149		
CCCC	ATTGAC	GTCAAT	GGG	−133/−95		
gggC	Aa TGAC	Gc a AAT	GGG	−91/−73		
t t CC	ATTGAC	GTa AAT	GGG	−70/−52		
Ca CC	ATTGAC	GTCAAT	GGc	−236/−218	MCMV IE enhancer	DORSCH-HÄSLER et al. 1985
g CCC	ATTGAC	GTCAt T	GGt	11752/11770	pTI plasmid of *Agrobacterium tumefaciens*, *tml* gene	GIELEN et al. 1984
a a	ATTGAC	GTCAt g	Gt a	−128/−111	Human chorionic gonadotropin α-subunit	SILVER et al. 1987

and −50 (JEANG et al. 1987) (Table 1). A remarkable similarity exists with the sequence upstream of the *tml* promoter of the Ti plasmid in *Agrobacterium tumefaciens*; this sequence is a functional eukaryotic promoter in plant cells (GIELEN et al. 1984). The inner palindromic core of the HCMV 19-bp repeat also corresponds to a transcription regulatory element of the human chorionic gonadotropin α-unit promoter which is a cAMP-response element (CRE) for transcription enhancement (SILVER et al. 1987). Other CREs with core sequences identical or very similar to the 8-bp core palindrome of the HCMV 19-bp repeat (TGACGTCA) have been found in the upstream gene sequences of the hormone somatostatin (MONTMINY et al. 1986) and vasoactive intestinal polypeptide (TSUKADA et al. 1985), of proenkephalin (TERAO et al. 1983; COMPB et al. 1987), of the protooncogene c-*fos* (van BEVEREN et al. 1983), and of the enzyme phosphoenolpyruvate carboxykinase (WYNSHAW-BORIS et al. 1986). This led to the question of whether the transcription-potentiating activity of the HCMV enhancer could be regulated by cAMP, an important cellular second messenger. Transient expression assays with CAT fusion genes proved that inducers of cAMP activate the HCMV IE-1 enhancer (STAMMINGER et al. 1989) (Fig. 6). cAMP treatment of the HCMV promoter itself (sequences downstream from nucleotide −65) did not result in significant levels of induction. One single 19-bp palindrome, however, was sufficient to mediate the cAMP effect. The stimulation of the HCMV enhancer by cAMP was found in a number of cell types including

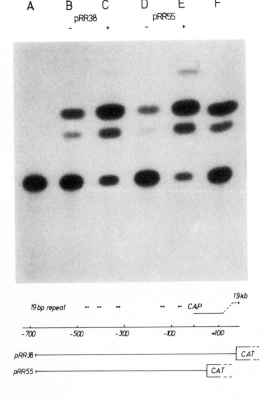

Fig. 6. Stimulation of the major enhancer/promoter of HCMV by cyclic AMP. Enhancer/CAT fusion genes derived from the plasmids pRR55 and pRR38 were transfected into HeLa cells. Stimulation was achieved by addition of 1 mM 8-bromo-cAMP to the culture medium 16 h before harvest. *Lane A*, mock transfected HeLa cells; *lane B*, HeLa cells transfected with 5 μg pRR 38, without addition of 8-bromo-cAMP; *lane C*, HeLa cells transfected with 5 μg pRR55 with addition of 8-bromo-cAMP; *lane D*, HeLa cells transfected with 5 μg pPR55 without addition of 8-bromo-cAMP; *lane E*, HeLa cells transfected with 5 μg pRR55 with addition of 8-bromo-cAMP; *lane F*, 0.1 units CAT enzyme as positive control

Table 2. Sequence homologies of the 19-bp repeat sequence to the consensus sequence of transcription factor AP-1

Sequence			Reference
cccATTGAC	GTCAATggg	HCMV IE enhancer 19-bp repeat	BOSHART et al. 1985
cTGAC	GTCAg	c-AMP-responsive element (CRE)	MONTMINY et al. 1986
TGA	C TCA	AP-1 consensus sequence	ANGEL et al. 1987 LEE et al. 1987
ATGA	C TCTT	GCN-4 and c-*jun*	HILL et al. 1986
ATGA	C TCTT		STRUHL 1987

lymphoid cells (STAMMINGER et al. 1989). In view of the known similarities between the target sequences for the CRE-binding proteins (MONTMINY and BILEZIKIJIAN 1987), for transcription factor AP-1 (ANGEL et al. 1987; LEE et al. 1987), and for the c-*jun* oncoprotein (STRUHL 1987), common binding characteristics were studied (Table 2). A synthetic oligonucleotide in which the center of the 19-bp repeat was turned into an AP-1 consensus sequence was retarded in gels to the same position as the native palindrome. Protein complexing of the AP-1 consensus sequence oligonucleotide could be competed by the canonical palindrome. This suggested that a protein of the AP-1 group is able to bind the 19-bp element of the HCMV IE-1 enhancer. Since AP-1 can be induced by tetradecanoylphorbolacetate (TPA) (ANGEL et al. 1987; LEE et al. 1987), a plasmid containing a single 19-bp repeat upstream of the promoter was tested for induction by TPA, a phorbolester known to stimulate protein kinase C. Significant stimulation indicated that the 19-bp element is involved in the TPA response that had been described before for the entire HCMV enhancer (LEBKOWKSI et al. 1987). Thus, two different cellular signal transmission pathways are able to regulate transcription through one response element.

The 18-bp repeat element which occurs four times in the HCMV IE-1 enhancer appears also to be relevant for the constitutive function, as competition for binding protein by homologous synthetic oligonucleotides strongly reduced enhancer strength. A deletion variant of SV40/HCMV enhancer recombinant containing the 18-bp and 19-bp repeats, each as a single copy respectively, was fairly strong in enhancer activity. An 11-nucleotide core sequence of the 18-bp repeat from the HCMV IE upstream region finds complete homology with multiple repeats of the IE upstream region of the MCMV (DORSCH-HÄSLER et al. 1987) (Table 3). A similar sequence was found in the HCMV U$_s$ IE-enhancer (WESTON 1988). It is not present in the functionally equivalent upstream region of SCMV (JEANG et al. 1987), and it could not be found in any other herpesvirus. In comparison, sequence homology between the HCMV 18-bp repeat and a sequence motif of the pseudorabies IE upstream region, as suggested by CAMPBELL and PRESTON (1987), is rather weak and probably not significant. The 18-bp repeat, however, nicely matches with the GT-1

Table 3. Sequence Homologies to the 18-bp repeat

Sequence		Localization nt	Gene	Reference
CCaAta	GGGACTTTCCA t			
CCTtAt	GGGACTTTCC t A			
ACTcAC	GGG g a TTTCCA A			
AtcAAC	GGGACTTTCCA A			
cAc	c G t ACTTTCC c A			
AcC	GGGACTTTCC g c	−428/−411		
AcC	GGGACTTT t CA c	−277/−260		
AcC	GGGACTTTCCA c	−172/−155		
tAC	GG t ACTTTCC g t	−109/−92		
	GGGACTTTCCA	−761/−744	MCMV	DORSCH-
	GGGACTTTCCA	−668/−651	IE enhancer	HÄSLER
	GGGACTTTCCA	−575/−558		et al. 1985
	GGGACTTTCCA	−482/−465		
	GGGACTTTCCA	−390/−373		
	GGGACTTTCCA	158/ 175	SV40 enhancer	WEIHER
	GGGACTTTCCA	230/ 247		et al. 1983
	CTTTCC		GT-I core	
	GGGACTTTCC g	344/ 361	HIV-1, 5′LTR	RATNER
	GGGACTTTCCA	358/ 375		et al. 1985
	GGGACTTTCC g	9459/9476	3′LTR	
	GGGACTTTCCA	9473/9490		
	GGGACTTTCCA	9390/9400	HIV-2, 3′LTR	GUYADER et al. 1987
	GGGACTTTCCA	519/ 536	Mouse endogeneous retrovirus 3′LTR	IKEDA et al. 1985
	GGGACTTTCCA	306/ 323	Murine leukemia virus, 3′LTR	YOSHIMURA et al. 1985
	GGGACTTTCCA	153/ 170	Mink cell focus-forming virus	KHAN et al. 1982
	GGGACTTTCC g	247/ 264	κ-Ig enhancer	PICARD and SCHAFFNER 1984

core consensus sequence of the SV40 enhancer (WEIHER et al. 1983; DAVIDSON et al. 1986). Perfect sequence matching over 11 nt was found with sequence motifs in regulatory domains of various onco- and lentiviruses such as human immunodeficiency viruses (HIV-1/2) (RATNER et al. 1985; GUYADER et al. 1987) and over 10 bp with the NF-κ-B-binding site of the κ IgG enhancer (PICARD and SCHAFFNER 1984; SEN and BALTIMORE 1986; ATCHISON and PERRY 1987). Thus, the transcription factor NF-κ-B may activate immunoglobulin transcription in B cells, HIV gene expression, and HCMV IE transcription from the same type of sequence elements (NABEL and BALTIMORE 1987). This, however, does not rule out that the transcription activators from other cell types, e.g., HeLa cells, binding to the 18-bp repeat of HCMV are distinct from NF-κ-B. Thus far, it is a matter of speculation if the shared sequence motif of HIV LTR and the 18-bp repeat of HCMV are functionally related to the known cross-activation of the viruses (DAVIS et al. 1987; SKOLNIK et al. 1988). An octameric DNA sequence, present in three of the 18-bp repeats, resembles the cellular heat shock element core consensus. It was suggested that this element might be involved in transcriptional activation of IE-1 gene expression following heat shock in a cell line harboring several stably integrated copies of the IE-1 gene (BOOM et al. 1986; GEELEN et al. 1987).

Repeats of 17 bp and 21 bp form a combined strong binding site for another protein from HeLa cell extracts (GHAZAL et al. 1987). A SV40/HCMV enhancer recombinant which had a single 21-bp motif without any other repeat sequences retained activity, suggesting that it is sufficient, though not required, for enhancer activity (FICKENSCHER and STAMMINGER, unpublished). Computer searches did not find any significant homology to the 21-bp repeat within all entries of the National Biological Research Foundation (NBRF) gene library. The 17-bp repeat is not necessary for enhancer activity, as it is missing in a number of replication competent SV40-type deletion mutants. By computer compilation, the 17-bp repeat of the HCMV enhancer was found to be identical with a nonrepetitive sequence between nt -253 and -237 upstream of the major IE promoter from the Colburn strain of SCMV (JEANG et al. 1987) (Table 4). A sequence element similar to the 17-bp repeat of HCMV and SCMV is not present within the IE region of MCMV (DORSCH-HÄSLER et al. 1987; KEIL et al. 1987) or within the entire genomes of varicella-zoster virus (α-herpesvirus) (DAVISON and SCOTT 1986) and Epstein-Barr virus (γ-herpesvirus) (BAER et al. 1984). Similarity was detected between the 17-bp element and an 11-bp consensus core which is part of the hepatitis B virus enhancer region (SHAUL et al. 1985). However, no other homology greater than 60% became apparent with any other of the eukaryotic entries in the NBRF gene library.

The peculiar organization of the HCMV enhancer with its pattern of repeat elements and protein-binding sites, respectively, gives a plausible model for the modular organization of eukaryotic enhancers where multiple sequence elements are often redundant (SCHAFFNER 1985; SERFLING et al. 1985). Regulated and constitutive elements of different tissue specificity are combined in a single complex functional unit (SCHIRM et al. 1987). One class of repeats may be missing, still leaving sufficient activity at reduced level. The architecture of β-herpesvirus IE enhancers also infers that some defined elements are not required for function; the 17-bp repeat

Table 4. Sequence homologies to the 17-bp repeat

Sequence	Localization nt	Gene	Reference
ACTT GGCAGTA CATCAA	$-373/-357$	HCMV major	BOSHART
ACTT GGCAGTA CATCt A	$-260/-244$	IE enhancer	et al. 1985
t t TT GGCAGTA CATCAA	$-209/-193$		
ACTT GGCAGTA CATCAA	$-273/-253$	SCMV	JEANG
ACTT GGCAGTA CATt Ac	$-204/-221$	IE enhancer	et al. 1987
a			
Ag TT GGCAGTA CAg Cc t	$1387/-1401$	Hepatitis B virus, downstream of enhancer sequence	ONO et al. 1983 SHAUL et al. 1985

is lacking in MCMV, though present in the SCMV IE-regulatory region. Inversely, the 18-bp repeat is part of the MCMV enhancer, but is not found in SCMV (DORSCH-HÄSLER et al. 1985; JEANG et al. 1987). The total absence of those sequence elements in herpesviruses of other subgroups (α- and γ-herpesviruses) contributes to the general view that regulatory elements of herpesviruses diverge more than most protein-coding sequences. Strong constitutive enhancers of defined functions have been found only in cytomegalo type (β-) herpesviruses up to now. The adaptation of herpesviruses to various patterns of pathogenicity or host cell tropisms may have been more determined by evolutionary modification at the level of gene regulation than by mutations of structural protein-coding sequences.

Acknowledgments. We thank Walter Schaffner for stimulating discussions. Original work presented in this review was supported by the Deutsche Forschungsgemeinschaft.

References

Akrigg A, Wilkinson GWG, Oram JD (1985) The structure of the major immediate early gene of human cytomegalovirus AD169. Virus Res 2: 107–121

Angel P, Imagawa M, Chiu R, Stein B, Imbra RJ, Rahmsdorf HJ, Jonat C, et al. (1987) Phorbol ester-inducible genes contain a common *cis* element recognized by a TPA-modulated *trans*-acting factor. Cell 49: 729–739

Atchison ML, Perry RP (1987) The role of the kappa enhancer and its binding factor NF-kappa-B in the developmental regulation of kappa gene transcription. Cell 48: 121–128

Baer R, Bankier AT, Biggin MD, Deininger PL, Farrell PJ, Gibson TJ, Hatfull G, et al. (1984) DNA sequence and expression of the B95-8 Epstein-Barr virus genome. Nature 310: 207–211

Blanton RA, Tevethia MJ (1981) Immunoprecipitation of virus-specific immediate-early and early polypeptides from cells lytically infected with human cytomegalovirus strain AD169. Virology 112: 262–273

Boom R, Geelen JL, Sol CJ, Raap AK, Minnaar RP, Klaver BP, van der Noordaa J (1986) Establishment of a rat cell line inducible for the expression of human cytomegalovirus immediate-early gene products by protein synthesis inhibition. J Virol 58: 851–859

Boshart M, Weber F, Jahn G, Dorsch-Häsler K, Fleckenstein B, Schaffner W (1985) A very strong enhancer is located upstream of an immediate early gene of human cytomegalovirus. Cell 41: 521–530

Cameron JM, Preston CM (1981) Comparison of the immediate early polypeptides of human cytomegalovirus isolates. J Gen Virol 54: 421–424

Campbell MEM, Preston CM (1987) DNA sequences which regulate the expression of the pseudorabies virus major immediate early gene. Virology 157: 307–316

Comb M, Brinberg NC, Seasholtz A, Nerbert E, Goodman HM (1987) A cyclic AMP- and phorbol ester-inducible DNA element. Nature 323: 353–356

Davidson I, Fromental C, Augereau P, Wildeman A, Zenke M, Chambon P (1986) Cell-type specific protein binding to the enhancer of simian virus 40 in nuclear extracts. Nature 323: 544–548

Davis MG, Kenney SC, Kamine J, Pagano JS, Huang E-S (1987) Immediate-early gene region of human cytomegalovirus *trans* activates the promoter of human immunodeficiency virus. Proc Natl Acad Sci USA 84: 8642–8646

Davison A, Scott J (1986) The complete DNA sequence of varicella zoster virus. J Gen Virol 67: 1759–1816

Delegeane AM, Ferland LH, Mellon PL (1987) Tissue-specific enhancer of the human glycoprotein hormone alpha-subunit gene: dependence on cyclic AMP-inducible elements. Mol Cell Biol 7: 3994–4002

DeMarchi JM (1981) Human cytomegalovirus DNA: restriction enzyme cleavage maps and map locations for immediate-early, early, and late RNAs. Virology 114: 23–38

Dorsch-Häsler K, Keil GM, Weber F, Jasin M, Schaffner W, Koszinowski UH (1985) A long and complex enhancer activates transcription of the gene coding for the highly abundant immediate early mRNA in murine cytomegalovirus. Proc Natl Acad Sci USA 82: 8325–8329

Ellis JG, Llewellyn DJ, Walker JC, Dennis ES, Peacock WJ (1987) The *ocs* element: a 16 base pair palindrome element for activity of the octopine synthase enhancer. EMBO J 6: 3203–3208

Everett RD, Dunlop M (1984) *Trans* activation of plasmid-borne promoters by adenovirus and several herpes group viruses. Nucleic Acids Res 12: 5969–5978

Fickenscher H, Stamminger T, Rüger R, Fleckenstein B (1989) The role of a repetitive palindromic sequence element in the human cytomegalovirus major immediate early enhancer. J Gen Virol 70: 107–123

Föcking MK, Hofstetter H (1986) Powerful and versatile enhancer-promoter unit for mammalian expression vectors. Gene 45: 101–105

Geelen JLC, Boom R, Klaver GP, Minnaar RP, Feltkamp MCW, van Milligen FJ, Sol CJA, van der Noordaa J (1987) Transcriptional activation of the major immediate early transcription unit of human cytomegalovirus by heat-shock, arsenite and protein synthesis inhibitors. J Gen Virol 68: 2925–2931

Ghazal P, Lubon H, Fleckenstein B, Hennighausen L (1987) Binding of transcription factors and creation of a large nucleoprotein complex on the human cytomegalovirus enhancer. Proc Natl Acad Sci USA 84: 3658–3662

Ghazal P, Lubon H, Hennighausen L (1988a) Multiple sequence-specific transcription factors modulate cytomegalovirus enhancer activity in vitro. Mol Cell Biol 8: 1809–1811

Ghazal P, Lubon H, Hennighausen L (1988b) Specific interactions between transcription factors and the promoter-regulatory region of the human cytomegalovirus major immediate-early-gene. J Virol 62: 1076–1079

Gibson W (1981) Immediate-early proteins of human cytomegalovirus strains AD169, Davis, and Towne differ in electrophoretic mobility. Virology 112: 350–354

Gielen J, DeBeuckeleer M, Seurinck J, Deboeck F, DeGreve H, Lemmers M, van Montagu M, Schell J (1984) The complete nucleotide sequence of the TL-DNA of the *Agrobacterium tumefaciens* plasmid pTiAch5. EMBO J 3: 835–846

Guyader M, Emerman M, Sonigo P, Clavel F, Montagnier L, Alizon M (1987) Genome organization and transactivation of the human immunodeficiency virus type 2. Nature 326: 662–669

Hennighausen L, Fleckenstein B (1986) Nuclear factor 1 interacts with five DNA elements in the promoter region of the human cytomegalovirus major immediate early gene. EMBO J 5: 1367–1371

Hermiston TW, Malone CL, Witte PR, Stinski MF (1987) Identification and characterization of the human cytomegalovirus immediate-early region 2 gene that stimulates gene expression from an inducible promoter. J Virol 61: 3214–3221

Hill DE, Hope IA, Macke JP, Struhl K (1986) Saturation mutagenesis of the yeast his3 regulatory site: requirements for transcriptional induction and for binding by GCN4 activator protein. Science 234: 451–457

Honess RW, Roizman B (1974) Regulation of herpesvirus macromolecular synthesis. J Virol 14: 8–19

Honess RW, Roizman B (1975) Regulation of herpesvirus macromolecular synthesis: sequential transition of polypeptide synthesis requires functional viral polypeptides. Proc Natl Acad Sci USA 72: 1276–1280

Hope IA, Struhl K (1987) GCN4, a eukaryotic transcriptional activator protein, binds as a dimer to target DNA, EMBO J 6: 2781–2784

Ikeda H, Laigret F, Martin MA, Repaske R (1985) Characterization of a molecularly cloned retroviral sequence associated with Fv-4 resistance. J Virol 55: 768–777

Jahn G, Knust E, Schmolla H, Sarre T, Nelson JA, McDougall JK, Fleckenstein B (1984) Predominant immediate-early transcripts of human cytomegalovirus AD169. J Virol 49: 363–370

Jeang J-T, Rawlins DR, Rosenfeld PJ, Shero JH, Kelly TJ, Hayward GS (1987) Multiple tandemly repeated binding sites for cellular nuclear factor 1 that surround the major immediate-early promoters of simian and human cytomegalovirus. J Virol 61: 1559–1570

Khan AS, Repaske R, Garon CF, Chan HW, Rowe WP, Martin MA (1982) Characterization of proviruses cloned from mink cell focus-forming virus-infected cellular DNA. J Virol 41: 435–448

Keil GM, Ebeling-Keil A, Koszinowski UH (1987) Sequence and structural organization of murine cytomegalovirus immediate-early gene 1. J Virol 61: 1901–1908

LaFemina RL, Hayward G (1988) Differences in cell type-specific blocks to immediate early gene expression and DNA replication of human, simian and murine cytomegalovirus. J Gen Virol 69: 355–374

Lebkowski JS, McNally MA, Okarma TB, Lerch LB (1987) Inducible gene expression from multiple promoters by the tumor-promoting agent PMA. Nucleic Acids Res 15: 9043–9055

Lee W, Mitchell P, Tijan R (1987) Purified transcription factor AP-1 interacts with TPA-inducible enhancer elements. Cell 49: 741–752

Lubon H, Ghazal P, Hennighausen L, Reynolds-Kohler C, Lockshin C, Nelson JA (1989) Cell-specific activity of the modulator region in the human cytomegalovirus major immediate early gene. Mol Cell Biol 9: 1342–1345

MDonough S, Spector DH (1983) Transcription in human fibroblasts permissively infected by human cytomegalovirus strain AD169. Virology 125: 31–46

Michelson-Fiske S, Horodniceanu F, Guillon J-C (1977) Immediate early antigens in human cytomegalovirus infected cells. Nature 270: 615–617

Montminy MR, Bilezikijian LM (1987) Binding of a nuclear protein to the cyclic-AMP response element of the somatostatin gene. Nature 328: 175–178

Montminy MR, Sevarino KA, Wagner JA, Mandel G, Goodman RH (1986) Identification of a cyclic-AMP-responsive element within the rat somatostatin gene. Proc Natl Acad Sci USA 83: 6682–6686

Nabel G, Baltimore D (1987) An inducible transcription factor activates expression of human immunodeficiency virus in T cells. Nature 326: 711–713

Nelson JA, Groudine M (1986) Transcriptional regulation of the human cytomegalovirus major immediate-early gene is associated with induction of DNase I-hypersensitive sites. Mol Cell Biol 6: 452–461

Nelson JA, Fleckenstein B, Galloway DA, McDougall JK (1982) Transformation of NIH 3T3 cells with cloned fragments of human cytomegalovirus strain AD169. J Virol 43: 83–91

Nelson JA, Fleckenstein B, Jahn G, Galloway DA, McDougall JK (1984) Structure of the transforming region of human cytomegalovirus AD169. J Virol 49: 109–115

Nelson JA, Reynolds-Kohler C, Smith BA (1987) Negative and positive regulation of the human cytomegalovirus major immediate-early gene is associated with induction of DNAse I-hypersensitive sites. Mol Cell Biol 6: 4125-4129

Ono Y, Onda H, Sasada R, Igarashi K, Sugino Y, Nishioka K (1983) The complete nucleotide sequences of the cloned hepatitis B virus DNA; subtype adr and adw. Nucl Acids Res 11: 1747–1757

Parker CS, Topol J (1984) A Drosophila RNA polymerase II transcription factor binds to the regulatory site of an hsp 70 gene. Cell 37: 273–283

Picard D, Schaffner W (1984) A lymphocyte-specific enhancer in the mouse immunoglobulin kappa gene. Nature 307: 80–82

Plachter B, Traupe B, Albrecht J, Jahn G (1988) Abudant 5 kb RNA of human cytomegalovirus without a major translational reading frame. J Gen Virol 69: 2251–2266

Ptashne M (1986) A genetic switch. Blackwell, Oxford

Ratner L, Haseltine W, Patarca R, Livak KJ, Starich B, Josephs SF, Doran ER, et al. (1985) Complete nucleotide sequence of the AIDS virus, HTLV III. Nature 313: 277–284

Schaffner W (1985) Introduction. In: Gluzman Y (ed) Eukaryotic transcription. The role of cis- and trans-acting elements in initiation. Cold Spring Harbor Laboratory, New York pp 1–18 (Current communications in molecular biology)

Schirm S, Jiricny J, Schaffner W (1987) The SV40 enhancer can be dissected into multiple segments, each with a different cell type specificity. Genes Dev 1: 65–74

Sen R, Baltimore D (1986) Multiple nuclear factors interact with the immunoglobulin enhancer sequences. Cell 46: 705–716

Serfling E, Jasin M, Schaffner W (1985) Enhancers and eukaryotic gene transcription. Trends Genet 1: 224–230

Shaul Y, Rutter WJ, Laub O (1985) A human hepatitis B viral enhancer element. EMBO J 4: 427–430

Silver BJ, Bokar JA, Virgin JB, Vallen EA, Milsted A, Nilson JH (1987) Cyclic AMP regulation of the human glycoprotein hormone α-subunit gene is mediated by an 18-base-pair element. Proc Natl Acad Sci USA 84: 2198–2202

Sinclair JH (1987) The human cytomegalovirus immediate early gene promoter is a strong promoter in cultured Drosophila melanogaster cells. Nucleic Acids Res 15: 2392

Skolnik PR, Kosloff BR, Hirsch MS (1988) Bidirectional interactions between human immunodeficiency virus type 1 and cytomegalovirus. J Infect Dis 157: 508–514

Stamminger T, Fickenscher H, Fleckenstein B (1990) The cell type-specific induction of the major immediate early enhancer of human cytomegalovirus by cyclic AMP. J Gen Virol (in press)

Staprans SI, Spector DH (1986) 2.2-kilobase class of early transcripts encoded by cell-related sequences in human cytomegalovirus strain AD169. J Virol 57: 591–602

Stenberg RM, Depto AS, Fortney J, Nelson JA (1989) Regulated Expression of Early and Late RNAs and Proteins from the Human Cytomegalovirus Immediate-Early Gene Region. J Virol 63: 2699–2708

Stenberg RM, Thomsen DR, Stinski MF (1984) Structural analysis of the major immediate early gene of human cytomegalovirus. J Virol 49: 190–199

Stenberg RM, Witte PR, Stinski MF (1985) Multiple spliced and unspliced transcripts from human cytomegalovirus immediate-early region 2 and evidence for a common initiation site within immediate-early region 1. J Virol 56: 665–675

Stinski MF, Roehr TJ (1985) Activation of the major immediate early gene of human cytomegalovirus by cis-acting elements in the promoter-regulatory sequence and by virus-specific trans-acting components. J Virol 55: 431–441

Stinski MF, Thomsen DR, Stenberg RM, Goldstein LC (1983) Organization and expression of the immediate early genes of human cytomegalovirus. J Virol 46: 1–14

Struhl K (1987) The DNA-binding domains of the jun oncoprotein and the yeast GCN4 transcriptional activator protein are functionally homologous. Cell 50: 841–846

Takeda Y, Ohlendorf DH, Anderson WF, Matthews BW (1983) DNA-binding proteins. Science 221: 1020–1026

Terao M, Watanabe Y, Mishina M, Numa S (1983) Sequence requirement for transcription in vivo of the human preproenkephalin A gene. EMBO J 2: 2223–2228

Thomsen DR, Stenberg RM, Goins WF, Stinski MF (1984) Promoter-regulatory region of the major immediate early gene of human cytomegalovirus. Proc Natl Acad Sci USA 81: 659–663

Tsukada T, Horovitch SJ, Montminy MR, Mandel G, Goodman RH (1985) Structure of the human vasoactive intestinal polypeptide gene. DNA 4: 293–300

Van Beveren C, van Straaten F, Curran T, Müller R, Verma IM (1983) Analysis of FBJ-MuSV provirus and c-fos (mouse) gene reveals that viral and cellular fos gene products have different carboxy termini. Cell 32: 1241–1255

Wathen MW, Stinski MF (1982) Temporal patterns of human cytomegalovirus transcription: mapping the viral RNAs synthesized at immediate early, early, and late times after infection. J Virol 41: 462–477

Weber F, DeVilliers J, Schaffner W (1984) An SV40 "enhancer trap" incorporates exogenous enhancers or generates enhancers from its own sequences. Cell 36: 983–992

Weiher H, König M, Gruss P (1983) Multiple point mutations affecting the simian virus 40 enhancer. Science 219: 626–631

Weston K (1988) An enhancer element in the short unique region of human cytomegalovirus regulates the production of a group of abundant immediate early transcripts. Virology 162: 406–416

Wilkinson GWG, Akrigg A, Greenaway PJ (1984) Transcription of the immediate early genes of human cytomegalovirus strain AD169. Virus Res 1: 101–116

Wynshaw-Boris A, Short JM, Loose DS, Hanson RW (1986) Characterization of the phosphoenolpyruvate carboxykinase (GTP) promoter-regulatory region. J Biol Chem 261: 9714–9720

Yoshimura FK, Davison B, Chaffin K (1985) Murine leukemia virus long terminal repeat sequences can enhance gene activity in a cell-type-specific manner. Mol Cell Biol 5: 2832–2835

Human Cytomegalovirus Early Gene Expression

D. H. Spector, K. M. Klucher, D. K. Rabert, and D. A. Wright

1 Introduction   21
2 HCMV IE Gene Expression   24
3 Class of Transcripts and Family of Proteins Encoded by *Eco*RI Fragments R and d   26
4 Early Transcripts Encoded by the Long Repeat   33
5 Other HCMV Early Genes   37
6 Concluding Remarks   40
References   40

1 Introduction

Human cytomegalovirus (HCMV), a member of the herpesvirus group, is species specific and can establish both persistent and latent infections. The virus appears to be able to infect a number of cell types in vivo including epithelial cells, neural cells, endothelial cells, mesenchymal cells, and some subclasses of leukocytes, although viral gene expression may be limited in some of these cells. Within the past 30 years, this virus has been recognized as an important pathogen of man capable of causing disease that affects all age groups worldwide (for review, see Ho 1982; NANKERVIS and KUMAR 1978; RAPP 1983; SPECTOR 1985). In developed countries, it is the major viral cause of birth defects leading to mental retardation and deafness. Transmission of HCMV usually occurs via salivary secretions, sexual contact, or blood, and it remains the most common transfusion-related pathogen. Although primary infection may be asymptomatic or result in a mononucleosis-like syndrome in the immunocompetent individual, severe and sometimes fatal HCMV infections frequently develop in immunocompromised persons, particularly premature infants, organ transplant recipients, and AIDS patients. In AIDS, HCMV is a serious opportunistic infection (DREW et al. 1982; MACHER et al. 1983; MARCHEVSKY et al. 1985; SPECTOR et al. 1984; SPECTOR and SPECTOR 1985) and is frequently implicated as a possible cofactor in the development or progression of the disease.

HCMV has a double-stranded DNA genome 240 kilobase pairs (kbp) in length, consisting of two covalently linked segments, L (long) and S (short), each bounded by inverted repeats (DEMARCHI et al. 1978; FLECKENSTEIN et al. 1982; GEELEN et al.

Department of Biology and Center for Molecular Genetics, University of California, San Diego, La Jolla, California 92093, USA

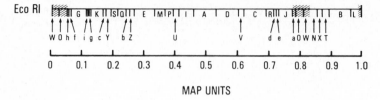

Eco RI

WOhf   igcY   bZ   U   V   d e   aOWNXT

0   0.1   0.2   0.3   0.4   0.5   0.6   0.7   0.8   0.9   1.0

MAP UNITS

Fig. 1. *Eco*RI restriction endonuclease map of the HCMV strain AD169 genome (SPECTOR et al. 1982). Only the prototype orientation is shown. The long and short inverted repeat sequences are indicated by the *slanting lines.* HCMV *Eco*RI fragment H equals the junction of *Eco*RI fragments W plus N. HCMV *Eco*RI fragment F equals the junction of *Eco*RI fragments W plus L in the inverted orientation

1978; GREENAWAY et al. 1982; LAFEMINA and HAYWARD 1980; LAKEMAN and OSBORN 1979; ORAM et al. 1982; SPECTOR et al. 1982; STINSKI et al. 1979; WESTSTRATE et al. 1980). The L and S segments can invert relative to one another, giving rise to four possible genome orientations in a viral population. For reference, the *Eco*RI restriction endonuclease map of HCMV strain AD169 in the prototype orientation is shown in Fig. 1 (SPECTOR et al. 1982).

Given the large size of the HCMV genome, it has been estimated that greater than 100 proteins can be encoded; however, less than half of the potential gene products have been mapped and characterized (ANDERS and GIBSON 1988; BECK and BARRELL 1988; CRANAGE et al. 1986, 1988; DAVIS and HUANG 1985; DAVIS et al. 1984; GRETCH et al. 1988b; HEILBRONN et al. 1987; HUTCHINSON and TOCCI 1986; JAHN et al. 1987; KEMBLE et al. 1987; KOUZARIDES et al. 1987a,b, 1988; MACH et al. 1986; MARTINEZ et al. 1989; MEYER et al. 1988; MOCARSKI et al. 1985, 1988; NOWAK et al. 1984; PANDE et al. 1984; RUGER et al. 1987; STINSKI et al. 1983; WESTON and BARRELL 1986; WRIGHT et al. 1988). Although only a few of the viral functions involved in HCMV infection of its host have been identified, we do know that HCMV, like other herpesviruses, undergoes a sequential order of gene expression following the permissive infection of human fibroblasts in tissue culture (DEMARCHI 1981; DEMARCHI et al. 1980; MCDONOUGH and SPECTOR 1983; STINSKI 1977, 1978; WATHEN and STINSKI 1982; WATHEN et al. 1981). In the case of HCMV, both transcriptional and posttranscriptional control mechanisms appear to govern the pattern of gene expression (DEMARCHI 1983; GEBALLE et al. 1986a,b; GEBALLE and MOCARSKI 1988; GOINS and STINSKI 1986; HERMISTON et al. 1987; KOUZARIDES et al. 1988; SPAETE and MOCARSKI 1985; STAPRANS et al. 1988; STENBERG et al. 1985; STINSKI and ROEHR 1985; WATHEN and STINSKI 1982; WRIGHT and SPECTOR 1989).

Production of herpes virus-encoded gene products has been broadly classified into three temporal classes: immediate-early (α), early (β), and late (γ). The immediate-early (IE) gene products are those synthesized immediately after infection. Experimentally, the IE RNAs are those transcribed in the presence of protein synthesis inhibitors, and the IE proteins are those synthesized immediately upon release of the cell from translational inhibition. Early RNA and protein synthesis begin before the onset of viral DNA replication (which occurs about 16-24 h postinfection in the case of HCMV) and are dependent on the prior expression of one or more IE genes. Finally, the late genes are transcribed in abundance after the commencement of viral DNA synthesis and are encoded by a major fraction of the genome. A fourth temporal class, designated delayed early or leaky-late, is sometimes included in this grouping. The initiation of transcription of this class of RNA is not absolutely dependent upon viral DNA replication, but its abundance does increase markedly as the viral template is amplified during late times in the infection. In practice, it has often been difficult to distinguish between the delayed early and true late transcripts, and the designation of a transcript to a particular class has depended upon the sensitivity of the methodology used for its detection. By analogy with other herpesviruses, it is likely that many of the early gene products will be involved in viral DNA replication as well as the activation and repression of specific viral (and perhaps cellular) promoters, while a major fraction of the late gene products will function in the packaging of viral DNA and the formation of mature virus particles.

Studies on HCMV gene expression initially focused on identifying the regions of the viral genome which were transcriptionally active at IE, early, and late times in the infection. To measure the rate of accumulation of viral transcripts, pulse-labeled whole cell, nuclear, or cytoplasmic RNA was hybridized to dot blots of cloned subgenomic fragments or Southern blots of viral DNA cleaved with restriction endonucleases and fractionated by gel electrophoresis (DeMarchi 1981, 1983; DeMarchi et al. 1980; McDonough and Spector 1983; Wathen and Stinski 1982; Wathen et al. 1981). In complementary experiments, the size and abundance of various RNAs were determined by hybridization of radiolabeled viral DNA or cloned subgenomic fragments to dot blots or Northern blots of RNA isolated at various times in the infection (DeMarchi 1983; McDonough and Spector 1983; Wathen and Stinski 1982). Two important points emerged from these studies. First, there appeared to be no clustering of RNA transcripts according to their temporal expression. Furthermore, some HCMV early gene expression appeared to be subject to posttranscriptional controls which governed either the transport of RNA from the nucleus to the cytoplasm or the stability of the RNA in the cytoplasm. These early studies, which provided information on the relative abundance, size, and temporal expression of the RNAs, have become the framework for more detailed analysis of individual transcription units and the underlying mechanisms which regulate their expression.

This article focuses on human cytomegalovirus early gene expression with emphasis on the sequence requirements and *trans*-acting functions necessary for the regulated expression of this complex class of genes. Included in this review are several transcription units which could be classified as delayed early but which we will refer to as early. As we begin to elucidate the molecular mechanisms of this regulation, we open a unique window on the cell's own molecular machinery, with visions of how the virus is selectively utilizing this machinery for its own needs as the infection proceeds. Indeed, the progress of the viral infection and the changes in the pattern of gene expression are in many ways analogous to the types of changes one sees as part of tissue-specific or developmental regulation of gene expression. In higher eukaryotes, control of gene expression involves multiple regulatory mechanisms operating at the level of initiation of RNA transcription, RNA processing and transport, translation, and mRNA and protein stability. Complex processing pathways are the norm in eukaryotic cells, and, even within a single transcription unit, multiple mRNAs may be generated by differential utilization of sites of initiation or cleavage and polyadenylation, and by alternative exon splicing. It has been argued that the utilization of these complex pathways by viruses allows for genomic economy, but it is likely that these pathways are equally important for the regulation of the viral infection. The challenge is to determine how the complex interplay of viral and host functions relates to the in vivo pathogenesis of the virus.

Studies in our laboratory have been directed at understanding the regulation and function of three early transcription units: the major 2.7-kb and 1.2-kb transcripts encoded by the repeat bounding the long unique segment of the genome (McDonough et al. 1985) and a family of transcripts (originally designated the 2.2-kb RNAs) encoded by HCMV strain AD169 EcoRI fragments R and d in the long unique segment of the genome (map units 0.682–0.713; Staprans and Spector 1986). Although all of these transcripts appear at early times, they appear to be subject to different regulatory controls. The steady-state concentration of the 2.7-kb RNA increases greatly between 8 h and 14 h postinfection (p.i.), while the steady-state concentration of the 1.2-kb RNA shows a major increase between 28 h and 72 h p.i. These patterns are in contrast to the family of transcripts encoded by EcoRI fragments R and d, whose steady-state levels remain about the same after 8 h p.i. In this review, we will primarily discuss these three transcription units and summarize what is currently known about several other early genes.

2 HCMV IE Gene Expression

We begin with a brief discussion of HCMV IE gene expression since the activation of early gene transcription requires the prior synthesis of at least some IE proteins. The reader is directed to other chapters in this volume for a more in-depth treatment of this topic.

In HCMV, IE gene expression is diverse and originates from multiple regions within the genome. In strain AD169 of HCMV, the predominant site of IE transcription is located within a region of the long unique segment defined by HindIII fragment E which contains EcoRI fragments J, e, d, and R (Jahn et al. 1984a, b; McDonough and Spector 1983; Wilkinson et al. 1984). This site is located in a homologous position in both the Davis and Towne strains of HCMV (DeMarchi 1981; Stinski et al. 1983), and encodes at least three related IE transcription units designated IE1, IE2, and IE3 (Hermiston et al. 1987; Stenberg et al. 1984, 1985; Wathen and Stinski 1982; Wathen et al. 1981). A fourth IE transcription unit which generates a 5.0-kb RNA also initiates from within this region (DeMarchi 1983; Jahn et al. 1984a, b; Plachter et al. 1988; Wathen and Stinski 1982). Additional IE gene expression arises within a region corresponding to the EcoRI Q fragment of strain AD169 (DeMarchi 1981; McDonough and Spector 1983; Wathen and Stinski 1982; Wilkinson et al. 1984). Three transcripts appear to be specified by this region, including a spliced 3.4-kb RNA present only at

IE times which may encode a membrane glycoprotein, a 1.7-kb unspliced RNA which is present throughout the infection, and a 1.65-kb spliced RNA which increases in abundance at late times and is 3' coterminal to the 3.4-kb RNA (KOUZARIDES et al. 1988). Another region of IE transcription originates within the short unique region of HCMV at an open reading frame designated HQLF1 (within HCMV strain AD169 *Eco*RI fragment L) and encodes at least four differentially spliced mRNAs (WESTON 1988; WESTON and BARRELL 1986). This transcription unit accounts for part of the IE expression arising from the AD169 L-S junction fragment *Eco*RI F (W + L) initially described by MCDONOUGH and SPECTOR (1983). We have also found that additional transcription from the region *Eco*RI F, as well as that seen from the L-S junction fragment *Eco*RI H (W + N), initiates from within the short repeats and extends into both the left and right ends of the short unique segment generating transcripts of 2.7 and 3.5 kb (RASMUSSEN and SPECTOR, unpublished observations). The positions of these transcripts correspond well with open reading frames found by sequence analysis of this region (WESTON and BARRELL 1986). Finally, other regions of IE transcription which have not been well characterized include *Eco*RI fragment B within the short unique segment and *Eco*RI fragments A and D within the long unique segment (MCDONOUGH and SPECTOR 1983).

The predominant IE RNA of HCMV, designated IE1, is a 1.9-kb spliced mRNA (DEMARCHI 1981; JAHN et al. 1984a, b; STENBERG et al. 1984) which encodes a 72-kDa nuclear phosphoprotein (GIBSON 1981; STINSKI et al. 1983). The high level of expression of IE1 has been attributed to a viral *trans*-acting factor (SPAETE and MOCARSKI 1985; STINSKI and ROEHR 1985) in addition to an extremely strong enhancer/promoter (BOSHART et al. 1985; STINSKI and ROEHR 1985). The enhancer element of IE1 contains multiple subsets of partially conserved repeats of 17, 18, 19, and 21 bp. The 18-bp repeats, which are imperfectly repeated four times, contain a core element (5'GGGGACTTTCC3') which is present in the enhancer of the immunoglobulin κ light-chain gene and which is the recognition sequence for the factor NF-$\kappa\beta$ (PICARD and SCHAFFNER 1984; SEN and BALTIMORE 1986). Regions homologous to the 18-bp repeats have been identified in another IE enhancer located in the short unique region upstream of the open reading frame HQLF1 discussed above (WESTON and BARRELL 1986; WESTON 1988). Enhancer elements homologous to the 18-bp repeats are also found in the HIV enhancer (NABEL and BALTIMORE 1987), in the SV40 enhancer (DAVIDSON et al. 1986; WILDEMAN et al. 1986; ZENKE et al. 1986), and within the major IE promoter of murine cytomegalovirus (DORSCH-HASLER et al. 1985). The 19-bp repeats are found in five partially conserved copies, four of which contain the consensus sequence, 5'A/TCGTCA3', for binding of the cellular transcription factor designated ATF (LEE et al. 1987). This sequence is nested within the cyclic AMP response element (CRE) (MONTMINY et al. 1986; SILVER et al. 1987), and it is likely that the factors ATF and the CRE-binding protein (CREB) are identical or closely related. The ATF sequence has been found in a variety of adenovirus E1A-dependent promoters (LEE and GREEN 1987; LEE et al. 1987) and is also contained within several HCMV early promoters including a region of the HCMV 2.2-kb early RNA promoter that has been shown to be essential for transcription (STAPRANS et al. 1988). This will be discussed below.

Immediately downstream of IE1 is the IE2 region which appears to encode at least five protein products (86-, 55-, 40-, 27-, and 23-kDa) generated by alternative splicing events and sites of initiation (HERMISTON et al. 1987; STENBERG et al. 1989). Expression of the IE2 region is very complex and has been reported to occur by initiation from the IE1 promoter and linkage of the upstream exon(s) of IE1, or by initiation from an IE2 promoter. Recent studies suggest that region 2 mRNAs may be differentially expressed at early and late times in the infection (STENBERG et al. 1989). IE 3 lies downstream of IE 2 and has not yet been investigated in detail.

Clearly, IE transcription in HCMV is complex and involves many factors, both viral and cellular. Many of the putative IE gene products have not yet been identified, and the precise functions of even the known IE proteins have not been determined. Regulation of various early transcription units by IE factors most likely involves different IE gene products, alone or in combination, and probably in concert with host cellular factors as well. Whether the IE gene products interact directly with the viral DNA or modulate gene expression by interaction with host cellular factors at the transcriptional or posttranscriptional level are important questions to be answered. However, given the absolute dependence of HCMV early gene expression on prior expression of the IE genes, the full characterization of these gene products is essential for understanding the complex program of HCMV early transcription.

3 Class of Transcripts and Family of Proteins Encoded by *Eco*RI Fragments R and d

A major focus of research in our laboratory has been directed toward understanding the regulation and function of a class of early transcripts (originally designated the 2.2-kb class of RNAs; STAPRANS and SPECTOR 1986) arising from the adjacent *Eco*RI fragments R and d (map units 0.682–0.713), located at the right end of the long unique segment of the HCMV strain AD169 genome (see Fig. 2). Our analyses have revealed that gene expression from this region of the genome is regulated at multiple levels, involving both transcriptional and posttranscriptional mechanisms. RNA transcripts from this region are detected by 8 h p.i. and include two fully processed species (2.1 kb and 2.2 kb) with a complex spliced structure consisting of invariable 5′ and internal exons and alternative 3′ exons with coterminal 3′ ends (STAPRANS and SPECTOR 1986). As the infection progresses from early to middle and late times, there is an increase in the complexity of transcription from this region. As will be discussed below, part of this increase in complexity results from a change in the splicing patterns of the primary transcription unit, generating two additional transcripts, one of 2.5 kb which has spliced out only the first intron and a second completely unspliced transcript of 2.65 kb (STAPRANS and SPECTOR 1986; WRIGHT and SPECTOR 1989). The other late RNAs arise from transcription of the opposite strand (RASMUSSEN and SPECTOR, unpublished results).

The position of the 5′ end of this class of RNA transcripts was determined by S₁ nuclease analysis (STAPRANS and SPECTOR 1986). At early times in the infection, a

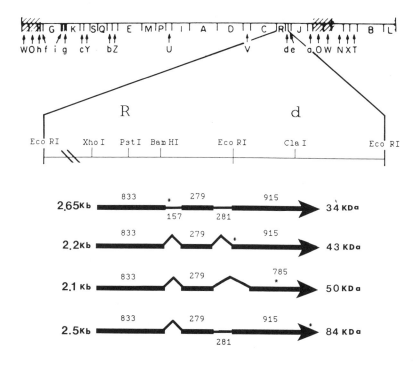

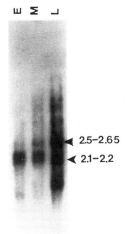

Fig. 2. The *Eco*RI restriction profile of HCMV strain AD 169 is shown along with an expanded map of the R/d region encoding the family of early RNAs. Not all *Bam*HI and *Xho*I sites are shown. The positions of the component exons and introns of the RNAs are summarized below, with sizes given in nucleotides. The *asterisks* represent in-frame stop codons for each RNA. The size of the RNA (kb) is shown *on the left*, and the protein specified by each RNA is shown *on the right*. The Northern analysis *at the bottom* is an adaptation from STAPRANS and SPECTOR (1986). Cytoplasmic polyadenylated RNA (5 μg) from uninfected cells or from infected cells at 8 h (E), 28 h (M), or 72 h (L) postinfection was electrophoresed on a denaturing formaldehyde gel, transferred to diazotized paper, and hybridized to the ^{32}P-labeled HCMV R-d fusion fragment

single initiation site was detected. If one assigns the 5′ terminus as position 1 on the DNA sequence, a 5′-TATAAA-3′ sequence is present at nucleotide −27 through −22. At late times, a second transcription start site also appeared to be used. This site maps 60 bp upstream of the early site. Just upstream of this second initiation site are two sequences which resemble a TATA box: a 5′-TAATAAA-3′ sequence which appears 42 bp upstream and a 5′-TTTAA-3′ sequence which appears 28 bp upstream. The latter sequence is similar to the 5-TTTAAAAA-3′ sequence which appears to be the functional TATA box of the herpes simplex virus type 1 glycoprotein D gene promoter (EVERETT 1984).

To define functionally important upstream regulatory elements of this early gene, a hybrid plasmid containing 5' promoter sequences (-694 to $+35$) fused to the *Escherichia coli* chloramphenicol acetyltransferase (CAT) gene was tested in transient expression assays in human fibroblast cells, both in the absence and presence of HCMV infection (STAPRANS et al. 1988). This promoter-CAT hybrid gene generated a low basal level of activity in uninfected cells which was significantly induced within 6 h after HCMV infection, consistent with the expectation for an early gene. The RNA start site for the hybrid mRNA corresponded to the major early start site of the viral RNA, at least up to 28 h p.i. Whether the second upstream site is used for the hybrid gene at late times in the infection has not been determined. By sequential deletions of the 5' end of the promoter, several regions were found to be functionally important for the regulation of this gene at early times. For full induction by HCMV infection, 323 bp of upstream sequence was necessary. With further successive deletions, a stepwise reduction in the inducible CAT activity was noted, with plasmids containing 224, 113, and 58 bp of 5' sequences showing 2- to 3-fold 4- to 6-fold, and 25- to 50-fold reductions, respectively, of CAT activity. A construct containing only the TATA box and three additional bp upstream (-30) was still minimally inducible, but deletion of the TATA sequence resulted in a total loss of activity. These results suggested that this HCMV early promoter consists of multiple elements, the sum total of which results in full inducibility.

By visual inspection and computer-assisted homology searches against a number of viral early gene promoters and known cellular transcription-factor-binding sites, the promoter sequence was analyzed for potential regulatory sequences (STAPRANS et al. 1988). Three major structural features in the promoter sequence were revealed by this analysis. The first *cis* element is a nine-base direct repeat (GCGGAAAGG) starting at positions -244 and -218, which is referred to as DR2. The second feature is also a nine-base direct repeat (ACGTTGTTT) that is located at positions -193 and -69 and is designated DR1. The third important region is a "TATA" box starting at position -27. Close inspection of the sequence (TGACGTTGTTT) that overlaps the DR1 element at position -69 (but not the DR1 at -193) reveals that there is a 10 out of 11 base match with a sequence in an important regulatory region of the adenovirus E2 promoter (IMPERIALE et al. 1985; MURTHY et al. 1985; SIVARAMAN and THIMMAPPAYA 1987; SIVARAMAN et al. 1986). Within this region is the consensus sequence (in the inverted orientation) for the binding site [(T/A)CGTCA] of the cellular transcription factor ATF/CREB (LEE and GREEN 1987; LEE et al. 1987; MONTMINY et al. 1986; SILVER et al. 1987). It is likely that the region surrounding and including the DR1 at -69 plays a major role in the regulation of the 2.2-kb RNA gene, since the greatest reduction in activity of the hybrid gene occurs with the deletion of -113 to -58. To verify that these sequence elements are important for promoter activity, it will be necessary to demonstrate specific protein-DNA interactions at these sites, as well as to define precisely the critical sequences within these regions by site-directed mutagenesis.

In concert with the analysis of the *cis*-acting regions necessary for induction of this promoter at early times, studies have also been directed toward the identification of the essential *trans*-acting factors interacting with this promoter. As discussed above, it has been assumed that one or more HCMV IE gene products would play an important role in the regulation of early gene expression. Several previous studies attempted to identify the IE gene(s) of HCMV that could *trans*-activate other genes, and focused on the major IE region encoded in *Hin*dIII fragment E. Using transient expression assays, *Everett* (1984) first demonstrated that the HCMV *Hin*dIII fragment E, encoding the IE1, IE2, and IE3 genes, could stimulate transcription from a herpes simplex virus early gene promoter. HERMISTON et al. (1987) subsequently found that IE2a was sufficient to activate heterologous promoters, although this activity could be augmented by the addition of IE1. In contrast, PIZZORNO et al. (1988) and DAVIS et al. (1987) have shown that the minimum IE region required for *trans*-activation of heterologous promoters is the first three exons of IE1 linked to IE2a in the genomic configuration. The difficulty in interpreting these data is that each study used different promoters and performed the transient expression assays in different cells. In the studies by STAPRANS et al. (1988), the question of which IE genes are specifically required for *trans*-activating HCMV early genes in cells fully permissive for HCMV viral replication was first addressed. For these analyses, human foreskin fibroblasts were cotransfected with constructs containing the major IE region or subclones thereof, and one of the hybrid gene constructs (i.e., viral promoter linked to CAT). It was found that the minimal IE region capable of activating this early gene promoter is IE1 and IE2a linked in the genomic configuration.

Although it is clear that IE gene products specified by the IE1 and IE2a regions are essential for induction of HCMV early gene expression, how they participate in this regulation remains enigmatic. From a comparison of this HCMV early promoter with that of other CMV and HSV early promoters (see below), it appears that, other than the TATA sequence, relatively little sequence homology is shared between them. This sequence diversity suggests viral gene regulation is mediated through multiple *cis*-acting regulatory sequences and *trans*-acting factors. Additionally, it is expected that most of these *trans*-acting factors will be normal host factors either induced or modified by viral IE genes. The challenge is to identify these factors and determine the basis of their regulation.

The above studies showed that the genetic unit encoded by *Eco*RI fragments R and d was regulated at the level of transcription by IE gene products. However, as described below, subsequent analysis of the pattern of expression of the specific mRNAs and their corresponding protein products suggested additional levels of regulation.

To first identify the proteins encoded by this genetic unit, antisera directed against a synthetic peptide corresponding to the predicted amino terminus of the proteins was generated (WRIGHT et al. 1988). With this antisera, it was possible to show that the class of transcripts specified by this region in strain AD169 encodes four nuclear phosphoproteins of 84, 50, 43, and 34 kDa. The proteins are highly conserved among other HCMV strains and have been identified in the laboratory strain, Towne, as well as in two recent, independent clinical isolates (WRIGHT and SPECTOR 1989). From a comparison of the tryptic peptide maps of the [^{35}S] methionine-labeled 84-, 50-, 43-, and 34-kDa infected cell proteins, it was apparent that all four proteins shared a common amino terminus which corresponds to exon 1 (WRIGHT et al. 1988). We also compared their tryptic peptide maps to an in vitro polypeptide derived from a synthetic RNA beginning upstream of the first initiating AUG codon and extending into the 3' exons. The first in-frame stop codon for this in vitro product occurred 48 bases downstream of the putative splice donor site. We found that the in vitro and in vivo proteins were similar in size (~ 34 kDa) and generated identical tryptic maps. This led us to suggest that the 34-kDa protein could be encoded from a transcript which had failed to splice out the first intron.

Analysis of the kinetics of expression of the proteins in short-term labeling experiments revealed that all four proteins could be detected by 8 h p.i. (WRIGHT et al. 1988). The 43-kDa protein was the most abundantly translated throughout the infection. Its rate of synthesis was maximal by 8 h p.i. and only decreased slightly at late times. The 84- and 50-kDa proteins displayed a low level of synthesis at 8 h p.i. and increased in rate as the infection progressed. The 34-kDa protein was barely detectable at 8 h p.i. and its rate of synthesis increased significantly between 24 and 72 h p.i. Analysis of steady-state levels of the proteins by Western blot analysis showed a major increase in the accumulation of all four proteins as the infection progressed to late times.

To further address the posttranscriptional regulatory mechanisms involved in the generation of these proteins, we have subsequently utilized cDNA cloning and transient expression assays in COS-7 cells to correlate each protein product with a specific mRNA (WRIGHT and SPECTOR 1989). Four classes of cDNAs were identified. One class of cDNAs corresponded to the unspliced 2.65-kb genomic transcript, which, as noted above, increased in abundance as the infection proceeded to late times. When this genomic clone was transfected into COS-7 cells, all four of the proteins were synthesized in proportions similar to that seen in AD169-infected cells at late times in the infection. Two other classes of cDNAs corresponded to the fully processed transcripts of 2.1 and 2.2 kb, which we previously identified as the predominant early RNAs (STAPRANS and SPECTOR 1986). The group which had spliced the two common 5' exons to the larger of the two 3' heterologous exons and which corresponded to the 2.2-kb RNA encoded the 43-kDa protein. The other class, which had spliced the two common exons to the shorter 3' exon and thus corresponded to the 2.1-kb RNA, encoded the 50-kDa protein. The final group of cDNAs had spliced out only the first intron and corresponded to the 2.5-kb transcript, which also does not appear in abundance until late times in the infection. In transient expression assays, this cDNA class specified predominantly the 84-kDa protein and small amounts of the 43- and 50-kDa proteins, which were probably generated by secondary splicing events in the COS-7 cells. Our finding that the 34-kDa protein was not generated by any clone which had removed the first intron further supported our previous suggestion, which was based on a comparison of tryptic peptide maps of an in vitro synthesized polypeptide with the in vivo 34-kDa protein, that a full-length transcript could encode the 34-kDa protein (WRIGHT et al. 1988).

The above data, as well as previous analysis of the kinetics of accumulation and relative rates of synthesis of this family of proteins as a function of time (WRIGHT et al. 1988), suggested that this transcription unit was regulated posttranscriptionally by alternative RNA splicing as the infection progresses. This type of posttranscriptional regulatory mechanism generating alternatively spliced RNAs from the same genetic unit, although not commonly used by herpesviruses, has been noted for several other HCMV genes. For example, the multiple HCMV RNAs arising from the IE1- and IE2-coding units likely arise, at least in part, from alternative splicing (HERMISTON et al. 1987; STENBERG et al. 1985). Alternative processing is also seen for the IE RNAs originating from the open reading frame designated HQLF1 located within EcoRI fragment L in the short unique region of HCMV strain AD169 (WESTON 1988; WESTON and BARRELL 1986), as well as for the IE RNAs arising from EcoRI fragment Q located in the long unique segment of the AD169 genome (KOUZARIDES et al. 1988). The general trend in these alternative splicing mechanisms is the transition from highly spliced RNAs to less-processed RNAs as the infection progresses to late times. This is the same pattern we see for the family of RNAs encoded by EcoRI fragments R and d described above. An exception to this trend is the RNA of a proposed late gene product which is transcribed at early times, but does not accumulate in the cytoplasm until late in the infection (GOINS and STINSKI 1986). In this case, the appearance of the transcripts in the cytoplasm correlates with differential processing of the 3' ends either by alternative 3'-terminal cleavage and polyadenylation or by differential splicing. The mechanisms responsible for the differential splicing patterns of HCMV RNAs have yet to be elucidated, but their identification and characterization should provide important insights into the host cell splicesome as well as the posttranscriptional regulatory mechanisms utilized by HCMV.

With assignment of the 84-, 50-, 43-, and 34-kDa proteins to individual transcripts, it was then possible to compare the pattern of expression of the RNAs with that of the proteins. The pattern of expression of the 84- and 34-kDa proteins correlated well with that of their corresponding mRNAs. The appearance of the 43-kDa protein as the most abundant protein at early times was also consistent with the finding that the fully processed 2.2-kb transcript was most abundant by 8 h p.i. (STAPRANS and SPECTOR 1986). In contrast, however, the 2.1-kb RNA was only slightly less abundant than the 2.2-kb RNA at all times in the infection, and yet the synthesis of the 50-kDa protein was barely detectable at 8 h p.i., and its rate of synthesis only increased as the infection progressed (WRIGHT et al. 1988). These results suggested that expression of the 50-kDa protein was subject to additional posttranscriptional controls. One possible explanation for the lack of correlation between the concentration of the 2.1-kb RNA and the synthesis of the 50-kDa protein is that at early times in the infection the 2.1-kb RNA, although located in the cytoplasm, is blocked in transport to polysomes or not translated efficiently. Alternatively, the 50-kDa protein might be highly unstable and quickly degraded. This latter explanation, however, is difficult to reconcile with previous pulse-chase analysis, which showed that when infected cell monolayers at 8 h p.i. were pulsed for 10 min with [^{35}S]methionine and chased for up to 120 min the 50-kDa protein was as stable as the 43-kDa protein (WRIGHT et al. 1988). It is also possible that the 50-kDa protein is transiently unstable either during or immediately after translation, and that only after localization to the nucleus does it become stabilized.

An additional level of regulation of this class of HCMV early RNAs appears to be related to viral DNA replication (WRIGHT and SPECTOR 1989). In particular, when viral DNA replication is inhibited, the steady-state concentration of these transcripts is reduced. It should be noted that in the absence of inhibitors the overall abundance of the class of RNAs analyzed in this study does not increase at late times despite a large amplification of template. Therefore, this pseudodependence on DNA replication is more likely the result of this true early transcription unit being greatly downregulated as viral template levels increase, giving the appearance of a relatively constant level of RNA production. Whether this downregulation is the result of a decrease in positive regulatory factor(s), or an increase in negative regulatory factor(s), remains an important question yet to be addressed.

Although the overall production of this family of RNAs and their protein products was diminished when viral DNA replication was inhibited, we also observed differential susceptibility of the proteins to this inhibition. In the absence of viral DNA replication, there was a disproportional loss of the 2.2-kb transcript encoding the 43-kDa protein. Despite the decrease in abundance of the 2.2-kb RNA, the 43-kDa protein still accumulated to higher levels than the other proteins. These data support the previous results, which indicated that the 2.2-kb RNA was most efficiently translated at early times, and imply that this mechanism is retained when the infection is held in an "early" state by inhibition of viral DNA replication. In contrast, although the concentration of the 2.1-kb RNA decreased somewhat in the absence of viral DNA replication, the 50-kDa protein was markedly sensitive to inhibition of viral DNA replication and decreased in abundance to levels below detection. These results lend support to the idea that the posttranscriptional processes which allow accumulation of the 50-kDa protein at late times are blocked when viral DNA replication is inhibited, and that these functions are not required for production of the other proteins.

A final mechanism of posttranscriptional processing of this family of proteins was found to operate at the level of differential phosphorylation (WRIGHT and SPECTOR 1989). This differential phosphorylation was not due to phosphorylation of different amino acids, since all four proteins contained only phosphoserine. The tryptic maps of all four proteins showed unique patterns of phosphorylation with only a single common phosphopeptide. The shared phosphopeptide contained the most abundant site of phosphorylation for the 43-kDa protein and was present in lesser amounts in each of the other proteins. The functional significance of the alternative sites of phosphorylation in the HCMV proteins is not clear. In this regard, we have recently initiated experiments further to characterize the biochemical properties of these proteins (WRIGHT and SPECTOR, unpublished results). All four proteins have been shown to bind to both ssDNA and dsDNA in vitro with a higher affinity for ssDNA. The proteins are concentrated in nuclear inclusions and colocalize with the 52-kDa major DNA-binding protein from human cytomegalovirus (GIBSON 1984; GIBSON et al. 1981; WRIGHT and SPECTOR, unpublished results).

A key question yet to be answered concerns the role of these proteins in HCMV replication. Attention was first drawn to this region in studies which showed that

*Eco*RI fragment R (specifically the region corresponding to exon 1 of the above-described transcripts) and, to a lesser extent, *Eco*RI fragment d in HCMV strain AD169 hybridized to uninfected cell DNA of human, murine, and sea urchin origin (SHAW et al. 1985). From the DNA sequence, it is clear that some of the observed virus-cell homology is likely due to the high $G + C$ content of both this HCMV region and the corresponding cell sequences, which include the 28S ribosomal DNA locus (SHAW et al. 1985; STAPRANS and SPECTOR 1986). Of special note is the high glycine content of the first exon. Preliminary DNA sequence analysis of the remainder of the coding region for these proteins also shows that the proteins are basic, are glycine and proline rich, and contain numerous stretches of polyglycine and polyalanine (WRIGHT et al., unpublished data). In many respects, these proteins resemble the Epstein-Barr-virus-encoded nuclear antigen designated EBNA 1 (REEDMAN and KLEIN 1973), which plays an important role in the maintenance and replication of Epstein–Barr virus (EBV) when it is in an episomal form (YATES et al. 1985). EBNA 1 has been identified as an ssDNA-binding phosphoprotein (HEARING and LEVINE 1985), which contains a repeated amino acid domain, composed of glycine and alanine, that is encoded by repeated DNA sequences (termed IR3) with homology to moderately reiterated and interspersed sequences in mouse and human DNA (HELLER et al. 1982, 1985; HEARING et al. 1984; HENNESSEY and KIEFF 1983). These homologies to EBNA 1, along with the evolutionary conservation and nuclear localization of these HCMV early DNA-binding phosphoproteins, suggest that they may perform an important role in the regulation of viral DNA replication or gene expression.

In summary, these studies have revealed that this family of proteins has multiple levels of regulation. Transcription from this early gene is highly regulated and is dependent upon IE gene expression for induction and an unknown mechanism for downregulation late in the infection. Production of the proteins is regulated by alternative RNA splicing, which varies as the infection progresses to late times by decreasing the overall levels of splicing. The relative abundance of the proteins is also determined by differential translation or protein stability, which allows increased levels of the 50-kDa protein to be produced at late times. Finally, the presence of alternative phosphorylation patterns for each of the proteins, despite significant regions of homology, reveals yet another level of posttranscriptional regulation involved in their synthesis. Further analysis of the biochemical character-istics of these proteins and the regulatory mechanisms involved in their production should allow identification of the function of this family of highly regulated and evolutionarily conserved DNA-binding phosphoproteins from HCMV.

4 Early Transcripts Encoded by the Long Repeat

In initial studies on the transcription pattern of HCMV strain AD169, the major early transcription site was localized to a region within the repeat sequences bounding the long unique segment of the genome (MCDONOUGH and SPECTOR

1983). A similar transcription pattern was described for Towne, Eisenhardt, and Davis strains of HCMV, except that the major early transcription site of the Davis strain is located in the long segment adjacent to the repeat (DeMarchi 1981, 1983; Wathen and Stinski 1982; Hutchinson et al. 1986).

The nature of this site of abundant transcription was investigated by Northern blot and nuclease protection analyses, and two major noncontiguous RNAs of 1.2 kb and 2.7 kb were identified (McDonough et al. 1985; Hutchinson et al. 1986). The RNAs were unspliced and were transcribed in the same direction with the 3′ terminus of the 1.2-kb RNA mapping 1.7 kb upstream from the 5′ terminus of the 2.7-kb RNA. In strain AD169, the 1.2-kb RNA maps entirely within *Eco*RI fragment O, while the 2.7-kb RNA is transcribed from the *Eco*RI fragment O into *Eco*RI fragment W. This region also encodes a minor transcript of 2.0 kb which increases somewhat in abundance as the infection progresses (McDonough et al. 1985; Hutchinson et al. 1986). The 2.0-kb RNA is transcribed from the opposite strand and maps with its 5′ end very close to the 5′ end of the 2.7-kb RNA and its 3′ end overlapping the 3′ end of the 1.2-kb RNA by approximately 250 bases (Hutchinson et al. 1986). The two major RNAs, although both detected at early times, appear to be subject to different regulatory controls. The 2.7-kb RNA is greatly amplified between 8 and 27 h after infection, with the major increase in abundance occurring between 8 and 14 h, whereas the 1.2-kb RNA is amplified later, between 27 and 72 h after infection (McDonough et al. 1985).

Spaete and Mocarski (1985) first showed that a hybrid gene consisting of 1000 bp of promoter-proximal and 142 bp of transcribed sequences of the gene encoding the 2.7-kb RNA fused to an indicator gene was induced in a temporally authentic manner in transient assays. Subsequent studies (Geballe et al. 1986b; Geballe and Mocarski 1988) revealed that within the 5′ leader sequence (+ 62 to + 142) was a *cis*-acting signal which acted at the translational level to regulate expression of the hybrid gene. This translational control appears to be mediated by either of the two upstream AUG codons located within the leader sequence (Geballe and Mocarski 1988). Each of these AUG codons is followed by a short open reading frame (ORF), 7 and 35 codons in length, which would terminate before the initiation codon of the indicator gene. To identify the important *cis*-acting sequences important for the specific regulation of this gene at the transcriptional level, we proceeded to construct hybrid plasmids in which 5′ promoter sequences plus only 54 bp of putative leader sequence (lacking the upstream AUG codons) were fused to the CAT gene. These hybrid plasmids were then tested in transient expression assays in human fibroblasts (Klucher et al. 1989). Initially, we found that 651 bp of sequence upstream of the RNA start site was sufficient for HCMV-inducible CAT activity. By incubating these cells in the presence of phosphonoacetic acid, a specific inhibitor of viral DNA replication, we also were able to compare the hybrid CAT transcript to viral RNA produced from a nonreplicating template. Under these conditions, the steady-state accumulation of RNA expressed from the hybrid CAT gene closely paralleled that seen for the viral 2.7-kb RNA. In contrast, however, when viral DNA replication was allowed to proceed normally, the temporal accumulation of the hybrid CAT RNA paralleled that of the viral transcript until 26 h p.i., but then decreased threefold between 26 and

48 h p.i. During this latter period, the viral transcript increased approximately 1.5-fold. It should be noted that this difference occurs during the time interval when the viral template is undergoing 50- to 100-fold amplification. Thus, although the concentration of the 2.7 kb RNA is undergoing a slight increase at this time, it is also likely that there is either a relative decrease in positive regulatory factors or an accumulation of negative factors.

DNA sequence analysis of the region upstream of the start site of the 2.7-kb RNA showed a number of promoter-like features including homology to known cellular transcription factor-binding sites, G-C rich regions, and a TATA box sequence (GREENAWAY and WILKINSON 1987). To define important cis-acting signals within this promoter, a series of 5'-promoter deletion mutants were constructed and analyzed in transient expression assays (KLUCHER et al. 1989). A promoter containing 213 bp of upstream sequence was found to have full inducible activity, while deletion of sequences down to -13 completely abolished it. Reductions in inducible activity between these sequences occurred in a stepwise manner, analogous to what was described above for the family of RNAs transcribed from EcoRI fragments R and d. Analysis of the sequences contained within these defined regions showed a number of interesting features. Deletion of the region between -114 and -95 relative to the RNA start site resulted in approximately a two- to threefold decrease in HCMV-inducible activity. Within this region, we noted the presence of a palindromic octamer TCACGTGA (-112 to -105), which matches seven of eight nucleotides within the consensus binding site for MLTF/USF located in the promoter of the adenovirus major late gene (CARTHEW et al. 1985; SAWADAGO and ROEDER 1985). Also located within this region was the sequence TCGTCAC (-115 to -109), which contains within it the core sequence for CRE/ATF (LEE and GREEN 1987; LEE et al. 1987; MONTMINY et al. 1986; SILVER et al. 1987). The importance of this latter sequence is questionable, however, since it is also repeated in a region (-85 to -79) that does not appear to be necessary for inducible activity in transient expression assays. Other sequences important in the transient assays included a non-SPI (BRIGGS et al. 1986) G-C-rich region found between -53 and -39 (GTCAGCCCGCGCTCG) and the TATA box (-26 to -19).

Experiments have also recently been initiated to analyze the important upstream regulatory elements of the gene encoding the 1.2-kb RNA. Preliminary transient expression studies show that hybrid plasmids containing approximately 400 bp of upstream sequence and 42 bp of leader linked to the CAT gene are induced at early times following HCMV infection of transfected cells (RABERT et al., unpublished data). Within this upstream region at position -29 is a sequence (CATAAAA) resembling the TATA box (GREENAWAY and WILKINSON 1987). Further upstream, at position -74, is the consensus sequence for the binding site of the transcription factor AP1 (ANGEL et al. 1987; LEE et al. 1987a, b) and at position -211 is the consensus sequence for the binding site of CREB/ATF. The functional importance of these latter two sequences, if any, as well as other upstream regions are currently under investigation.

In studies analogous to those conducted above for the promoter directing the synthesis of the family of transcripts from EcoRI fragments R and d, we have also examined specific IE gene transactivation for the hybrid constructs containing the 1.2-kb and 2.7-kb RNA promoters (KLUCHER et al. 1989; RABERT et al., unpublished results). In both cases, we found that the minimum requirement for *trans*-activating hybrid promoters was cotransfection with a construct containing the IE1 and IE2 genes in a genomic configuration, but the level of transactivation was considerably less than that seen following HCMV infection. This is in contrast to the studies described in Sect. 3 where contransfection of the same IE gene construct with the chimaeric gene containing the *Eco*RI fragments R/d RNA promoter resulted in only a slightly lower level of transactivation than that seen following HCMV infection. These results are compatible with the temporal accumulation of the RNAs and suggest that full activation of the 2.7-kb and 1.2-kb RNA promoters requires additional viral or viral-induced cellular factors as the infection progresses.

In an effort to study the interactions of *trans*-acting factors with the regions defined by transient assays, we have recently prepared nuclear protein extracts and used these extracts in gel shift and DNase protection assays (KLUCHER et al. 1989; KLUCHER and SPECTOR, manuscript in preparation). In a series of experiments, using a probe that contained sequences from -213 to $+56$ of the 2.7-kb RNA promoter, specific DNA-protein complexes were seen with extracts from uninfected HeLa cells as well as uninfected and HCMV-infected human fibroblasts. The formation of these complexes could be specifically competed with sequences from -114 to $+56$ but not with sequences from -94 to $+56$. These specific complexes could also be formed with a probe containing sequences from -114 to $+56$ but not with sequences from -94 to $+56$. Therefore, it would appear that a specific protein-DNA interaction is occurring between a normal cellular protein and a segment of the DNA spanning nucleotides -114 to -95. This is one of the regions that we had defined as important for promoter activity in transient expression assays. When DNase footprinting was used to determine protein-DNA interactions, a single protected region was seen, which extended from -116 to -101 (ATCGTCACGTGAAATA) and which contains, at position -112 to -105, the previously described MLTF/USF-binding site (CARTHEW et al. 1985; SAWADAGO and ROEDER 1985). Further mutational analyses, competition studies with the adenovirus major late promoter, and in vitro transcription assays will be required to determine the exact nature and functional importance of this site.

The nature of the gene products specified by these two major RNAs have yet to be identified. DNA sequence analysis of the Eisenhardt strain of HCMV suggests that the 1.2-kb mRNA could encode a basic polypeptide of 30 kDa, and in vitro translation of infected cell mRNA which has been hybrid selected with a probe specific to this region yields a product which has an apparent size of 37 kDa (HUTCHINSON and TOCCI 1986). Yet, from the published DNA sequence of strain AD169, the region coding for the 1.2-kb mRNA contains multiple short ORFs (GREENAWAY and WILKINSON 1987). In the case of the 2.7-kb RNA, DNA sequencing has also shed little light on the product(s) of this gene, since, in strain AD169, it also contains multiple short ORFs, the longest of which could encode a polypeptide of 170 amino acids (GREENAWAY and WILKINSON 1987).

It may be that these short ORFs do serve a posttranscriptional regulatory function. For the 2.7-kb RNA, the ORF of 170 amino acids in length is preceded by two very short ORFs. As described above, analysis in transient assays of chimeric constructs containing these upstream AUG codons has shown that these upstream codons effectively inhibit translation from the downstream ORF (GEBALLE et al. 1986b; GEBALLE and MOCARSKI 1988). Whether CMV utilizes these upstream AUG codons to modulate the expression of any protein products encoded by this gene awaits the identification and kinetic characterization of the gene products actually specified by the 2.7-kb RNA in the infected cell. Although there is no direct evidence that CMV does utilize upstream AUG codons and short ORFs to regulate posttranscriptionally the abundance of any gene product, upstream AUG codons are also present in the genes encoding DNA polymerase (KOUZARIDES et al. 1987a,b), the pp150 phosphoprotein (JAHN et al. 1987), the gB envelope glycoprotein (KOUZARIDES et al. 1987a), and a 67-kDa tegument protein (DAVIS and HUANG 1985).

5 Other HCMV Early Genes

In this section, we briefly describe the properties of several additional early genes which have been mapped and characterized. For ease of presentation, they will be discussed according to their map position on the HCMV genome proceeding from left to right in the prototype organization.

CHANG et al. (1989) have analyzed an early transcription unit which is within the long unique segment adjacent to the long terminal repeat at the left end of the genome. Three unspliced coterminal RNAs of approximately 1.7 kb are transcribed from left to right from three separate initiation sites. Although all three promoters can be activated by IE2 alone when driven by a strong promoter or by IE1 and IE2 in transient expression assays, the three promoters appear to be regulated differentially during the infection such that the upstream promoter is used only at late times. As discussed above, a similar situation was noted for the family of transcripts encoded by *Eco*RI fragments R and d which also utilize an upstream promoter at late times. Upstream of the major early start site is the consensus sequence for the CCAAT-box binding factors, and just upstream of the initiation site used at late times is the consensus sequence for ATF/CRE.

Within *Eco*RI fragments Z, b, and Q is the coding unit for the major 52-kDa DNA-binding phosphoprotein designated ICP36 (GIBSON 1983, 1984; GIBSON et al. 1981; MOCARSKI et al. 1985). To localize the gene, MOCARSKI et al. (1985) screened a λgt11 expression library of random HCMV DNA fragments with a mixture of monoclonal antibodies directed against this specific protein (PEREIRA et al. 1982). The DNAs from positive plaques were then used as hybridization probes to map the coding sequences on the HCMV genome and to identify the major 4.8-kb transcript encoded by this region. The RNA is transcribed from right to left, but its precise 5′ and 3′ domains have not been defined. Preliminary analysis does suggest, however, that the 5′ end is heterogeneous with one major initiation site and two minor start sites just downstream of the major one (GEBALLE et al. 1986a). The observation that this transcript is present in high concentrations at early times in the infection, but the protein does not accumulate to its highest abundance until late times, has led to the suggestion that full expression of this gene is also controlled posttranscriptionally (GEBALLE et al. 1986a).

The region encoding the HCMV 140-kDa polymerase was identified on the basis of hybridization studies and DNA sequence analysis (KOUZARIDES et al. 1987a.b; HEILBRONN et al. 1987). In the course of sequencing a large region including *Eco*RI fragment M and parts of adjoining *Eco*RI fragments P and E within the long unique segment of HCMV strain AD169, KOUZARIDES et al. (1987a, b) noted an open reading frame which showed extensive amino acid homology to the polymerases of herpes simplex virus type 1 and Epstein-Barr virus. In a complementary approach, HEILBRONN et al. (1987) used a DNA fragment corresponding to the herpes simplex virus type 1 DNA polymerase gene as a probe and low stringency conditions of hybridization to identify cross-hybridizing sequences with the HCMV genome. The HCMV DNA polymerase gene is located within *Eco*RI fragment M and is transcribed from right to left into an RNA of approximately 5 kb. A single initiation site at the 5′ end has been mapped, but the presence of several S1-nuclease discontinuities at the 3′ end has precluded precise determination of the termination site. This transcript is present at early times in the infection but undergoes a major increase in abundance between early and late times p.i., analogous to the situation described for the 1.2-kb RNA encoded by the long repeat. Upstream of the RNA initiation site is the consensus sequence for ATF/CRE. It is interesting to note that preceding the *pol* open reading frame in the RNA is a 383-nucleotide leader segment that contains three AUG codons leading to short ORFs. The contribution, if any, of these ORFs to the regulation of expression of this RNA is unknown.

Upstream of the *pol* gene and transcribed in the same direction is the gene encoding a family of antigenically related glycoproteins initially designated gA (PEREIRA et al. 1984) but now designated gB because of the homology of the gene to the herpes simplex virus gB gene (CRANAGE et al. 1986; MACH et al. 1986; KOUZARIDES et al. 1987a). The ORF from this region is 906 amino acids in length and specifies a protein with a predicted size of 102 kDa and 16 possible N-linked glycosylation sites (KOUZARIDES et al. 1987a). The synthesis of the members of this family of glycoproteins appears to involve glycosylation of the primary translation product (p95) to form a high-mannose, simple N-linked protein of 158 kDa which is subsequently processed to form gp138, gp130, gp93, and gp55 (BRITT and AUGER 1986; FARRAR and GREENAWAY 1986; GRETCH et al. 1988a; RASMUSSEN et al. 1985). Using a probe from the gB-coding region, three transcripts can be detected including an unspliced 3.7-kb transcript and two longer transcripts of over 7.5 kb (KOUZARIDES et al. 1987a). The longer transcripts may be generated by read-through of an inefficient cleavage/polyadenylation site which is positioned immediately after the gB ORF and within the coding region of the DNA polymerase gene. These transcripts can be detected at early times but show a major increase in abundance at late times in the infection. There appears to be a single initiation site for the gB mRNA, and the RNA contains a 361-nucleotide leader with an AUG codon and a 16-amino-acid ORF preceding the gB ORF. Upstream of the gB RNA start site is the consensus sequence for ATF/CRE, although the functional significance of either this site or the one upstream of the *pol* gene has not yet been addressed.

KEMBLE et al. (1987) and ANDERS and GIBSON (1988) have mapped the HCMV homolog of the major DNA-binding protein of herpes simplex virus designated ICP8. This protein is 135–140 kDa in size and is expressed early in the infection, localizes to the nucleus, and binds to ssDNA in vitro (ANDERS and GIBSON 1988; ANDERS et al. 1986, 1987; KEMBLE et al. 1987). The large 10- to 12-kb RNA encoding this protein is transcribed from right to left and its 3' end maps at the right end of the region corresponding to EcoRI fragment P in HCMV strain AD169. As has already been discussed for other HCMV early genes, the transcript is present at high levels at early times (24 h p.i.), but the protein product accumulates to highest abundance at late times in the infection. Although the function of this HCMV DNA-binding protein is unknown, by analogy with its HSV counterpart ICP8 it is expected that it will play an important role in the replication of the viral DNA and in the regulation of gene expression (CONLEY et al. 1981; GODOWSKI and KNIPE 1983, 1985, 1986; O'DONNELL et al. 1987; ORBERG and SCHAFFER 1987; RUYECHAN 1983; RUYECHAN and WEIR 1984; RUYECHAN et al. 1986; SCHAFFER et al. 1976; WELLER et al. 1983).

Within a region corresponding to the left end of the EcoRI fragment I in the HCMV genome is an early transcription unit which is regulated posttranscriptionally by mechanisms which affect either the transport of the viral transcripts from the nucleus to the cytoplasm or the stability of the RNAs in the cytoplasm at early times after infection (GOINS and STINSKI 1986). At early times in the infection, high molecular weight RNAs from this region were transcribed from left to right and could be detected in abundance only in the nucleus. Beginning at 24 h p.i., two species, a minor RNA of 2.5 kb and a major RNA of 1.9 kb, could be detected in the cytoplasm and their steady-state concentration continued to increase as the infection progressed. A posttranscriptional processing event, occurring only after viral DNA replication, appears to alter the 3' end of the transcript, allowing either the export of the message into the cytoplasm or stabilization of the mRNA once in the cytoplasm. This differential processing of the 3' end of the transcript involves either alternative 3'-terminal cleavage and polyadenylation or differential splicing.

The region corresponding to EcoRI fragment B in the short unique segment of the HCMV strain AD169 genome is a site of extensive transcription at early times (MCDONOUGH and SPECTOR 1983). One gene contributing to this early transcription pattern corresponds to the HWLF1 reading frame (WESTON and BARRELL 1986). MOCARSKI et al. (1988) have shown that a major 2.4-kb RNA is synthesized from this region at early times and reaches maximal steady-state levels by 4–8 h p.i. This is analogous to the kinetics seen for the family of early RNAs synthesized by EcoRI fragments R and d discussed above. However, other than a TATA box, there appears to be no sequence homology in the putative promoter region. Interestingly, this gene encodes a 76-kDa nuclear phosphoprotein, originally designated ICP22 (PEREIRA and HOFFMAN 1986), which is released from cells as a soluble protein at both early and late times in the infection.

A second region transcribed at early times within EcoRI fragment B encodes a component of the virion envelope designated the gcII family or gp47–52 (GRETCH et al. 1988b, c; KARI et al. 1986). Within this region is a multigene family designated HXLF (WESTON and BARRELL 1986) consisting of five tandem ORFs with varying degrees of homology. By Northern blot analysis, a major 1.6-kb bicistronic transcription product of HXLF1 and 2 was detected at early times in the infection (GRETCH et al. 1988b). Analogous to the family of transcripts encoded by *Eco*RI fragments R and d, the abundance of the 1.6-kb transcript decreased somewhat as the infection progressed, and within the putative promoter region of this transcript are two sequences corresponding to the consensus binding site for ATF/CREB. Less-abundant transcripts of 1.0 and 0.8 kb, were also detected at early times. On the basis of amino acid and immunoprecipitation analysis it appears that this family of glycoproteins is most likely the product of the HXLF1 and HXLF2 genes. As has been noted for other early genes discussed in this review, the glyco-proteins specified by the HXLF gene family did not accumulate to highest abundance until late in the infection.

6 Concluding Remarks

The increasing awareness of the serious medical problems associated with HCMV infections has made it essential to focus research efforts toward understanding the molecular biology of this virus and its interaction with the host. The multiple pathogenic effects of HCMV are likely manifested through complex alterations in the biological and biochemical pathways of infected cells, involving not only viral gene products but also induced and repressed cellular gene functions. HCMV early gene expression clearly plays a pivotal role in this scheme. The molecular cloning and restriction endonuclease mapping of the HCMV genome have provided the basis of studying genome structure, viral replication, gene expression, and the nature and function of specific virus-encoded gene products. RNA analysis with defined probes, and protein analysis with specific monoclonal and polyclonal antibodies, have further contributed to our knowledge of HCMV gene expression. Much of the 240-kbp viral genome has already been sequenced, and with the expectation that this task will be completed soon the cataloguing of RNA transcripts and their respective protein products should proceed rapidly. The challenge remains to identify the role of HCMV gene products in viral replication and pathogenesis and to understand the complex regulatory mechanisms governing their expression.

References

Anders DG, Gibson W (1988) Location, transcript analysis, and partial nucleotide sequence of the cytomegalovirus gene encoding an early DNA-binding protein with similarities to ICP8 of Herpes simplex virus Type 1. J Virol 62: 1364–1372

Anders DG, Irmiere A, Gibson W (1986) Identification and characterization of a major early cytomegalovirus DNA-binding protein. J Virol 58: 253–262

Anders DG, Kidd JR, Gibson W (1987) Immunological characterization of an early cytomegalovirus single-strand DNA binding protein with similarities to the HSV major DNA-binding protein. Virology 161: 579–588

Angel P, Imagawa M, Chiu R, Stein B, Imbra RJ, Rahmsdorf HJ, Jonat C, et al. (1987) Phorbol ester-inducible genes contain a common *cis* element recognized by a TPA-modulated *trans*-acting factor. Cell 49: 729–739

Beck S, Barrell BG (1988) Human cytomegalovirus encodes a glycoprotein homologous to MHC class-I antigens. Nature 331: 269–272

Boshart M, Weber F, Jahn G, Dorsch-Hasler K, Fleckenstein B, Schaffner W (1985) A very strong enhancer is located upstream of an immediate early gene of human cytomegalovirus. Cell 41: 521–530

Briggs MR, Kadonaga JT, Bell SP, Tjian R (1986) Purification and biochemical characterization of the promoter-specific transcription factor, Spl Science 234: 47–52

Britt WJ, Auger D (1986) Synthesis and processing of the envelope gp55–116 complex of human cytomegalovirus. J Virol 58: 185–191

Carthew RW, Chodosh LA, Sharp PA (1985) An RNA polymerase II transcription factor binds to an upstream element in the adenovirus major late promoter. Cell 43: 439–448

Chang C-P, Malone CL, Stinski MF (1989) A human cytomegalovirus early gene has three inducible promoters that are regulated differentially at various times after infection. J Virol 63: 281–290

Conley AJ, Knipe DM, Jones PC, Roizman B (1981) Molecular genetics of herpes simplex virus. VII. Characterization of a temperature-sensitive mutant produced by in vitro mutagenesis and defective in DNA synthesis and accumulation of α polypeptides. J Virol 37: 191–206

Cranage MP, Kouzarides T, Bankier AT, Satchwell S, Weston K, Tomlinson P, Barrell B et al. (1986) Identification of the human cytomegalovirus glycoprotein B gene and induction of neutralizing antibodies via its expression in recombinant vaccinia virus. EMBO J 5: 3057–3063

Cranage MP, Smith GL, Bell SE, Hart H, Brown C, Bankier AT, Tomlinson P et al. (1988) Identification and expression of a human cytomegalovirus glycoprotein with homology to the Epstein-Barr virus BXLF2 product, varicella-zoster virus gpIII, and herpes simplex virus Type 1 glycoprotein H. J Virol 62: 1416–1422

Davidson I, Fromental C, Augereau P, Wildeman A, Zenke M, Chambon P (1986) Cell-type specific protein binding to the enhancer of simian virus 40 in nuclear extracts. Nature 323:544–548

Davis MG, Huang E-S (1985) Nucleotide sequence of a human cytomegalovirus DNA fragment encoding a 67-kilodalton phosphorylated viral protein. J Virol 56: 7–11

Davis MG, Mar E-C, Wu Y-M, Huang E-S (1984) Mapping and expression of a human cytomegalovirus major viral protein. J Virol 52: 129–135

Davis MG, Kenney S, Kamine J, Pagano JS, Huang E-S (1987) Immediate-early gene region of human cytomegalovirus *trans*-activates the promoter of human immunodeficiency virus. Proc Natl Acad Sci USA 84: 8642–8646

DeMarchi JM (1981) Human cytomegalovirus DNA: restriction enzyme cleavage and map locations for immediate early, early and late RNAs. Virology 114: 23–28

DeMarchi JM (1983) Posttranscriptional control of human cytomegalovirus gene expression. Virology 124: 390–402

DeMarchi JM, Blankenship ML, Brown GD, Kaplan AS (1978) Size and complexity of human cytomegalovirus DNA. Virology 89: 643–646

DeMarchi JM, Schmidt CA, Kaplan AS (1980) Patterns of transcription of human cytomegalovirus in permissively infected cells. J Virol 35: 277–286

Dorsch-Hasler K, Keil GM, Weber F, Jasin M, Schaffner W, Koszinowski UH (1985) A long and complex enhancer activates transcription of the gene coding for the highly abundant immediate early mRNA in murine cytomegalovirus. Proc Natl Acad Sci USA 82: 8325–8329

Drew WL, Miner RC, Ziegler JL, Gullett JH, Abrams DI, Conant MA, Huang E-S, et al. (1982) Cytomegalovirus and Kaposi's sarcoma in young homosexual men. Lancent 2: 125–127

Everett RD (1984) A detailed analysis of an HSV-1 early promoter: sequences involved in *trans*-activation by viral immediate-early gene products are not early-gene specific. Nucleic Acids Res 12: 3037–3056

Farrar GJ, Greenaway PJ (1986) Characterization of glycoprotein complexes present in human cytomegalovirus envelopes. J Gen Virol 67: 1469–1473

Fleckenstein B, Muller I, Collins J (1982) Cloning of the complete human cytomegalovirus genome in cosmids. Gene 18: 39–46

Geballe AP, Mocarski ES (1988) Translation control of cytomegalovirus gene expression is mediated by upstream AUG codons. J Virol 62: 3334–3340

Geballe AP, Leach FS, Mocarski ES (1986a) Regulation of cytomegalovirus late gene expression: γ genes are controlled by posttranscriptional events. J Virol 57: 864–874

Geballe AP, Spaete RR, Mocarski ES (1986b) A *cis*-acting element within the 5′ leader of a cytomegalovirus β transcript determines kinetic class. Cell 46: 865–872

Geelen JLMC, Walig C, Wertheim P, van der Noordaa J (1978) Human cytomegalovirus DNA I. Molecular weight and infectivity. J Virol 26: 813–816

Gibson W (1981) Immediate-early proteins of human cytomegalovirus strains AD169, Davis, and Towne differ in electrophoretic mobility. Virology 112: 350–354

Gibson W (1983) Protein counterparts of human and simian cytomegaloviruses. Virology 128: 391–406

Gibson W (1984) Synthesis, structure, and function of cytomegalovirus major nonvirion nuclear protein. UCLA Symp Mol Biol 21: 423–440

Gibson W, Murphy T, Roby C (1981) Cytomegalovirus-infected cells contain a DNA-binding protein. Virology 111: 251–262

Godowski PJ, Knipe DM (1983) Mutations in the major DNA-binding protein gene of herpes simplex virus type 1 result in increased levels of viral gene expression. J Virol 47: 478–486

Godowski PJ, Knipe DM (1985) Identification of a herpes simplex virus function that represses late gene expression from parental viral genomes. J Virol 55: 357–365

Godowski PJ, Knipe DM (1986) Transcriptional control of herpesvirus gene expression: gene functions required for positive and negative regulation. Proc Natl Acad Sci USA 83: 256–260

Goins WF, Stinski MF (1986) Expression of a human cytomegalovirus late gene is posttranscriptionally regulated by a 3'-end-processing event occurring exclusively late after infection. Mol Cell Biol 6: 4202–4213

Greenaway PJ, Wilkinson GWG (1987) Nucleotide sequence of the most abundantly transcribed early gene of human cytomegalovirus strain AD169. Virus Res 7: 17–31

Greenaway PJ, Oram JD, Downing RG, Patel K (1982) Human cytomegalovirus DNA: *Bam*HI, *Eco*RI and *Pst*I restriction endonuclease cleavage maps. Gene 18: 355–360

Gretch DR, Gehrz RC, Stinski MF (1988a) Characterization of a human cytomegalovirus glycoprotein complex (gcI). J Gen Virol 69: 1205–1215

Gretch DR, Kari B, Gehrz RC, Stinski MF (1988b) A multigene family encodes the human cytomegalovirus glycoprotein complex gcII (gp 47–52 complex). J Virol 62: 1956–1962

Gretch DR, Kari B, Rasmussen L, Gehrz R, Stinski MF (1988c) Identification and characterization of three distinct families of glycoprotein complexes in the envelopes of human cytomegalovirus. J Virol 62: 875–881

Hearing JC, Levine AJ (1985) The Epstein-Barr virus nuclear antigen (*Bam*HI K antigen) is a single-stranded DNA binding phosphoprotein. Virology 145: 105–116

Hearing JC, Nicolay J-C, Levine AJ (1984) Identification of Epstein-Barr virus sequences that encode a nuclear antigen expressed in latently infected lymphocytes. Proc Natl Acad Sci USA 81: 4373–4377

Heilbronn R, Jahn G, Burkle A, Fresse U-K, Fleckenstein B, zur Hausen H (1987) Genomic localization, sequence analysis, and transcription of the putative human cytomegalovirus DNA polymerase gene. J Virol 61: 119–124

Heller M, van Santen V, Kieff E (1982) Simple repeat sequence in Epstein-Barr virus DNA is transcribed in latent and productive infections. J Virol 44: 311–320

Heller M, Flemington E, Kieff E, Deininger P (1985) Repeat arrays in cellular DNA related to the Epstein-Barr virus IR3 repeat. Mol Cell Biol 5: 457–465

Hennessey K, Kieff E (1983) One of two Epstein-Barr virus nuclear antigens contains a glycine-alanine copolymer domain. Proc Natl Acad Sci USA 80: 5665–5669

Hermiston TW, Malone CL, Witte PR, Stinski MF (1987) Identification and characterization of the human cytomegalovirus immediate-early region 2 gene that stimulates gene expression from an inducible promoter. J Virol 61: 3214–3232

Ho M (1982) Cytomegalovirus: biology and infection. Plenum, New York

Hutchinson NI, Tocci MJ (1986) Characterization of a major early gene from human cytomegalovirus long inverted repeat; predicted amino acid sequence of a 30-kDa protein encoded by the 1.2 kb mRNA. Virology 155: 172–182

Hutchinson NI, Sondermeyer RT, Tocci MJ (1986) Organization and expression of the major genes from the long inverted repeat of the human cytomegalovirus genome. Virology 155: 160–171

Imperiale MJ, Hart RP, Nevins JR (1985) An enhancer-like element in the adenovirus E2 promoter contains sequences essential for uninduced and EIA-induced transcription. Proc Natl Acad Sci USA 82: 381–385

Jahn G, Knust E, Schmolla H, Sarre T, Nelson JA, McDougall JK, Fleckenstein B (1984a) Predominant immediate-early transcripts of human cytomegalovirus AD169. J Virol 49: 363–370

Jahn G, Nelson JA, Plachter B, McDougall JK, Fleckenstein B (1984b) Transcription of a human cytomegalovirus DNA region which is capable of transforming rodent cells. UCLA Symp Mol Cell Biol 21: 455–463

Jahn G, Kouzarides T, Mach M, Schol B-C, Plachter B, Traupe B, Preddie E, et al. (1987) Map position and nucleotide sequence of the gene for the large structural phosphoprotein of human cytomegalovirus. J Virol 61: 1358–1367

Kari B, Lussenhop N, Goertz R, Wabuke-Burot M, Radeke M, Gehrz R (1986) Characterization of monoclonal antibodies reactive to several biochemically distinct human cytomegalovirus glycoprotein complexes. J Virol 60: 345–352

Kemble GW, McCormick AL, Pereira L, Mocarski ES (1987) A cytomegalovirus protein with properties of herpes simplex virus ICP8; partial purification of the polypeptide and map position of the gene. J Virol 61: 3143–3151

Klucher KM, Rabert DK, Spector DH (1989) Sequences in the human cytomegalovirus 2.7-Kilobase promoter which mediate its regulation as an early gene. J Virol 63: 5334–5343

Kouzarides T, Bankier AT, Satchwell AC, Weston K, Tomlinson P, Barrell BG (1987a) Large-scale rearrangement of homologous regions in the genomes of HCMV and EBV. Virology 157: 397–413

Kouzarides T, Bankier AT, Satchwell AC, Weston K, Tomlinson P, Barrell BG (1987b) Sequence and transcription analysis of the human cytomegalovirus DNA polymerase gene. J Virol 61: 125–133

Kouzarides T, Bankier AT, Satchwell SC, Preddy E, Barrell BG (1988) An immediate early gene of human cytomegalovirus encodes a potential membrane glycoprotein. Virology 165: 151–164

LaFemina RL, Hayward GS (1980) Structural organization of the DNA molecules from human cytomegalovirus. ICN UCLA Symp Mol Cell Biol 18: 39–55

Lakeman AD, Osborn JE (1979) Size of infectious DNA from human and murine cytomegaloviruses. J Virol 30: 414–416

Lee KAW, Green MR (1987) A cellular transcription factor E4F1 interacts with an EIA-inducible enhancer and mediates constitutive enhancer function in vitro. EMBO J 6: 1345–1353

Lee KAW, Hai TY, SivaRaman L, Thimmappaya B, Hurst HC, Jones NC, Green MR (1987) A cellular protein, activating transcription factor, activates transcription of multiple EIA-inducible adenovirus early promoters. Proc Natl Acad Sci USA 84: 8355–8359

Lee W, Haslinger A, Karin M, Tjian R (1987a) Activation of transcription by two factors that bind promoter and enhancer sequences of the human metallothionein gene and SV40. Nature 325: 368–372

Lee W, Mitchell P, Tjian R (1987b) Purified transcription factor AP-1 interacts with TPA-inducible enhancer elements. Cell 49: 741–752

Mach M, Utz U, Fleckenstein B (1986) Mapping of the major glycoprotein gene of human cytomegalovirus. J Gen Virol 67: 1461–1467

Macher AM, Reichert CM, Straus SE, Longo DL, Parillo J, Lane HC, Fauci AS, et al. (1983) Death in the AIDS patient: role of cytomegalovirus. N Engl J Med 309: 1454

Marchevsky A, Rosen MJ, Chrystal G, Kleinerman J (1985) Pulmonary complications of the acquired immunodeficiency syndrome. Hum Pathol 16: 659–670

Martinez J, Lahijani RS, St Jeor SC (1989) Analysis of a region of the human cytomegalovirus (AD169) genome coding for a 25-kilodalton virion protein. J Virol 63: 233–241

McDonough SH, Spector DH (1983) Transcription in human fibroblasts permissively infected by human cytomegalovirus strain AD169. Virology 125: 31–46

McDonough SH, Staprans SI, Spector DH (1985) Analysis of the major transcripts encoded by the long repeat of human cytomegalovirus strain AD169. J Virol 53: 711–718

McKnight S, Tjian R (1986) Transcriptional selectivity of viral genes in mammalian cells. Cell 46: 795–805

Meyer H, Bankier AT, Landini MP, Brown CM, Barrell BG, Ruger B, Mach M (1988) Identification and procaryotic expression of the gene coding for the highly immunogenic 28-kilodalton structural phosphoprotein (pp28) of human cytomegalovirus. J Virol 62: 2243–2250

Mocarski ES, Pereira L, Michael N (1985) Precise localization of genes on large animal virus genomes: use of λgt11 and monoclonal antibodies to map the gene for a cytomegalovirus protein family. Proc Natl Acad Sci USA 82: 1266–1270

Mocarski ES, Pereira L, McCormick AL (1988) Human cytomegalovirus ICP22, the product of HWLF1 reading frame, is an early nuclear protein that is released from cells. J Gen Virol 69: 2613–2621

Montminy MR, Sevarino KA, Wagner JA, Mandel G, Goodman RH (1986) Identification of a cyclic-AMP responsive element within the rat somatostatin gene. Proc Natl Acad Sci USA 83: 6682–6686

Murthy SCS, Bhat GP, Thimmappaya B (1985) Adenovirus EIA promoter: transcriptional control elements and induction by the viral pre-early EIA gene, which appears to be sequence independent. Proc Natl Acad Sci USA 82: 2230–2234

Nabel G, Baltimore D (1987) An inducible transcription factor activates expression of human immuno-deficiency virus in T cell. nature 326: 711–713

Nankervis GA, Kumar ML (1978) Diseases produced by cytomegaloviruses. Med Clin North Am 62: 1021–1035

Nowak B, Gmeiner A, Sarnow P, Levine AJ, Fleckenstein B (1984) Physical mapping of human cytomegalovirus genes: identification of DNA sequences coding for a virion phosphoprotein of 71 kDa and a viral 65-kDa polypeptide. Virology 134: 91–102

O'Donnell ME, Elias P, Funnell BE, Lehman IR (1987) Interaction between the DNA polymerase and single-stranded DNA-binding protein (infected cell protein 8) of herpes simplex virus 1. J Biol Chem 262: 4260–4266

Oram JD, Downing RG, Akrigg A, Dollery AA, Duggleby CJ, Wilkinson GWG, Greenaway PJ (1982) Use of recombinant plasmids to investigate the structure of the human cytomegalovirus genome. J Gen Virol 59: 111–129

Orberg PK, Schaffer PA (1987) Expression of herpes simplex virus type 1 major DNA-binding protein, ICP8, in transformed cell lines: complementation of deletion mutants and inhibition of wild-type virus. J Virol 61: 1136–1146

Pande H, Baak WS, Riggs AD, Clark BR, Shively JE, Zaia JA (1984) Cloning and physical mapping of a gene fragment coding for a 64-kilodalton major late antigen of human cytomegalovirus. Proc Natl Acad Sci USA 81: 4965–4969

Pereira L, Hoffman M (1986) Immunology of human cytomegalovirus glycoproteins. In: Lopez C, Roizman B (eds) Human herpesvirus. Raven, New York, pp 69–92

Pereira L, Hoffman M, Gallo D, Cremer N (1982) Monoclonal antibodies to human cytomegalovirus: three surface membrane proteins with unique immunological and electrophoretic properties specify cross-reactive determinants. Infect Immun 36: 924–932

Pereira L, Hoffman M, Tatsuno M, Dondero D (1984) Polymorphism of human cytomegalovirus glycoproteins characterized by monoclonal antibodies. Virology 139: 73–86

Picard D, Schaffner W (1984) A lymphocyte specific enhancer in the mouse immunoglobulin kappa gene. Nature 307: 80–82

Pizzorno MC, O'Hare P, Sha L, LaFemina RL, Hayward GS (1988) Trans-activation and autoregulation of gene expression by immediate-early region 2 gene products of human cytomegalovirus. J Virol 62: 1167–1179

Plachter B, Traupe B, Albrecht J, Jahn G (1988) Abundant 5 kb RNA of human cytomegalovirus without a major translational reading frame. J Gen Virol 69: 2251–2266

Rapp F (1983) The biology of cytomegaloviruses. In: Roizman B (ed.) The herpesviruses. Plenum, New York, pp 1–66

Rasmussen L, Mullenax J, Nelson R, Merigan TC (1985) Viral polypeptides detected by a complement-dependent neutralizing monoclonal antibody to human cytomegalovirus. J Virol 55: 274–280

Reedman BM, Klein G (1973) Cellular localization of an Epstein-Barr virus (EBV)-associated complement-fixing antigen in producer and non-producer lymphoblastoid cell lines. Int J Cancer 11: 499–520

Ruger B, Klages S, Walla B, Albrecht J, Fleckenstein B, Tomlinson P, Barrell B (1987) Primary structure and transcription of genes coding for the two virion phosphoproteins pp65 and pp71 of human cytomegalovirus. J Virol 61: 446–453

Ruyechan WT (1983) The major herpes simplex virus DNA-binding protein holds single-stranded DNA in an extended conformation. J Virol 46: 661–666

Ruyechan WT, Weir AC (1984) Interaction with nucleic acids and stimulation of the viral DNA polymerase by the herpes simplex virus type 1 major DNA-binding protein. J Virol 52: 727–733

Ruyechan WT, Chytil A, Fisher CM (1986) In vitro characterization of a thermolabile herpes simplex virus DNA binding protein. J Virol 59: 31–36

Sawadago M, Roeder RG (1985) Interaction of a gene-specific transcription factor with the adenovirus major late promoter upstream of the TATA box region. Cell 43: 165–175

Schaffer PA, Bone DR, Courtney RJ (1976) DNA negative temperature-sensitive mutants of herpes simplex virus type 1: patterns of viral DNA synthesis after temperature shift up. J Virol 17: 1043–1048

Sen R, Baltimore D (1986) Multiple nuclear factors interact with the immunoglobulin enhancer sequences. Cell 46: 705–716

Shaw SB, Rasmussen RD, McDonough SH, Staprans SI, Vacquier JP, Spector DH (1985) Cell-related sequences in the DNA genome of human cytomegalovirus strain AD169. J Virol 55: 843–848

Silver BJ, Bokar JA, Virgin JB, Vallen EA, Milsted A, Nilson JH (1987) Cyclic AMP regulation of the human glycoprotein hormone α subunit gene is mediated by an 18-basepair element. Proc Natl Acad Sci USA 84: 2198–2202

SivaRaman L, Thimmappaya B (1987) Two promoter-specific host factors interact with adjacent sequences in an EIA-inducible adenovirus promoter. Proc Natl Acad Sci USA 84: 6112–6116

SivaRaman L, Subramanian S, Thimmappaya B (1986) Identification of a factor in HeLa cells specific for an upstream transcriptional control sequence of an EIA-inducible adenovirus promoter and its relative abundance in infected and uninfected cells. Proc Natl Acad Sci USA 83: 5914–5918

Spaete RR, Mocarski ES (1985) Regulation of cytomegalovirus gene expression: α and β promoters are trans-activated by viral functions in permissive fibroblasts. J Virol 56: 135–143

Spector DH (1985) Molecular studies on the cytomegaloviruses of mice and men. In: Setlow JK, Hollaender A (eds) Genetic engineering: principles and methods. Plenum, New York, pp 199–234

Spector DH, Hock L, Tamashiro JC (1982) Cleavage maps for human cytomegalovirus DNA strain AD169 for restriction endonucleases EcoRI, BglII, and HindIII. J Virol 42: 558–582

Spector DH, Shaw SB, Hock LJ, Abrams D, Mitsuyasu RT, Gottlieb MS (1984) Association of human cytomegalovirus with Kaposi's sarcoma. UCLA Mol Cell Biol [New Ser] 6: 109–126

Spector SA, Spector DH (1985) The use of DNA probes in studies of human cytomegalovirus. Clin Chem 31: 1514–1520

Staprans SI, Spector DH (1986) 2.2-kilobase class of early transcripts encoded by human cytomegalovirus strain AD169. J Virol 57: 591–602

Staprans SI, Rabert DK, Spector DH (1988) Identification of sequence requirements and trans-acting functions necessary for regulated expression of a human cytomegalovirus early gene. J Virol 62: 3463–3473

Stenberg RM, Thomsen DR, Stinski MF (1984) Structural analysis of the major immediate early gene of human cytomegalovirus. J Virol 49: 190–199

Stenberg RM, Witte PR, Stinski MF (1985) Multiple spliced and unspliced transcripts from human cytomegalovirus immediate-early region 2 and evidence for a common initiation site within immediate-early region 1. J Virol 56: 665–675

Stenberg RM, Depto AS, Fortney J, Nelson JA (1989) Regulated expression of early and late RNAs and proteins from the human cytomegalovirus immediate-early gene region. J Virol 63: 2699–2708

Stinski MF (1977) Synthesis of proteins and glycoproteins in cells infected with human cytomegalovirus. J Virol 23: 751–767

Stinski MF (1978) Sequence of protein synthesis in cells infected by human cytomegalovirus: early and late virus induced polypeptides. J Virol 26: 686–701

Stinski MF, Roehr TJ (1985) Activation of the major immediate early gene of human cytomegalovirus by cis-acting elements in the promoter-regulatory sequence and by virus-specific trans-acting components. J Virol 55: 431–441

Stinski MF, Mocarski ES, Thomsen DR (1979) DNA of human cytomegalovirus: size heterogeneity and defectiveness resulting from serial undiluted passage. J Virol 31: 231–239

Stinski MF, Thomsen DR, Stenberg RM, Goldstein LC (1983) Organization and expression of the immediate early genes of human cytomegalovirus. J Virol 46: 1–14

Wathen MW, Stinski MF (1982) Temporal patterns of human cytomegalovirus transcription: mapping the viral RNAs synthesized at immediate early, early, and late times after infection. J Virol 41: 462–477

Wathen MW, Thomsen DR, Stinski MF (1981) Temporal regulation of human cytomegalovirus transcription at immediate early and early times after infection. J Virol 38: 446–451

Weller SK, Lee KJ, Sabourin DJ, Schaffer PA (1983) Genetic analysis of temperature-sensitive mutants which define the gene for the major herpes simplex virus type 1 DNA-binding protein. J Virol 45: 354–366

Weston K (1988) An enhancer element in the short unique region of human cytomegalovirus regulates the production of a group of abundant immediate early transcripts. Virology 162: 406–416

Weston K, Barrell BG (1986) Sequence of the short unique region, short repeats, and part of the long repeats of human cytomegalovirus. J Mol Biol 192: 177–208

Weststrate MW, Geelen JLMC, van der Noordaa J (1980) Human cytomegalovirus DNA: physical maps for the restriction endonucleases BglIII, HindIII, and XbaI. J Gen Virol 49: 1–21

Wildeman AG, Zenke M, Schatz C, Wintzerith M, Grundstrom T, Matthes H, Takahasi K, Chambon P (1986) Specific protein binding to the Simian Virus 40 enhancer in vitro. Mol Cell Biol 6: 2098–2105

Wilkinson GWG, Akrigg A, Greenaway PJ (1984) Transcription of the immediate early genes of human cytomegalovirus strain AD169. Virus Res 1: 101–116

Wright DA, Spector DH (1989) Posttranscriptional regulation of a class of human cytomegalovirus phosphoproteins encoded by an early transcription unit. J Virol 63: 3117–3127

Wright DA, Staprans SI, Spector DH (1988) Four phosphoproteins with common amino termini are encoded by human cytomegalovirus AD169. J Virol 62: 331–340

Yates J, Warren N, Sugden B (1985) Stable replication of plasmids derived from Epstein-Barr virus in various mammalian cells. Nature 313: 812–815

Zenke M, Grundstrom T, Matthes H, Wintzerith M, Schatz C, Wildeman A, Chambon P (1986) Multiple sequence motifs are involved in SV40 enhancer function. EMBO J 5: 387–397

Molecular Genetic Analysis of Cytomegalovirus Gene Regulation in Growth, Persistence and Latency

E. S. Mocarski, Jr., G. B. Abenes, W. C. Manning, L. C. Sambucetti, and J. M. Cherrington

1   Introduction 47
1.1   General Biology 48
1.2   Host Range and Similarity to Other Herpesviruses 48
2   Pathogenesis and Latency 50
2.1   Acute Infection 50
2.2   Immune Response 51
2.3   Latent Infection 53
3   Regulation of Gene Expression 54
3.1   Background 54
3.2   α-Gene Regulation and Function 55
3.2.1 Role of IE-1 in Control of α-Gene Expression 58
3.3   Viral Mutants in α-Genes 61
3.3.1 Other Herpesviruses 61
3.3.2 Murine CMV Gene Function in Persistence and Latency 62
4   Concluding Remarks 67
References 68

1 Introduction

For the great number of RNA and DNA viruses that persist in the host following primary infection, two common tenets emerge: viral gene expression is generally downregulated or altered during persistent infection, and the host immune response fails to detect and clear virus-infected cells (OLDSTONE 1989). While evasion of immune surveillance is important in all persistence, viral gene products may play a direct role as regulatory functions in certain persistent viruses. Herpesvirus latency is associated with a dramatic restriction of viral replication and gene expression, suggesting that these viruses encode gene products that downregulate replication functions in certain target tissues (STEVENS 1980; JORDAN 1983; ROIZMAN and SEARS 1987; BAICHWAL and SUGDEN 1988). The best candidates for latency-regulatory genes are in the α (immediate early) class (LEIB et al. 1989) as well as genes that are expressed during latent infection (STROOP et al. 1984; CROEN et al. 1987; STEVENS et al. 1987; ROCK et al. 1987; BAICHWAL and SUGDEN, 1988).

Department of Microbiology and Immunology, Stanford University School of Medicine, Stanford, California 94305, USA

Current Topics in Microbiology and Immunology, Vol. 154
© Springer-Verlag Berlin · Heidelberg 1990

1.1 General Biology

Human cytomegalovirus (CMV, human herpesvirus five) is a ubiquitous human pathogen causing a broad range of clinical illness primarily in very young or immunocompromised hosts and is the prototype member of a larger group of biologically related herpesviruses, the β-herpesviruses (STINSKI 1983; SPECTOR and SPECTOR 1984; ALFORD and BRITT 1985; GRIFFITHS and GRUNDY 1987). Representatives of the β-herpesvirus subfamily, all cytomegaloviruses, are found throughout nature in many animal species (PLUMMER 1973). As is characteristic of all herpesviruses, CMV persists in the host following primary infection and remains latently associated with infected individuals for life (JORDAN 1983; Ho 1982). The precise sites and mechanism of CMV latency remain unclear, although latent virus appears to have a broad tissue distribution as indicated by the transmission of CMV following transplantation of different organs. Salivary gland, blood cells, spleen, and kidney are suspected tissue targets. Very little is known about the molecular events or viral functions that control persistence and latency. Given the extreme difficulty in studying these processes with human CMV in humans, cell culture models of human CMV persistence and animal studies (particularly with murine and guinea pig CMV) have been pursued with the expectation that they might provide insights into the human CMV-host interactions.

In humans as well as in animal species, the respective CMV silently infects an overwhelming majority of the population before adulthood but causes little or no overt illness in most individuals (Ho 1982; ALFORD and BRITT 1985). Each of the different CMVs replicates in salivary gland, and, because of persistent and recurrent replication in this organ, oral secretions seem to be a primary source of high-titered virus for dissemination within the population. In humans and other species the virus causes only mild symptoms during primary infection and remains an inocuous passenger in the immunocompetent individual. Human CMV reveals its pathogenic capabilities in the developing fetus, in the newborn, or in immunocompromised individuals. Even though the virus can spread efficiently during primary infection, persistent and latent virus appears to be a major contributor to CMV disease. A latently infected mother may reactivate virus and pass it to her fetus. Blood transfusion, from latently infected seropositive donors, is a major source of CMV transmission in hospitalized patients. Latent virus (either within an individual or introduced along with a transplant) is usually the infectious source in CMV-related illness during immunosuppression or immunodeficiency. Thus, the molecular basis of CMV persistence and latency is of central importance to our understanding of CMV pathogenesis.

1.2 Host Range and Similarity to Other Herpesviruses

CMV is highly restricted in its host range in cell culture. Only differentiated cells appear to be permissive; undifferentiated or transformed cell lines are nonpermissive

(STINSKI 1983; GONCZOL et al. 1984, 1985; NELSON and GROUDINE 1986; LAFEMINA and HAYWARD 1986, 1988; DUTKO and OLDSTONE 1981). Most studies on human CMV have been carried out in human fibroblast (HF) cell culture just as studies on murine CMV have used mouse embryo fibroblast or immortal (3T3) fibroblast cell lines. Other differentiated cell types have been found to be permissive for growth of virus (MICHELSON-FISKE et al. 1975; KNOWLES 1976; FIGUEROA et al. 1978; WROBLEWSKA et al. 1981; TUMILOWICZ et al. 1985; REISER et al. 1986); however, none yields levels of virus comparable to the fibroblast. In nonpermissive cells, the block to viral replication appears to be postpenetration; viral gene expression either does not occur or is limited to the earliest kinetic class(es) of gene products if it occurs at all (DEMARCHI 1983; STINSKI 1983; NELSON and GROUDINE 1986; LAFEMINA and HAYWARD 1986, 1988). Viral DNA replication and expression of the full complement of viral gene products only occurs in permissive cells (STINSKI 1983). Infection of permissive or nonpermissive cells with human CMV causes stimulation of host cell DNA, RNA and protein synthesis. The viral functions responsible for stimulation are not as yet identified (RAPP 1983). Following or during the stimulation, viral DNA replication begins. The switch from early to late gene expression during human CMV replication occurs between 24 and 36 h post-infection (hpi) (STINSKI 1983; MOCARSKI 1988). Progeny virions accumulate by 48 hpi and reach maximal levels by 72–96 hpi. Because cellular metabolism continues unabated during CMV replication, peak protein synthesis and production of virus continues for more than 1 week (STINSKI 1977).

Although the cytomegalovirus group has many members with similar biological properties, the species specificity, slow growth, and requirement for differentiated host cells (generally restricted to the species of origin) have combined to limit the amount of information on this group in general and on human CMV in particular. Although human CMV shares little nucleotide sequence homology with the other human herpesviruses, the available sequence data and comparative studies (CRANAGE et al. 1986; KOUZARIDES et al. 1987a, b; RUGER et al. 1987; JAHN et al. 1987; HEILBRONN et al. 1987; KEMBLE et al. 1987; CHEE et al. 1989; see CHEE et al. this volume) suggest that it is related to the other herpesviruses both in primary amino acid sequence of individual gene products (particularly those involved in virion structure or DNA replication) and in genome organization. The presence of nearly three times the number of genes in human CMV compared with herpes simplex virus (HSV), Epstein-Barr virus (EBV), or varicella zoster virus (VZV) serves to reinforce its complicated biology. Even though the nucleotide sequence of the genomes of other members of the CMV group is far from complete, our knowledge of genome size, organization of certain genes and regulatory signals, and general biology suggests that representatives from human, simian, equine, bovine, and rodent sources are remarkably similar (WELLER 1971a, b; PLUMMER 1973; OSBORN 1982; STINSKI 1983; LUDWIG 1983; RAPP 1983; O'CALLAGHAN et al. 1983; GRIFFITHS and GRUNDY 1987).

2 Pathogenesis and Latency

2.1 Acute Infection

Infection with CMV is usually by contact with contaminated bodily secretions, primarily saliva, urine, and milk (REYNOLDS et al. 1973; JORDAN 1983; ALFORD and BRITT 1985). CMV may also be spread by sexual contact and by transfusion or transplantation. Only a small proportion of individuals worldwide escape CMV infection; in most populations the incidence of infection approaches 100% (SAROV et al. 1982; PECKHAM et al. 1983). CMV infection is usually clinically inapparent, even in congenitally infected infants where disease can be most severe (ALFORD and BRITT 1985). Most people develop serological evidence of CMV infection by early adulthood. In immunocompetent adults, primary infection can be associated with a form of infectious mononucleosis, but immunocompromised individuals are by far the most likely group to suffer clinical disease. Infection with CMV is commonly associated with a prolonged period of virus shedding during primary infection and intermittent shedding throughout life (REYNOLDS et al. 1973; ALFORD and BRITT 1985). While bodily excretions contain both cell-free and cell-associated virus, the cell-associated viremia that occurs during acute infection is localized to polymorphonuclear leukocytes and monocytes (GARNETT 1982; SALTZMAN et al. 1988; TURTINEN et al. 1987). Cellular immune mechanisms are believed to be responsible for eventually controlling virus excretion (KOSZINOWSKI et al. 1987b; GRIFFITHS and GRUNDY 1987).

The tissue distribution of CMV growth depends to a significant degree on the immune status and age of the host. Congenital transmission during the first half of pregnancy may result in widespread growth and disease (ALFORD and BRITT 1985). Pathologically, the salivary gland and kidney are the two prominent target organs during acute infection in all individuals. Human CMV has been isolated from salivary gland even in unselected autopsies on young children, with an incidence ranging from 8% to 32%. The most frequently infected gland is the parotid, with the submandibular and sublingual glands less often involved. Cytomegaly (and virus isolation) is almost always associated with the ductal epithelium. In situ hybridization analysis has reinforced earlier viral isolation and histopathological work in identifying epithelial, endothelial, and fibroblast cells as targets for human CMV replication (MYERSON et al. 1984). In different organs, the following cell types are most frequently involved (HO 1982): in the intestines, the mucous epithelium and submucosal endothelial cells; in the liver, bile ductal epithelium, capillary endothelium and portal areas; in the lungs, alveolar and bronchial epithelium; in the pancreas, ductal epithelium; and in the kidneys, endothelial cells and monocytes. Other organs that have been observed to be infected during primary infection include ovaries, skin, bone marrow, brain, and placenta.

Different CMVs may exhibit apparently distinct characteristics such as the observed growth of murine CMV in acinar cells, rather than ductal epithelium, of the salivary gland (OSBORN 1982; JORDAN 1983). While some investigators have stressed the importance of these differences, the overwhelming similarity in their tissue tropism, persistence, and latency as well as in their structural and biological characteristics suggests that the different members of the group should be studied comparatively.

Murine CMV has been the subject of reviews by PLUMMER (1973), HUDSON (1979), OSBORN (1982), and GRIFFITHS and GRUNDY (1987) that provide a useful background. Like its human relative, acute infection with murine CMV is most often observed in young mice, generally less than 3 weeks old. Also, acute infection is more severe and can be initiated with lower doses of virus in immunodeficient or immunosuppressed animals (OSBORN 1982). A persistent form of acute infection is observed in certain resistant strains of mice and after sublethal inoculation of susceptible strains of mice and typically results in prolonged excretion of virus in saliva (QUINAN et al. 1978; SHELLAM et al. 1985; MERCER and SPECTOR 1986). The pathological form of infection depends upon the strain and passage history of the virus, the dose and route of inoculation, and the strain, age, and immune status of the host animal. Many strains of mice have been tested, with the BALB/c mouse, which is susceptible to acute disease, and the C3H mouse, which is more resistant, being popular strains for study (MERCER and SPECTOR 1986). In a natural setting it is believed that murine CMV, like human CMV, is spread by the oral route following direct contact with infectious body fluids (saliva, milk, urine), a situation made clear in very early studies (MANNINI and MEDEARIS 1961). The best-tested route of experimental inoculation is intraperitoneal (i.p.) usually using at least 10^4 plaque-forming units (PFUs) of virus per dose to induce acute infection in the normal BALB/c mouse (although other routes, particularly subcutaneous, have also been used). In immunodeficiency models, which have relied on either genetic immunodeficiency or lethal γ-irradiation-induced immunosuppression, murine CMV causes a pneumonitis (HO 1982; JORDAN et al. 1982; SHANLEY et al. 1982; GRUNDY et al. 1985; REDDEHASE et al. 1985; MUTTER et al. 1988), a pathology which is also observed in a variety of immunodeficiency states in CMV-infected humans. Interestingly, it appears that pathogenesis of acute CMV disease in the irradiated mouse is due to a virus-induced deficiency in hematopoietic stem cell regeneration rather than pneumonitis (MUTTER et al. 1988).

2.2 Immune Response

The immunology of CMV infection has been the subject of recent reviews (KOSZINOWSKI et al. 1987b; GRIFFITHS and GRUNDY 1987). The virus is cleared by immune surveillance, but this is a complex process because CMV itself may cause immunosuppression and can interact with cells of the immune system. The mouse has provided a wealth of information on host defense against CMV. Neutralizing antibodies do not seem to play a role in the recovery from primary CMV infection since the infection generally resolves before antibody levels rise. Administration of neutralizing antibodies, though, will protect animals from disease (ARAULLO-CRUZ et al. 1978; SHANLEY et al. 1981) and this appears to occur naturally in newborns that suckle immune mothers (MEDEARIS and PROKAY 1978). In humans,

CMV can be transmitted despite the presence of passively acquired antibody (STAGNO et al. 1977, 1980) although CMV disease may be moderated by administration of antibody (WINSTON et al. 1982; BLACKLOCK et al. 1985).

Both cytotoxic T cells (STARR and ALLISON 1977; QUINAN et al. 1978; HO 1980; KOSZINOWSKI et al. 1987b) and natural killer (NK) cells have been implicated in protective immunity (QUINAN and MANISCHEWITZ 1979; BANCROFT et al. 1981). One type of genetically determined resistance in mice (SELGRADE and OSBORN 1974; CHALMER et al. 1977) seems to be determined by the major histocompatibility complex (MHC), and H-2^k mice are more resistant. Another type of resistance is not MHC linked (CHALMER et al. 1977) and may not even be immune mediated (QUINAN and MANISCHEWITZ 1987). Strains of mice lacking NK cell activity are more susceptible to murine CMV. BUKOWSKI et al. (1984) demonstrated that administration of anti-asialo-G_{M1} antibody increases the level to which the virus replicates in tissues. The production of interferon is higher in resistant strains of mice and may provide a basis for the differences in NK cell activity following CMV infection. Though less well documented, NK cell activity has also been demonstrated against human CMV-infected cells (BORYSIEWICZ et al. 1985). The central importance of cell-mediated immunity to the control of CMV infection is suggested by the observation that individuals with deficiencies in this arm of the immune system are at risk of CMV disease. Furthermore, CMV-reactive cytotoxic T cells have been observed in mice and humans (QUINNAN et al. 1978, 1981; SETHI and BRANDIS 1979; HO 1980; BORYSIEWICZ et al. 1983).

KOSZINOWSKI et al. (1987a, b) and REDDEHASE and KOSZINOWSKI (1984) have completed the most detailed investigation into the basis of the cytotoxic T cell response to murine CMV. Studying infected BALB/c mice, they detected peak cytotoxic T cell frequencies of approximately 1/5000 cells between days 4 and 8 (using high-dose virus inoculum). Adoptive transfer of $CD8^+$, but not $CD4^+$, cells into an immunodeficiency model prevented CMV death (REDDEHASE et al. 1987a; KOSZINOWSKI et al. 1987b). Surprisingly, a majority of the responding cells recognized α-gene products, with the remainder recognizing late antigens and structural proteins. The target of approximately 50% of the cytotoxic T cells in the BALB/c mouse was identified as the IE-1 gene product, an 89 000 molecular weight nuclear phosphoprotein and the major α-gene product (REDDEHASE and KOSZINOWSKI 1984; KOSZINOWSKI et al. 1987b). Negative selection experiments were initially used to show that the protective cell population was specific for α-gene products, most likely IE-1 (REDDEHASE et al. 1987a), and, more recently, a vaccinia recombinant expressing IE-1 (and no other CMV proteins) was shown to be capable of protecting mice from lethal challenge (JONJIC et al. 1988). Recent work has shown a single dominant cytotoxic T-cell epitope predominates on IE-1, between amino acids 136 and 249 of this 595 amino acid protein, and one well-characterized T-cell clone, IE-1 (REDDEHASE et al. 1987b; DEL VAL et al. 1988), reacts with an epitope centering on a pentapeptide between amino acids 170 and 174 (REDDEHASE et al. 1989). Thus, in an inbred mouse strain, reactivity of cytotoxic T cells with a restricted region of one α-gene product can be crucial to attaining clearance of CMV. Interestingly, some studies indicate that humans carry cytotoxic T cells α-gene products (RODGERS et al. 1987; BORYSIEWICZ et al. 1988).

2.3 Latent Infection

Many groups have addressed the general parameters and biology of CMV persistence and latency over the past 30 years (MANNINI and MEDEARIS 1961; WELLER 1971a, b; PLUMMER 1973; OSBORN 1982; JORDAN 1983; GRIFFITHS and GRUNDY 1987; MERCER et al. 1988). Because therapeutic immunosuppression leads to activation of CMV replication in such a high percentage of seropositive individuals, it appears that CMV establishes latent infection in most or all of the infected individuals in the population (GLENN 1981). General insights into the requirement for permissive cells to allow for the expression of all kinetic classes of viral genes and for viral DNA replication have come from cell culture models of persistence and latency (MOCARSKI and STINSKI 1979; DUTKO and OLDSTONE 1981; GONCZOL et al. 1984, 1985; NELSON and GROUDINE 1986; LaFEMINA and HAYWARD 1986, 1988). With so little known about the process of latency in the naturally infected host, cell culture models of latency remain of undetermined significance. Investigators have therefore sought to investigate the nature and extent of human CMV gene expression in infected tissues, particularly during viral persistence (JORDAN 1983; SCHRIER et al. 1985; SALTZMAN et al. 1988). Alternative related members of the CMV group, particularly rodent CMVs, have been the subject of investigations in their respective hosts. The emphasis on murine and guinea pig CMV in this regard is due to their degree of biological similarity to human CMV as well as the ease of manipulating their respective host species. The level of understanding of the mouse immune system also stimulates the number of investigations on murine CMV.

In herpesviruses, including CMV, latency is operationally defined as the ability to reactivate virus from cells of infected tissues following cocultivation with permissive cells in culture without being able to detect virus directly in disrupted tissues (OLDING et al. 1975; JORDAN and MAR 1982; JORDAN et al. 1982). In murine CMV, evidence has been presented for latency in a wide variety of tissues, including spleen, salivary gland, blood, skin, prostate, and testes (OLDING et al. 1975; MIMS and GOULD 1978a; WU and HO 1979; BRAUTIGAM et al. 1979; JORDAN and MAR 1982; JORDAN et al. 1982; HO 1982; OSBORN 1982; GRIFFITHS and GRUNDY 1987). The capacity to persist and latently infect a variety of tissues in the host rather than one specific tissue target, as in the case for HSV-1 which infects sensory ganglia, makes interpretation of studies on murine CMV latency difficult. Latent infections of leukocytes and spleen have been studied and sometimes conflicting evidence has been presented for viral latency in macrophages, monocytes, B cells, T cells, and splenic stromal cells (OLDING et al. 1975; MIMS and GOULD 1978a; WU and HO 1979; BRAUTIGAM et al. 1979; JORDAN and MAR 1982; JORDAN et al. 1982; HO 1982; MERCER et al. 1988). The most commonly studied site of latency has been spleen and recent studies by MERCER et al. (1988) have served to clarify the nature of murine CMV-spleen interactions. Through double detection of viral antigens and transcripts, these investigators demonstrated the central role of sinusoidal-lining cell of the red pulp in acute infection and the likelihood that a stromal cell, rather than a T-cell, B-cell, or monocyte, is critical for CMV latency in spleen. It appears that virus must replicate in a particular tissue during the acute phase of infection for the subsequent detection of latent virus in that tissue (Mims and Gould 1978b; Wu and Ho 1979; Shanley and Pesanti 1983).

3 Regulation of Gene Expression

3.1 Background

The control of gene expression during CMV growth in cultured cells has general features common to other herpesviruses. During viral growth, CMV gene expression is both coordinately regulated and sequentially ordered (Mocarski 1988). Viral gene expression can be divided into at least three different kinetic classes, α (immediate early), β (delayed early) and γ (late), which occur over a period of approximately 72 h (Stinski 1978, 1983; Wathen and Stinski 1982). The first genes expressed, the α-genes, are transcriptionally regulated through promoter proximal *cis* signals that confer responsiveness to a *trans*-acting virion protein (Spaete and Mocarski 1985; Stinski and Roehr 1985) and to both positive and negative regulation by α-gene products themselves (Pizzorno et al. 1988; Cherrington and Mocarski 1989; Sambucetti et al. 1989). In addition, the CMV α-enhancer is among the strongest transcriptional enhancers that have been characterized (Thomsen et al. 1984; Boshart et al. 1985; Dorsch-Hasler et al. 1985) and is subject to positive and negative regulation in different cell types (Nelson et al. 1987; Lubon et al. 1989). The subsequent expression of β- and γ-genes falls under the control of α-gene products (Staprans et al. 1988; Depto and Stenberg 1989). Transcriptional activation by α gene products is important in the regulation of β- and γ-genes with the initiation of DNA replication influencing the β- to γ-transition. Transcriptional activation of β- and γ-genes appear to occur via many different types of transcription factors available in cells. There does not seem to be a common set of factors used to activate coordinately regulated sets of genes. Human CMV makes use of multiple, differentially regulated promoters in expression of certain genes (Chang et al. 1989; Leach and Mocarski 1989).

Posttranscriptional events appear to be responsible for a delay in the full expression of transcriptionally active genes (Chua et al. 1981; Wathen and Stinski 1982; DeMarchi 1983; Geballe et al. 1986a, b; Goins and Stinski 1986; Geballe and Mocarski 1988). To date two types of posttranscriptional regulatory events have been observed:

(a) delay in the transport of transcripts from the nucleus to cytoplasm possibly due to 3'-end processing changes (Goins and Stinski 1986) and
(b) delay in translation of transcripts due to short open reading frames in the 5' leader region of a transcript (Geballe et al. 1986b; Geballe and Mocarski 1988).

Two powerful molecular genetic approaches that have been used to identify and investigate viral regulatory genes: transient assay of gene functions, and construction of null and conditional viral mutants. To date, studies on human CMV have concentrated on the former, while studies on murine CMV have used both.

3.2 α-Gene Regulation and Function

The α-class of viral gene products might be expected to play some role in the cell-type-specific regulation of viral gene expression in infected tissues because they are the first to be expressed and generally carry out regulatory activities. Evidence for long-term expression of α-transcripts in human tissues, particularly blood cells, has been presented even in the absence of detectable virus growth (SCHRIER et al. 1985). Three α gene regions have been mapped on the human CMV genome, with one (0.728 to 0.751 map units) much more abundantly expressed than the others (MOCARSKI, 1988). This region consists of at least three distinct genes: 1, 2, and 3 (IE-1, IE-2, and IE-3), diagrammed in Fig. 1a, whose expression is under the control of the strong α promoter-enhancer (THOMSEN et al. 1984; STENBERG et al. 1984; STENBERG et al. 1985; HERMISTON et al. 1987; STINSKI, personal communication). Viral genes that encode regulatory functions have been identified by ability to transactivate expression from viral (or nonviral) promoters in transient trans-fection assays which have revealed that both positive and negative regulatory functions are encoded in the α-gene cluster (HERMISTON et al. 1987; PIZZORNO et al. 1988; CHERRINGTON and MOCARSKI 1989). In HF cells, the α-promoter-enhancer is clearly subject to both positive and negative regulation during virus replication and is transactivated by both unidentified virion proteins (SPAETE and MOCARSKI 1985; STINSKI and ROEHR 1985) as well as an α-gene product, IE-1 (CHERRINGTON and MOCARSKI 1989). The α promoter is repressed by α-gene products encoded in the IE-2 region (PIZZORNO et al. 1988), a region whose products also act as trans-activators of β- and possibly even γ-gene expression. Human CMV IE-2 gene products act as nonspecific transactivators that are active on a variety of non-CMV promoters (HERMISTON et al. 1987; PIZZORNO et al. 1988). IE-1 and IE-2 together have the capacity to transactivate CMV β-promoter-regulators (STAPRANS et al. 1988; DEPTO and STENBERG 1989). In murine CMV, the α-gene products IE-1 and IE-3 act together as transactivators (KOSZINOWSKI et al. 1986; KOSZINOWSKI, personal communication).

The human CMV promoter-enhancer is very active even in uninfected cells (THOMSEN et al. 1984; BOSHART et al. 1985) and consists of a mixed series of repeated 16-, 18-, 19-, and 21-base pair (bp) sequence motifs which contain binding sites for cellular transcription factors such as a cAMP-responsive element (CRE; also called an ATF element) within the 19-bp element and nuclear factor κB (NF-κB) and AP-1 sites within 18-bp elements (GHAZAL et al. 1987, 1988a, b; SAMBUCETTI et al. 1989). Murine CMV also has a very strong transcriptional enhancer controlling α gene expression (DORSCH-HASLER et al. 1985). The human and murine CMV enhancers share sequence homology in the 18 and 19 bp repeat elements that appear to play a role in transcriptional regulation (BOSHART et al. 1985; GHAZAL et al. 1987; STINSKI and ROEHR 1985; CHERRINGTON and MOCARSKI 1989; SAMBUCETTI et al.

Human CMV

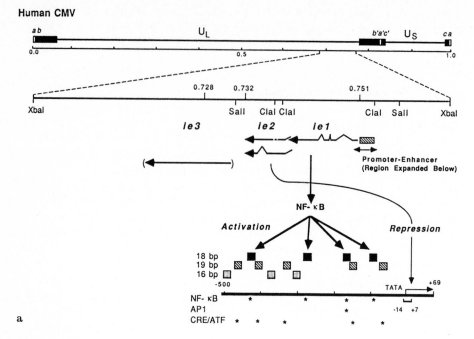

Murine CMV

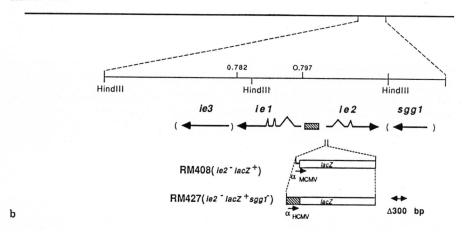

Fig. 1a, b. The structure of the α-gene region in human and murine CMV. **a** Human CMV α-promoter-enhancer and summary of regulation. The 235-kbp genome is depicted with inverted repeat sequences as *large boxes*. The *b* repeats bracket the unique sequences of the L component (U_L) and the *c* repeats bracket the unique sequences of the S component (U_S). An *a* sequence is present as a direct repeat at the genomic ends and in inverted orientation at the L-S junction. The expanded region is an *Xba*I fragment from the CMV (Towne) genome that carries the locus of most abundantly expressed α-genes (along with map coordinates defining the region). This region is expressed from an enhancer-promoter (*hatched rectangle*) that drives the expression of regions 1 (IE-1), 2 (IE-2), and 3 (IE-3) through differential splicing (STINSKI et al. 1983; WILKINSON et al. 1984; THOMSEN et al. 1984; STENBERG and STINSKI 1985; HERMISTON et al. 1987; reviewed in MOCARSKI 1988). IE-1 is a 491-amino-acid nuclear phosphoprotein that is also known as the "major immediate protein" and is responsible for transactivation of the α-promoter-

1989). The NF-κB sites within 18 bp repeat elements have homology to elements found in a number of enhancers including SV40.

Cellular transcription factors are likely to be necessary for constitutive as well as induced expression of this promoter and cells contain a number of α-enhancer-binding proteins (HENNIGHAUSEN and FLECKENSTEIN 1986; GHAZAL et al. 1987, 1988a, b). Furthermore, CMV infection of HF apparently cells induces transcription factors that bind to AP-1 within one 18 bp repeat element and ATF sites within the 19 bp repeat elements (SAMBUCETTI et al. 1989). Human CMV IE-1 trans-activates the α promoter-enhancer via on NF-κB site within the 18 bp repeat element (CHERRINGTON and MOCARSKI, 1989; SAMBUCETTI et al. 1989).

The structure and expression of α-genes has also been extensively studied in murine CMV. The α-gene cluster in murine CMV is roughly colinear with that of the human CMV genome and is characterized by some common structural features (Fig. 1). Within the α-gene cluster, both human and murine CMV have at least three separate regions (JAHN et al. 1984; KEIL et al. 1984, 1987a, b; MARKS et al. 1983; STENBERG et al. 1984, 1985; STINSKI et al. 1983; WILKINSON et al. 1984), diagrammed in Fig. 1. The IE-1 region is structurally similar in both viruses, having a common splicing pattern (KEIL et al. 1987a; STENBERG et al. 1984) and encodes the predominant α-gene product, which in both viruses is a nuclear phosphoprotein. The IE-1 products themselves share little amino acid homology (KEIL et al. 1985, 1987a; STENBERG et al. 1984). The major murine CMV α-transcript (2.75 kb) encodes a 595-amino acid phosphoprotein, whereas the major human CMV α-transcript (1.95 kb) encodes a 491-amino acid phosphoprotein. Both viruses have a very strong transcriptional enhancer controlling α-gene expression (BOSHART et al. 1985; DORSCH-HASLER et al. 1985). In the murine virus, IE-1 is transcribed immediately down-regulated at early times and expressed again at late times in infection (REDDEHASE et al. 1986). Transcription of human CMV IE-1 is similar (STENBERG et al. 1989). Furthermore, in human CMV, the entire α-gene cluster is positioned to one side of the enhancer (HERMISTON et al. 1987; STENBERG et al. 1984; STINSKI et al. 1983), whereas, in murine CMV, one gene (IE-2) is transcribed

---

enhancer via the NF-κB site in the 18-bp repeat. The IE-2 region is responsible for expression of four different proteins, 579, 440, 424, and 255 amino acids in size. While this region encodes a powerful nonspecific transactivator, it is responsible for repression of α-gene expression via a short sequence overlapping the transcription start site (−14 to +7). The α-promoter-enhancer region is expanded and the figure depicts the position of the 18-bp (with an NF-κB site), 19-bp (with a CRE or ATF site), and 16-bp sequences (CHERRINGTON and MOCARSKI 1989; SAMBUCETTI et al. 1989). The *bold arrow* indicates the positive regulation by IE-1 and the *thin arrow* indicates negative regulation by IE-2. *Asterisks* denote the positions of various transcription-factor-binding sites within the enhancer repeats. **b** The murine CMV α-gene region and mutant viruses. The 240-kbp genome does not have repeated sequences and is depicted as *a line*. The expanded α-gene cluster (KEIL et al. 1987a, b; KEIL and KOSZINOWSKI, personal communication) and adjacent β-gene (*sgg1*) are shown along with the structure of RM408 (MANNING and MOCARSKI 1988) and RM427. The *lacZ* insert in RM408 and RM427 replaces IE-2 promoter sequences (−33 to +44 relative to the transcription start site). Neither RM408 nor RM427 encode any transcripts homologous to the IE-2 region. The 300-bp deletion in RM427 results in the disruption of *sgg1* transcription. The transcripts shown *in brackets* have not been fine mapped and are possibly spliced

in the opposite direction from the rest of the α-transcripts in this region, including IE-2 (Fig. 1). The IE-2 gene, which encodes a 391-amino acid protein (KEIL et al. 1987a; KEIL and KOSZINOWSKI, personal communication), appears to lack an obvious human CMV analog. Sequence analysis on the murine CMV IE-2 gene (KEIL and KOSZINOWSKI, personal communication) has indicated that this gene is not closely related to human CMV IE-1 or IE-2.

3.2.1 Role of IE-1 in Control of α-Gene Expression

Two types of experiments have been informative in understanding the role of different viral gene products and cellular proteins in the regulation of the α-promoter-enhancer: (a) transient assays carried out with viral α-genes in combination with indicator gene constructs [the α-promoter-enhancer, or derivatives, fused to indicator genes (the E. coli lacZ or chloramphenicol acetyltransferase genes); STENBERG and STINSKI 1985; SPAETE and MOCARSKI 1985; STINSKI and ROEHR 1985; HERMISTON et al. 1987; PIZZORNO et al. 1988; CHERRINGTON and MOCARSKI 1989] and (b) gel mobility shift and other DNA-binding assays carried out with probes representing portions of the α-promoter-enhancer (HENNIGHAUSEN and FLECKENSTEIN 1986; GHAZAL et al. 1987, 1988a, b; SAMBUCETTI et al. 1989). A number of human CMV α-enhancer-specific protein-DNA complexes have been detected in HeLa cell extracts, certain of which have been found to be specific for the different repeat elements within the ehancer. When double-stranded oligonucleotide probes corresponding to the 16-, 18-, and 19-bp repeat elements are examined directly, all of these sequences bind proteins in uninfected HF nuclear extracts (SAMBUCETTI et al. 1989), although the mobility of a number of these complexes is markedly different from those previously detected in HeLa cell extracts (GHAZAL et al. 1987, 1988a, b). Importantly, infection of HF cells with CMV induces the formation of complexes binding specifically to the 18- and 19-bp repeat elements that are absent (or greatly reduced) in uninfected HF or HeLa extracts. The time course of induction of these complexes gives some indication as to their potential significance in the regulation of α-gene expression (Fig. 2). There is a temporal difference in the activation of proteins that bind to different repeat elements. The predominant 18-bp specific complex is detected immediately after infection (at 3 h) and has been shown to bind to an NF-κB site in this element (SAMBUCETTI et al. 1989). This complex persists throughout infection and, based on time course of appearance, potentially plays a role in the activation of α-gene expression. An additional complex formed with an 18-bp element when it contained a consensus AP-1 site. This complex was also induced by 3 h after infection. The predominant 18-bp-specific complex contained protein with characteristics of NF-κB, a transcription factor first identified in B-lymphocytes (SEN and BALTIMORE 1986a, b) that has also been detected in other cell types, including T cells (LENARDO and BALTIMORE, 1989). The complex formed in CMV infected cells exhibits all established qualities of NF-κB, including activation by protein synthesis inhibitors, activation from cytoplasmic extracts by deoxycholate, competition with another known NF-κB site and lack of competition by 18-bp elements carrying point mutations in the NF-κB site (SAMBUCETTI et al. 1989). Consistent with the notion that NF-κB is

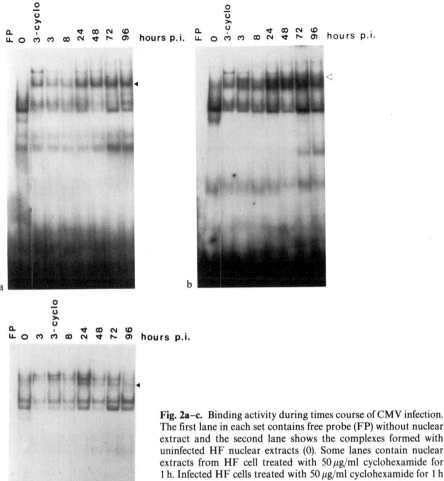

Fig. 2a–c. Binding activity during times course of CMV infection. The first lane in each set contains free probe (FP) without nuclear extract and the second lane shows the complexes formed with uninfected HF nuclear extracts (0). Some lanes contain nuclear extracts from HF cell treated with 50 µg/ml cyclohexamide for 1 h. Infected HF cells treated with 50 µg/ml cyclohexamide for 1 h prior to and 3 h during CMV infection (3-cyclo) and HF cells infected with CMV for 3, 8, 24, 48, 72, or 96 h (3, 8, 24, 48, 72, 96, respectively) are all indicated. **a** Binding to the 18R probe. **b** Binding to the AP18 probe. **c** Binding to the 19R probe. The *filled arrowhead* indicates the protein-DNA complex induced by CMV infection and shown to be specific by competition experiments similar to those depicted for the 18-bp complex in Fig. 3. In **b** the *open arrowhead* indicates the position of the NF-κB complex and the *filled arrowhead* indicates the AP-1 complex

part of this complex, an identical complex with the same properties was induced by treatment of T-lymphocytes (Jurkat) with phorbol ester in the presence of mitogen (Fig. 3). Thus, a similar 18-bp specific complex has been observed in CMV-infected HF cells and in stimulated T cells. Consistent with the mobility shift data, transient assays showed that the 18-bp element is the target of activation of the α-promoter-enhancer in both IE-1-transfected HF cells and stimulated T cells. Furthermore, using point mutations in the NF-κB site as well as an NF-κB site with different flanking sequences (from simian immunodeficiency virus) to replace the 18-bp motif, this transactivation has been shown to occur via the NF-αB site in the 18-bp element (SAMBUCETTI et al. 1989). These results suggest that NF-κB plays a role in regulation of the promoter-enhancer in two very different biological settings and two different cell types.

The cell specificity of IE-1 function has also been subsequently investigated (SAMBUCETTI et al., unpublished observation). Although IE-1 activated NF-κB in HF cells, it apparently lacked this activity in T cells. When nonstimulated Jurkat cells were transfected with the IE-1 gene along with α-promoter-enhancer indicator constructs the level of expression was no different from cells that received the indicator construct alone. Furthermore, even when Jurkat cells have been stimulated with phorbol ester and mitogen prior to transfection, no increase in the level of activation was observed in the presence of IE-1. Thus, IE-1 exhibited the qualities of a transactivator in HF cells but not in lymphocytes. One explanation for these results may be that IE-1 interacts differently with related cellular transcription factors in different cell types. The only work other than our own

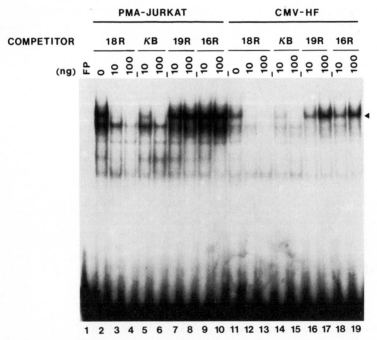

Fig. 3. Comparison of NF-κB recognition by extracts of Jurkat cells and CMV-infected HF cells. Gel mobility shift assays were performed with the 18R probe and extracts from either PMA-PHA-activated Jurkat cells (PMA-JURKAT) or HF cells infected with CMV for 48 h (CMV-HF). Specificity of the binding reaction was established by comparison of complexes formed without specific competitor (*lanes 2 and 11*) and after addition of 10 ng and 100 ng of either 18R (*lanes 3, 4 and 12, 13*), κB (*lanes 5, 6 and 14, 15*), 19R (*lanes 7, 8 and 16, 17*), or 16R (*lanes 9, 10 and 18, 19*)

that has attempted to assess IE-1 function had suggested that IE-1 could repress the α-promoter-enhancer in an African green monkey kidney cell line expressing SV40 T antigen (COS1 cells) (STENBERG and STINSKI 1985); even though IE-1 transactivates the α-promoter-enhancer in normal African monkey kidney (Vero) cells (CHERRINGTON and MOCARSKI 1989).

The behavior of IE-1 in HF cells and T cells may be of potential physiological significance in the CMV-host interaction. Considerable effort has gone into deciphering whether CMV can infect peripheral blood cells. Human CMV can apparently enter T cells in culture, although the infection is abortive (TOCCI and ST. JEOR 1979). In resting T cells, virus gene expression is apparently limited to the earliest kinetic classes of genes (EINHORN and OST 1984; RICE et al. 1984) with the infection blocked before viral DNA synthesis. When stimulated with mitogen, some T cells apparently support CMV replication (BRAUN and REISER 1986). Furthermore, as discussed above, one group has reportedly detected early gene expression in leukocytes from asymptomatic seropositive individuals (SCHRIER et al. 1985). Inability of IE-1 to transactivate the α-promoter-enhancer in lymphocytes may be related to the abortive infection that is observed with these cells and is consistent with antigen or mitogen stimulation leading to increased CMV growth through increased expression of α-gene products. The balance between viral activation (replication) and quiescence (latency) could depend upon the relative levels of activated NF-κB in these cells. Antigen stimulation or other immune phenomena could influence this balance and lead to activation of viral replication.

Finally, the expression of CMV α-gene products could influence interactions with other viruses, particularly human immunodeficiency virus (HIV). All primate immunodeficiency viruses, including HIV and simian immunodeficiency virus (SIV) have NF-κB elements within the LTR region of the proviral genome. Interactions between HIV and human CMV have been reported (SKOLNIK et al. 1988). CMV IE-1 may influence expression of HIV via NF-κB in lymphoid or nonlymphoid cells. It is now becoming clear that variants of HIV-1 are generated during infection of the host which are capable of infecting normal HF cells in culture (LEVY, personal communication). CMV and HIV may interact in host tissues with CMV IE-1 transactivating the HIV LTR and inducing HIV growth, replacing the role that antigen stimulation is thought to play in HIV growth in T-lymphocytes.

3.3 Viral Mutants in α-Genes

3.3.1 Other Herpesviruses

Construction of null mutants by insertion and deletion mutagenesis (POST and ROIZMAN 1981) is a powerful method of assigning gene function and may be useful in distinguishing genes important in viral growth from those more important in virulence, persistence, and latency. Using mutants, viral functions can be operationally divided into two categories: those essential and those dispensable for growth in cell culture. This approach has been successful in dissecting HSV-1 α-gene function and we have begun to apply it to murine CMV. Together with transient assays, null mutants can be instructive in assigning function to particular viral regulatory genes. For example, null mutations in a subset of HSV-1 α-genes (encoding αICP4 and αICP27) result in viruses incapable of growth in cell culture (DeLuca et al. 1985; McCarthy et al. 1989) whereas null mutations in the other α-genes (αICP0, αICP22, αICP47) are tolerated (Post and Roizman 1981; Longnecker and Roizman 1986; Sacks and Schaffer 1987). While these latter three functions are not apparently required for growth in cell culture under most conditions, subtle effects on overall virus yield and host range have been noted. Curiously, αICP0 scores as a transactivator in transient assays where it works in concert with αICP4 and αICP27 (O'Hare and Hayward 1985; Everett 1986), suggesting that it most likely plays a regulatory role at some level in the biology of the virus. Recent evidence (Leib et al. 1989) suggests that ICP0 plays a role in the establishment and reactivation of neuronal latency. Thus, null mutations can help establish the importance of genes in the viral life cycle, and those that are found to be dispensable in culture may be studied in the host animal to elucidate their functions.

Any gene that encodes a function that does not alter virus growth in cell culture might be expected to influence the virus/host interaction in some detectable way. Obviously, any of the different kinetic classes of viral gene products may be dispensable for growth. In HSV-1, envelope glycoproteins form the largest single group of genes that have been demonstrated to be dispensable for growth (Longnecker and Roizman 1987; Roizman and Sears 1987). Accessory DNA metabolic enzymes (thymidine kinase, ribonucleotide reductase, uracil glycosidase) form a second group (Field and Wildy 1978; Goldstein and Weller 1988; Mullaney et al. 1989). The reason for these enzymes being dispensable probably stems from the capacity of cultured cells to complement these enzymatic functions while cells in the host animal (such as neuronal cells in the case of HSV-1) do not. When it has been examined, these functions have been found to be important for growth in an intact animal host. By far the two most interesting groups of genes to study are α-genes, because of their apparent importance as regulatory genes, and genes that are expressed and may function during latent infection, because they may function during latent infection. Although the latency properties of ICP0 null mutants suggest that this α-gene may be important for viral gene expression in the neuronal cell (Leib et al. 1989), the principal latency-related gene of HSV-1 (Croen et al. 1987; Rock et al. 1987; Stevens et al. 1987) may be disrupted without any affect on establishment, maintenance, or explant reactivation from latency in a rodent model (Ho and Mocarski 1989).

3.3.2   Murine CMV Gene Function in Persistence and Latency

We have utilized insertion and deletion mutagenesis to investigate the functional importance of murine CMV α-genes for replication in fibroblast cells in culture as well as for growth, persistence, and latency in tissues of the inoculated BALB/c mouse. Although DNA from murine or human CMV was shown to be infectious long ago (Lakeman and Osborn 1979), progress on genetic manipulation of these viruses has only occurred recently (Manning and Mocarski 1988). The development of a modified *E. coli lacZ* gene as a genetic marker for insertion mutagenesis in human CMV (SPAETE and MOCARSKI 1987) has led to the successful disruption of murine CMV genes (MANNING and MOCARSKI 1988 and unpublished observations). The enzyme, β-galactosidase (β-gal), is not deleterious to viral growth and can be readily detected in mammalian cells and tissue sections with substrates already widely used in plasmid cloning and gene expression studies (SPAETE and MOCARSKI 1987; HO and MOCARSKI 1988). Using this technology, we have begun a systematic disruption of α-genes in the human and murine CMV genomes.

Initially, the role of the murine CMV IE-2 gene product has been investigated using a mutant RM408, which carries an insertion disrupting IE-2 expression (MANNING and MOCARSKI 1988). Studies on RM408, as well as other IE-2-deficient viruses (MANNING and MOCARSKI, unpublished observations), have established that IE-2 is dispensable for viral growth in cells in culture. RM408 carries a chimeric *lacZ* gene, with a CMV α-promoter (derived from murine CMV) driving expression of *lacZ* and terminated by an SV40-derived polyadenylation signal (Fig. 1b). This *lacZ* gene was inserted in place of IE-2 promoter sequences (-33 to $+44$ relative to transcription start site) in order to block expression of the IE-2 region. The IE-2$^-$ genotype did not affect viral growth in either mouse embryo or NIH3T3·fibroblast cell (MANNING and MOCARSKI 1988). Furthermore, the virus yield, the kinetics of expression of the other α-genes, IE-1 and IE-3, and the expression of the viral gene products were all unaffected by the mutation. Thus, the growth characteristics of this IE-2$^-$ virus was shown to be identical to parental wild-type murine CMV.

Another virus construct, RM427, carries a 300 bp deletion in a region adjacent to IE-2 in addition to the *lacZ* insertion into IE-2 (Fig. 1B). This region of the viral genome encodes a 1.5-kb transcript that can no longer be detected in RM427-infected fibroblasts (MANNING and MOCARSKI, unpublished observations). This gene, referred to as *sgg1* (salivary gland growth gene 1) is expressed with kinetics of a β-gene. In cell culture, growth characteristics of RM427 are similar to wild type murine CMV, indicating that the expression of IE-2 as well as *sgg1* are dispensable for growth in cell culture. The *sgg1* gene affects the expression of at least two abundant viral early proteins (MANNING and MOCARSKI, unpublished observations).

Transient assays in mouse fibroblast cells have ascribed regulatory function to the murine CMV IE-1 gene product (KOSZINOWSKI et al. 1986). Indeed, after more extensive analysis, it appears that IE-1 and IE-3 gene products act together for maximal transactivation of gene expression (KOSZINOWSKI, personal communication). Consistent with these observations, we have been unable to disrupt IE-1 or IE-3 by insertion mutagenesis (MANNING and MOCARSKI, unpublished observations). The IE-2 gene lacks detectable activity when assayed by transient contransfection or transformation assays (KOSZINOWSKI et al. 1986; KOSZINOWSKI, personal communication). To date, *sgg1* has not been subjected to an analysis of its regulatory activity in transient assays. Our observations that IE-2- and *sgg1*-deficient viruses replicate as well as wild-type virus in cell culture indicates that these genes are either unnecessary or encode functions that might only be revealed in certain cell types or tissues.

What function might be carried out by a gene that is dispensable for growth in cultured fibroblasts and has no obvious regulatory activity in transient assays?

Certainly, its function could be tissue specific and, therefore, unnecessary in fibroblasts. Even though IE-2 and *sgg1* are dispensable for growth in cell culture, we have found that viruses deficient in either of these two functions exhibit grossly altered replication and latency characteristics in certain tissues of the BALB/c mouse (ABENES, MANNING and MOCARSKI, unpublished observations). Significantly, RM408 and RM427 are specifically debilitated for salivary gland growth during the acute phase of infection in the mouse and RM408 is defective in spleen latency, although we do not yet know the precise role of IE-2 in either of these activities. When inoculated intraperitoneally with 10^6 PFUs, RM408 is capable of acute growth in peritoneal cells to the same level as wild-type virus (Fig. 4). The most striking differences are observed in the salivary gland, where IE-2-deficient virus RM408 replicates two to three orders of magnitude less efficiently and persists much longer than parental wild-type virus (Fig. 5). RM427 replicates 5–6 orders of magnitude less efficiently than wild type virus, suggesting the role of *sgg1* for efficient growth in this organ. In other organs, such as spleen and liver, RM408 and RM427 show less striking differences compared to wild type viruses.

RM408 also exhibits a striking difference in the time course of acute infection of the salivary gland (Fig. 5), persisting for twice as long as wild type (62 vs. 28 days). Interestingly, prolonged persistence of the mutant virus is only observed in salivary gland; RM408 is cleared from spleen, lungs, and liver at an even earlier time than wild type. Persistent replication in the salivary gland is a hallmark of CMV infection and, interestingly, cellular immune mechanisms responsible for clearance of virus from other tissues do not appear to be as effective in clearance from salivary gland (KOSZINOWSKI et al. 1987b). The increased persistence of RM408 appears to be under host control because animals that have been doubly infected with RM408 and wild-type virus exhibit peak salivary gland titers of each that are comparable to animals infected with each virus separately, but, in contrast to singly infected

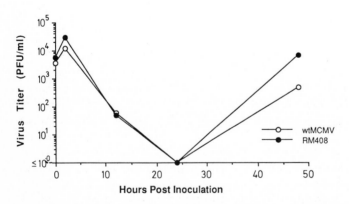

Fig. 4. Replication of wild-type murine CMV (wtMCMV) and RM408 in peritoneal exudate cells following inoculation of BALB/c mice with 10^6 PFUs. Cells recovered from peritoneal washes of mice inoculated with either virus were harvested at the indicated times, sonicated, and titered by plaque assay of NIH3T3 cell monolayers. Stock virus used for the inoculum was prepared on NIH3T3 cells in the culture. Each time point is the average of two animals

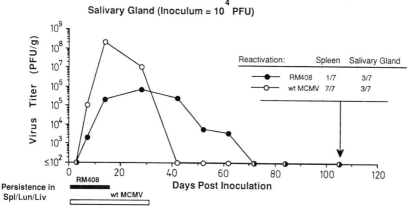

Fig. 5. Persistent infection and latency characteristics of wtMCMV and RM408 following intraperitoneal inoculation of 3-week-old BALB/c mice with 10^4 PFUs. Stock virus used for inoculation was prepared from BALB/c mouse salivary gland homogenates. Salivary glands were removed, pooled, and sonicated and the homogenates were titered by plaque assay on NIH3T3 cell monolayers at the times indicated. The results are expressed as PFUs/g sonicated tissue (prepared in each case as a 10% tissue suspension). Each time point is the average of two animals. Persistence of virus in the spleen (*Spl*), lungs (*Lun*), and liver (*Liv*) is summarized by the *bars* (RM408, *filled*; wtMCMV, *open*) below the graph. Reactivation of latent virus by explant culture was performed at 105 days postinoculation when virus was undetectable in sonicated tissues. Spleen or salivary gland was minced finely and cocultured with NIH3T3 cell cultures for a period of 1 month. Consistent with latent rather than low-level persistent infection, virus was detected in explanted tissues only after tissue fragments were in culture for longer than 10 days and not before

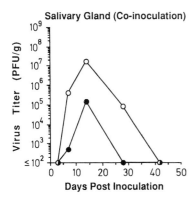

Fig. 6. Coinoculation of wtMCMV and RM408 restricts persistence of RM408 in the salivary gland. Following intraperitoneal inoculation of 3-week-old BALB/c mice with 10^4 PFUs RM408 and wtMCMV (mixed prior to injection), salivary gland was removed from duplicate animals and sonicated at the times indicated and titers were determined by plaque assay on NIH3T3 cell monolayers. Stock virus used for inoculation was prepared from salivary gland homogenates. The results are expressed as PFUs/g sonicated tissue (prepared in each case as a 10% tissue suspension) and each point represents the average of two animals

animals, the mutant virus is cleared well before wild type in doubly infected animals (Fig. 6). Thus, the lower level of viral replication in the salivary gland of RM408-inoculated animals apparently results in a slower immune recognition and clearance.

Even though it is less capable of replicating to high titers, RM408 can cause a lethal infection in 3-week-old BALB/c mice with an LD_{50} only slightly higher than wild-type virus (Fig. 7). At a uniformly lethal dose (3×10^7 PFUs) for 3-week-old BALB/c mice, there is a 10- to 100-fold difference in the levels of virus detected at 3 days postinoculation in the salivary gland, spleen, and kidneys, but little difference in the lungs and liver (Fig. 8). All animals infected with this dose of RM408 died on the 6th day postinoculation while animals infected with wild type all died on the 4th day. The cause of death in immunocompetent BALB/c mice is unknown, but, because of the short time course, is unlikely to be related to the stem cell depletion that occurs in CMV-infected, lethally irradiated BALB/c mice (MUTTER et al. 1988). The significance of the differences between RM408 and wild-type CMV end points remain unclear but are possibly related to the lower RM408 growth evident in all tissues at 3 days postinoculation.

Expression of β-galactosidase by RM408 during replication in cell culture is coordinate with other α-genes (MANNING and MOCARSKI 1988). In the RM408-infected animal, α-gene expression is readily demonstrated in salivary gland and spleen by staining fixed frozen sections with the β-galactosidase substrate, X-gal, using methods previously described for studies on recombinant herpes simplex virus

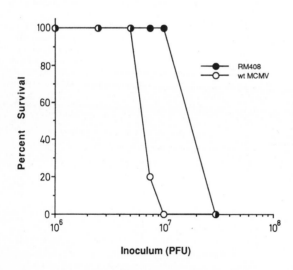

Fig. 7. LD$_{50}$ of RM408 compared with wtMCMV. Five 3-week-old BALB/c mice were inoculated with the indicated dose of RM408 or wtMCMV and observed twice daily for 1 week. All animals not succumbing within 1 week survived indefinitely. The calculated LD$_{50}$ for RM408 was approximately 2×10^7 PFUs and for wtMCMV was approximately 7×10^6 PFUs by the intraperitoneal route of inoculation. Stock virus used for inoculation was prepared in NIH3T3 cell cultures

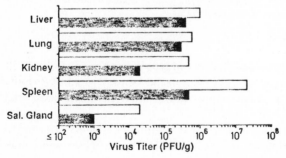

Fig. 8. Three-day titers of RM408 and wtMCMV after inoculation of 3-week-old BALB/c mice with a uniformly lethal dose of virus (3×10^7 PFUs stock virus prepared in NIH3T3 cell cultures). The results are expressed as PFUs/g sonicated tissue (prepared in each case as a 10% tissue suspension) and are the average of two animals

(Ho and MOCARSKI 1988, 1989). We have only been able to detect expression of β-galactosidase in acutely infected tissues, when virus can be detected directly in tissue sonicates. In an effort to determine whether murine CMV α-gene expression continues during latency, as has been suggested for human CMV (SCHRIER et al. 1985), we have examined spleen and salivary gland for evidence of β-galactosidase at various times during the acute and latent phases of infection. We have been unable to detect any α-gene expression during latent infection of either spleen or salivary gland at times when virus is readily reactivated from salivary gland by explant culture (ABENES et al. unpublished observations). Therefore, in this system it does not appear that α-gene expression continues during latent infection. This result may explain how murine CMV evades detection during latency given the well-documented presence of CMV α-protein-specific cytotoxic T cells in BALB/c mice (REDDEHASE and KOSZINOWSKI 1984; KOSZINOWSKI et al. 1987b).

By far the most striking characteristics of RM408 concern its latency phenotype (ABENES, MANNING and MOCARSKI, unpublished observations). Surprisingly, wild type and RM408 reactivate just as efficiently from explanted salivary gland even though peak RM408 titers during acute infection are at least 100-fold lower in this organ (see Fig. 5). Although RM408 appeared to grow well in spleen, latent infection in this organ is debilitated. At 4–6 months after inoculation of 10^4 PFUs, wild-type murine CMV is uniformly reactivated from BALB/c spleen using explant culture techniques (Fig. 5). Using a similar inoculum and after a similar time, RM408 is reactivated with a very low frequency from spleen (Fig. 5). This inefficient recovery by explant culture cannot be explained by the lower levels of virus growth in spleen during acute infection. When inocula that result in 100-fold higher acute phase titers of RM408 relative to wild-type virus are used (10^5 PFUs RM408 and 10^4 PFUs wild-type virus as shown in Fig. 6), RM408 reactivation from explants of spleen is still inefficient (1/4 vs 4/4 animals). Furthermore, animals that have been co-inoculated with 10^4 PFU of both RM408 and wild type virus yield efficient spleen reactivation of wild type virus (19/20 animals) but inefficient reactivation of mutant virus (3/20 animals) (ABENES, MANNING and MOCARSKI, unpublished observations). Therefore, the inability to reactivate RM408 from inoculated mice did not relate to differences in the immune status or level of virus replication in those animals.

4 Concluding Remarks

The complexities of CMV biology, and, as well, the large genome size, slow growth, species specificity, and different viruses represented in this group have contributed to the slow accumulation of knowledge on α-gene function in productive infection and in persistence. The combination of genetic and biochemical approaches outlined in this review provide the tools for systematic study of these genes and molecular genetic dissection of CMV persistence and latency. What we currently know about α-gene function and regulation already provides insights into CMV persistence and latency and also points the direction for future studies.

Acknowledgments. We sincerely appreciate the support of everyone in my laboratory who has directly or indirectly influenced this manuscript. We also thank Christine Martens for her comments on this manuscript. I acknowledge research support from the American Cancer Society and the Public Health Service.

References

Alford CA, Britt WJ (1985) Cytomegaloviruses. In: Fields B (ed) Virology. Raven, New York, pp 629–660

Allan JE, Shellam GR (1985) Characterization of interferon induction in mice of resistant and susceptible strains during murine cytomegalovirus infection. J Gen Virol 66: 1105–1112

Araullo Cruz TP, Ho M, Armstrong JA (1978) Protective effect of early serum from mice after cytomegalovirus infection. Infect Immun 21: 840–842

Baichwal VR, Sugden B (1988) Latency comes of age for herpesviruses. Cell 52: 787–789

Bancroft GJ, Shellam GR, Chalmer JE (1981) Genetic influences on the augmentation of natural killer (NK) cells during murine cytomegalovirus infection: correlation with patterns of resistance. J Immunol 126: 988–994

Blacklock HA, Griffiths P, Stirk P, Prentice HG (1985) Specific hyperimmune globulin for cytomegalovirus pneumonitis. Lancet 2: 152–153

Borysiewicz LK, Morris S, Page JD, Sissons JG (1983) Human cytomegalovirus-specific cytotoxic T lymphocytes: requirements for in vitro generation and specificity. Eur J Immunol 13: 804–809

Borysiewicz LK, Rodgers B, Morris S, Graham S, Sissons JG (1985) Lysis of human cytomegalovirus infected fibroblasts by natural killer cells: demonstration of an interferon-independent component requiring expression of early viral proteins and characterization of effector cells. J Immunol 134: 2695–2701

Borysiewicz LK, Hickling JK, Graham S, Sinclair J, Cranage MP, Smith GL, Sissons JG (1988) Human cytomegalovirus-specific cytotoxic T cells. Relative frequency of stage-specific CTL recognizing the 72-kD immediate early protein and glycoprotein B expressed by recombinant vaccinia viruses. J Exp Med 168: 919–931

Boshart M, Weber F, Jahn G, Dorsch-Hasler K, Fleckenstein B, Schaffner W (1985) A very strong enhancer is located upstream of an immediate early gene of human cytomegalovirus. Cell 41: 521–530

Braun RW, Reiser HC (1986) Replication of human cytomegalovirus in human peripheral blood T cells. J Virol 60: 29–36

Brautigam AR, Dutko FJ, Olding LB, Oldstone MB (1979) Pathogenesis of murine cytomegalovirus infection: the macrophage as a permissive cell for cytomegalovirus infection, replication and latency. J Gen Virol 44: 349–359

Bukowski JF, Woda BA, Welsh RM (1984) Pathogenesis of murine cytomegalovirus infection in natural killer cell-depleted mice. J Virol 52: 119–128

Chalmer JE, Mackenzie JS, Stanley NF (1977) Resistance to murine cytomegalovirus linked to the major histocompatibility complex of the mouse. J Gen Virol 37: 107–114

Chang CP, Malone CL, Stinski MF (1989) A human cytomegalovirus early gene has three inducible promoters that are regulated differentially at various times after infection. J Virol 63: 281–290

Chee M, Rudolph SA, Plachter B, Barrell B, Jahn G (1989) Identification of the major capsid protein gene of human cytomegalovirus. J Virol 63: 1345–1353

Cherrington JM, Mocarski ES (1989) Human cytomegalovirus ie1 transactivates the α promoter-enhancer via an 18-base pair repeat element. J Virol 63: 1435–1440

Chua CC, Carter TH, St Jeor S (1981) Transcription of the human cytomegalovirus genome in productively infected cells. J Gen Virol 56: 1–11

Cranage MP, Kouzarides T, Bankier AT, Satchwell S, Weston K, Tomlinson P, Barrell B, et al. (1986) Identification of the human cytomegalovirus glycoprotein B gene and induction of neutralizing antibodies via its expression in recombinant vaccinia virus. EMBO J 5: 3057–3063

Croen KD, Ostrove JM, Dragovic LJ, Smialek JE, Straus SE (1987) Latent herpes simplex virus in human trigeminal ganglia. Detection of an immediate early gene "anti-sense" transcript by in situ hybridization. N Engl J Med 317: 1427–1432

DeLuca NA, McCarthy AM, Schaffer PA (1985) Isolation and characterization of deletion mutants of herpes simplex virus type 1 in the gene encoding immediate-early regulatory protein ICP4. J Virol 56: 558–570

Del Val M, Volkmer H, Rothbard JB, Jonjic S, Messerle M, Schickedanz J, Reddehase MJ, Koszinowski UH (1988) Molecular basis for cytolytic T-lymphocyte recognition of the murine cytomegalovirus immediate-early protein pp89. J Virol 62: 3965–3972

DeMarchi JM (1983) Post-transcriptional control of human cytomegalovirus gene expression. Virology 124: 390–402

Depto AS, Stenberg RM (1989) Regulated expression of the human cytomegalovirus pp65 gene: octamer sequence in the promoter is required for activation by viral gene products. J Virol 63: 1232–1238

Dorsch-Hasler K, Keil GM, Weber F, Jasin M, Schaffner W, Koszinowski UH (1985) A long and complex enhancer activates transcription of the gene coding for the highly abundant immediate early mRNA in murine cytomegalovirus. Proc Natl Acad Sci USA 82: 8325–8329

Dutko FJ, Oldstone MB (1981) Cytomegalovirus causes a latent infection in undifferentiated cells and is activated by induction of cell differentiation. J Exp Med 154: 1636–1651

Einhorn L, Ost A (1984) Cytomegalovirus infection of human blood cells. J Infect Dis 149: 207–214

Everett RD (1986) The products of herpes simplex virus type-1 (HSV-1) immediate early genes 1, 2 and 3 can activate HSV-1 gene expression in trans. J Gen Virol 67: 2507–2513

Field HJ, Wildy P (1978) The pathogenicity of thymidine kinase-deficient mutants of herpes simplex virus in mice. J Hyg (Lond) 81: 267–277

Figueroa ME, Geder L, Rapp F (1978) Infection of human amnion cells with cytomegalovirus. J Med Virol 2: 369–375

Garnett HM (1982) Isolation of human cytomegalovirus from peripheral blood T cells of renal transplant patients. J Lab Clin Med 99: 92–97

Geballe AP, Leach FS, Mocarski ES (1986a) Regulation of cytomegalovirus late gene expression: γ genes are controlled by posttranscriptional events. J Virol 57: 864–874

Geballe AP, Spaete RR, Mocarski ES (1986b) A cis-acting element within the 5' leader of a cytomegalovirus β gene transcript determines kinetic class. Cell 46: 865–872

Geballe AP, Mocarski ES (1988) Translational control of cytomegalovirus gene expression is mediated by upstream AUG codons. J Virol 62: 3334–3340

Ghazal P, Lubon H, Fleckenstein B, Hennighausen L (1987) Binding of transcription factors and creation of a large nucleoprotein complex on the human cytomegalovirus enhancer. Proc Natl Acad Sci USA 84: 3658–3662

Ghazal P, Lubon H, Hennighausen L (1988a) Specific interactions between transcription factors and the promoter-regulatory region of the human cytomegalovirus major immediate gene. J Virol 62: 1076–1079

Ghazal P, Lubon H, Hennighausen L (1988b) Multiple sequence-specific transcription factors modulate cytomegalovirus enhancer activity in vitro. Mol Cell Biol 8: 1809–1811

Glenn J (1981) Cytomegalovirus infections following renal transplantation. Rev Infect Dis 3: 1151–1178

Goins WF, Stinski MF (1986) Expression of a human cytomegalovirus late gene is posttranscriptionally regulated by a 3'-end-processing event occurring exclusively late after infection. Mol Cell Biol 6: 4202–4213

Goldstein DJ, Weller SK (1988) Factor(s) present in herpes simplex virus type 1-infected cells can compensate for the loss of the large subunit of the viral ribonucleotide reductase: characterization of an ICP6 deletion mutant. Virology 166: 41–51

Gonczol E, Andrews PW, Plotkin SA (1984) Cytomegalovirus replicates in differentiated but not in undifferentiated human embryonal carcinoma cells. Science 224: 159–161

Gonczol E, Andrews PW, Plotkin SA (1985) Cytomegalovirus infection of human teratocarcinoma cells in culture. J Gen Virol 66: 509–515

Griffiths PD, Grundy JE (1987) Molecular biology and immunology of cytomegalovirus. Biochem J 241: 313–324

Grundy JE, Shanley JD, Shearer GM (1985) Augmentation of graft-versus-host reaction by cytomegalovirus infection resulting in interstitial pneumonitis. Transplantation 39: 548–553

Heilbronn R, Jahn G, Burkle A, Freese UK, Fleckenstein B, zur Hausen H (1987) Genomic localization, sequence analysis, and transcription of the putative human cytomegalovirus DNA polymerase gene. J Virol 61: 119–124

Hennighausen L, Fleckenstein B (1986) Nuclear factor 1 interacts with five DNA elements in the promoter region of the human cytomegalovirus major immediate early gene. EMBO J 5: 1367–1371

Hermiston TW, Malone CL, Witte PR, Stinski MF (1987) Identification and characterization of the human cytomegalovirus immediate-early region 2 gene that stimulates gene expression from an inducible promoter. J Virol 61: 3214–3221

Ho DY, Mocarski ES (1988) β-Galactosidase as a marker in the peripheral and neural tissues of the herpes simplex virus-infected mouse. Virology 167: 279–283

Ho DY, Mocarski ES (1989) Herpes simplex virus latent RNA (LAT) is not required for latent infection in the mouse. Proc Nat Acad Sci USA 86: 7596–7600

Ho M (1980) Role of specific cytotoxic lymphocytes in cellular immunity against murine cytomegalovirus. Infect Immun 27: 767–776

Ho M (1982) Cytomegalovirus biology and replication. Plenum, New York.

Hudson JB (1979) The murine cytomegalovirus as a model for the study of viral pathogenesis and persistent infections. Arch Virol 62: 1–29

Jahn G, Knust E, Schmolla H, Sarre T, Nelson JA, McDougall JK, Fleckenstein B (1984) Predominant immediate-early transcripts of human cytomegalovirus AD 169. J Virol 49: 363–370

Jahn G, Kouzarides T, Mach M, Scholl BC, Plachter B, Traupe B, Preddie E, et al. (1987) Map position and nucleotide sequence of the gene for the large structural phosphoprotein of human cytomegalovirus. J Virol 61: 1358–1367

Jonjic S, del Val M, Keil GM, Reddehase MJ, Koszinowski UH (1988) A nonstructural viral protein expressed by a recombinant vaccinia virus protects against lethal cytomegalovirus infection. J Virol 62: 1653–1658

Jordan MC (1983) Latent infection and the elusive cytomegalovirus. Rev Infect Dis 5: 205–215

Jordan MC, Mar VL (1982) Spontaneous activation of latent cytomegalovirus from murine spleen explants. Role of lymphocytes and macrophages in release and replication of virus. J Clin Invest 70: 762–768

Jordan MC, Takagi JL, Stevens JG (1982) Activation of latent murine cytomegalovirus in vivo and in vitro: a pathogenetic role for acute infection. J Infect Dis 145: 699–705

Keil GM, Ebeling-Keil A, Koszinowski UH (1984) Temporal regulation of murine cytomegalovirus transcription and mapping of viral RNA synthesized at immediate early times after infection. J Virol 50: 784–795

Keil GM, Fibi MR, Koszinowski UH (1985) Characterization of the major immediate-early polypeptides encoded by murine cytomegalovirus. J Virol 54: 422–428

Keil GM, Ebeling-Keil A, Koszinowski UH (1987a) Sequence and structural organization of murine cytomegalovirus immediate-early gene 1. J Virol 61: 1901–1908

Keil GM, Ebeling-Keil A, Koszinowski UH (1987b) Immediate-early genes of murine cytomegalovirus: location, transcripts, and translation products. J Virol 61: 526–533

Kemble GW, McCormick AL, Pereira L, Mocarski ES (1987) A cytomegalovirus protein with properties of herpes simplex virus ICP8: partial purification of the polypeptide and map position of the gene. J Virol 61: 3143–3151

Knowles WA (1976) In-vitro cultivation of human cytomegalovirus in thyroid epithelial cells. Arch Virol 50: 119–124

Koszinowski UH, Keil GM, Volkmer H, Fibi MR, Ebeling-Keil A, Munch K (1986) The 89,000-Mr murine cytomegalovirus immediate-early protein activates gene transcription. J Virol 58: 59–66

Koszinowski UH, Keil GM, Schwarz H, Schickedanz J, Reddehase MJ (1987a) A nonstructural polypeptide encoded by immediate-early transcription unit 1 of murine cytomegalovirus is recognized by cytolytic T lymphocytes. J Exp Med 166: 289–294

Koszinowski UH, Reddehase MJ, Keil GM, Volkmer H, Jonjic S, Messerle M, del Val M, et al. (1987b) Molecular analysis of herpesviral gene products recognized by protective cytolytic T lymphocytes. Immunol Lett 16: 185–192

Kouzarides T, Bankier AT, Satchwell SC, Weston K, Tomlinson P, Barrell BG (1987a) Large-scale rearrangement of homologous regions in the genomes of HCMV and EBV. Virology 157: 397–413

Kouzarides T, Bankier AT, Satchwell SC, Weston K, Tomlinson P, Barrell BG (1987b) Sequence and transcription analysis of the human cytomegalovirus DNA polymerase gene. J Virol 61: 125–133

LaFemina RL, Hayward GS (1983) Replicative forms of human cytomegalovirus DNA with joined termini are found in permissively infected human cells but not in non-permissive Balb/c-3T3 mouse cells. J Gen Virol 64: 373–389

LaFemina RL, Hayward GS (1986) Constitutive and retinoic acid-inducible expression of cytomegalovirus immediate-early genes in human teratocarcinoma cells. J Virol 58: 434–440

LaFemina RL, Hayward GS (1988) Differences in cell-type-specific blocks to immediate early gene expression and DNA replication of human, simian and murine cytomegalovirus. J Gen Virol 69: 355–374

Lakeman AD, Osborn JE (1979) Size of infectious DNA from human and murine cytomegaloviruses. J Virol 30: 414–416

Leach FS, Mocarski ES (1989) Regulation of cytomegalovirus late gene expression: differential use of three start sites in the transcriptional activation of ICP36 gene expression. J Virol 63:

Leib DA, Coen DM, Bogard CL, Hicks KA, Yager DR, Knipe DM, Tyler KL, Schaffer PA (1989) Immediate-early regulatory gene mutants define different stages in the establishment and reactivation of herpes simplex virus latency. J Virol 63: 759–768

Lenardo MJ, Baltimore, D (1989) NF-kB: A pleotropic mediator of inducible and tissue specific gene control. Cell 58: 227–229

Longnecker R, Roizman B (1986) Generation of an inverting herpes simplex virus 1 mutant lacking the L-S junction a sequences, an origin of DNA synthesis, and several genes including those specifying glycoprotein E and the α47 gene. J Virol 58: 583–591

Longnecker R, Roizman B (1987) Clustering of genes dispensable for growth in culture in the S component of the HSV-1 genome. Science 236: 573–576

Lubon H, Ghazal P, Hennighausen L, Reynolds-Kohler C, Lockshin C, Nelson J (1989) Cell-specific activity of the modulator region in the human cytomegalovirus major immediate early gene. Mol Cell Biol 9: 1342–1345

Ludwig H (1983) Bovine herpesviruses. In: Roizman B (ed) The herpesviruses, vol 2. Plenum, New York, pp 135–214

Manning WC, Mocarski ES (1988) Insertional mutagenesis of the murine cytomegalovirus genome: one prominent α gene (ie2) is dispensable for growth. Virology 167: 477–484

Mannini A, Medearis DN (1961) Mouse salivary gland virus infections. Am J Hyg 73: 329–343

Marks JR, Mercer JA, Spector DH (1983) Transcription in mouse embryo cells permissively infected by murine cytomegalovirus. Virology 131: 247–254

McCarthy AM, McMahan L, Schaffer PA (1989) Herpes simplex virus type 1 ICP27 deletion mutants exhibit altered patterns of transcription and are DNA deficient. J Virol 63: 18–27

Medearis DN Jr, Prokay SL (1978) Effect of immunization of mothers on cytomegalovirus infection in suckling mice. Proc Soc Exp Biol Med 157: 523–527

Mercer JA, Spector DH (1986) Pathogenesis of acute murine cytomegalovirus infection in resistant and susceptible strains of mice. J Virol 57: 497–504

Mercer JA, Wiley CA, Spector DH (1988) Pathogenesis of murine cytomegalovirus infection: identification of infected cells in the spleen during acute and latent infections. J Virol 62: 987–997

Michelson-Fiske S, Arnoult J, Febvre H (1975) Cytomegalovirus infection of human lung epithelial cells in vitro. Intervirology 5: 354–363

Mims CA, Gould J (1978a) The role of macrophages in mice infected with murine cytomegalovirus. J Gen Virol 41: 143–153

Mims CA, Gould J (1978b) Splenic necrosis in mice infected with cytomegalovirus. J Infect Dis 137: 587–591

Mocarski ES (1988) Biology and replication of cytomegalovirus. Transfusion Med Rev 2: 229–234

Mocarski ES, Stinski MF (1979) Persistence of the cytomegalovirus genome in human cells. J Virol 31: 761–775

Mullaney J, Moss HW, McGeoch DJ (1989) Gene UL2 of herpes simplex virus type 1 encodes a uracil-DNA glycosylase. J Gen Virol 70: 449–454

Mutter W, Reddehase MJ, Busch FW, Buhring HJ, Koszinowski UH (1988) Failure in generating hemopoietic stem cells is the primary cause of death from cytomegalovirus disease in the immunocompromised host. J Exp Med 167: 1645–1658

Myerson D, Hackman RC, Nelson JA, Ward DC, McDougall JK (1984) Widespread presence of histologically occult cytomegalovirus. Hum Pathol 15: 430–439

Nelson JA, Groudine M (1986) Transcriptional regulation of the human cytomegalovirus major immediate early gene is associated with induction of DNaseI-hypersensitivity sites. Mol Cell Biol 6: 452–461

Nelson JA, Reynolds-Kohler C, Smith BA (1987) Negative and positive regulation by a short segment in the 5'-flanking region of the human cytomegalovirus major immediate-early gene. Mol Cell Biol 7: 4125–4129

O'Callaghan DJ, Gentry GA, Randall CC (1983) The equine herpesviruses. In: Roizman B (ed) The herpesviruses, vol 2. Plenum, New York, pp 215–318

O'Hare P, Hayward GS (1985) Three trans-acting regulatory proteins of herpes simplex virus modulate immediate-early gene expression in a pathway involving positive and negative feedback regulation. J Virol 56: 723–733

Olding LB, Jenson FC, Oldstone MB (1975) Pathogenesis of cytomegalovirus infection. I. Activation of virus from bone marrow-derived lymphocytes by in vitro allogenic reaction. J Exp Med 141: 561–572

Oldstone MBA (1989) Viral persistence. Cell 56: 517–520

Osborn JE (1982) Cytomegalovirus and other herpesviruses. In: Foster HL, Small JD, Fox JG (eds) The mouse in biochemical research, vol 2. Academic, New York, pp 267–293

Peckham CS, Chin KS, Coleman JC, Henderson K, Hurley R, Preece PM (1983) Cytomegalovirus infection in pregnancy: preliminary findings from a prospective study. Lancet 1: 1352–1355

Pizzorno MC, O'Hare P, Sha L, LaFemina RL, Hayward GS (1988) *Trans*-activation and autoregulation of gene expression by the immediate-early region 2 gene products of human cytomegalovirus. J Virol 62: 1167–1179

Plummer G (1973) Cytomegalovirus of man and animals. Prog Med Virol 15: 92–125

Post LE, Roizman B (1981) A generalized technique for deletion of specific genes in large genomes: α gene 22 of herpes simplex virus 1 is not essential for growth. Cell 25: 227–232

Preece PM (1983) Cytomegalovirus infection in pregnancy: preliminary findings from a prospective study. Lancet 1: 1352–1355

Quinnan GV, Manischewitz JE (1979) The role of natural killer cells and antibody-dependent cell-mediated cytotoxicity during murine cytomegalovirus infection. J Exp Med 150: 1549–1554

Quinnan GV Jr, Manischewitz JF (1987) Genetically determined resistance to lethal murine cytomegalovirus infection is mediated by interferon-dependent and -independent restriction of virus replication. J Virol 61: 1875–1881

Quinnan GV, Manischewitz JE, Ennis FA, (1978) Cytotoxic T lymphocyte response to murine cytomegalovirus infection. Nature 273: 541–543

Quinnan GV Jr, Kirmani N, Esber E, Saral R, Manischewitz JF, Rogers JL, Rook AH, et al. (1981) HLA-restricted cytotoxic T lymphocyte and nonthymic cytotoxic lymphocyte responses to cytomegalovirus infection of bone marrow transplant recipients. J Immunol 126: 2036–2401

Rapp F (1983) The biology of cytomegalovirus. In: Roizman B (ed) The herpesviruses, vol 2. Plenum, New York, pp 1–66

Reddehase MJ, Koszinowski UH (1984) Significance of herpesvirus immediate early gene expression in cellular immunity to cytomegalovirus infection. Nature 312: 369–371

Reddehase MJ, Weiland F, Munch K, Jonjic S, Luske A, Koszinowski UH (1985) Interstitial murine cytomegalovirus pneumonia after irradiation: characterization of cells that limit viral replication during established infection of the lungs. J Virol 55: 264–273

Reddehase MJ, Fibi MR, Keil GM, Koszinowski UH (1986) Late-phase expression of a murine cytomegalovirus immediate-early antigen recognized by cytolytic T lymphocytes. J Virol 60: 1125–1129

Reddehase MJ, Mutter W, Munch K, Buhring HJ, Koszinowski UH (1987a) CD8-positive T lymphocytes specific for murine cytomegalovirus immediate-early antigens mediate protective immunity. J Virol 61: 3102–3108

Reddehase MJ, Zawatzky R, Weiland F, Buhring HJ, Mutter W, Koszinowski UH (1987b) Stable expression of clonal specificity in murine cytomegalovirus-specific large granular lymphoblast lines propagated long-term in recombinant interleukin 2. Immunobiology 174: 420–431

Reddehase MJ, Rothbard JB, Folkers G, Krug M, Koszinowski UH (1989) A pentapeptide as minimal antigenic determinant for MHC class I-restricted T lymphocytes. Nature 337: 651–653

Reiser H, Kuhn J, Doerr HW, Kirchner H, Munk K, Braun R (1986) Human cytomegalovirus replicates in primary human bone marrow cells. J Gen Virol 67: 2595–2604

Reynolds DW, Stagno S, Hosty TS, Tiller M, Alford CA Jr (1973) Maternal cytomegalovirus excretion and perinatal infection. N Engl J Med 289: 1–5

Rice GP, Schrier RD, Oldstone MB (1984) Cytomegalovirus infects human lymphocytes and monocytes: virus expression is restricted to immediate-early gene products. Proc Natl Acad Sci USA 81: 6134–6138

Rock DL, Nesburn AB, Ghiasi H, Ong J, Lewis TL, Lokensgard JR, Wechsler SL (1987) Detection of latency-related viral RNAs in trigeminal ganglia of rabbits latently infected with herpes simplx virus type 1. J Virol 61: 3820–3826

Rodgers B, Borysiewicz L, Mundin J, Graham S, Sissons P (1987) Immunoaffinity purification of a 72K early antigen of human cytomegalovirus: analysis of humoral and cell-mediated immunity to the purified polypeptide. J Gen Virol 68: 2371–2378

Roizman B, Sears AE (1987) An inquiry into the mechanisms of herpes simplex virus latency. Annu Rev Microbiol 41: 543–571

Ruger B, Klages S, Walla B, Albrecht J, Fleckenstein B, Tomlinson P, Barrell B (1987) Primary structure and transcription of the genes coding for the two virion phosphoproteins pp65 and pp71 of human cytomegalovirus. J Virol 61: 446–453

Saltzman RL, Quirk MR, Jordan MC (1988) Disseminated cytomegalovirus infection. Molecular analysis of virus and leukocyte interactions in viremia. J Clin Invest 81: 75–81

Sambucetti LC, Cherrington JM, Wilkinson GWG, Mocarski ES (1989) NF-kB activation of the cytomegalovirus enhancer is mediated by a viral transactivator and by T cell stimulation. EMBO J (in press)

Sarov B, Naggan L, Rosenzveig R, Katz S, Haikin H, Sarov I (1982) Prevalence of antibodies to human cytomegalovirus in urban, kibbutz, and Bedouin children in southern Israel. J Med Virol 10: 195–201

Schrier RD, Nelson JA, Oldstone MB (1985) Detection of human cytomegalovirus in peripheral blood lymphocytes in a natural infection. Science 230: 1048–1051

Selgrade MK, Osborn JE (1974) Role of macrophages in resistance to murine cytomegalovirus. Infect Immun 10: 1382–1390

Sen R, Baltimore D (1986a) Multiple nuclear factors interact with the immunoglobulin enhancer sequences. Cell 46: 705–716

Sen R, Baltimore D (1986b) Inducibility of kappa immunoglobulin enhancer-binding protein Nf-κB by a posttranslational mechanism. Cell 47: 921–928

Sethi KK, Brandis H (1979) Induction of virus specific and H-2 restricted cytotoxic T cells by UV inactivated murine cytomegalovirus. Arch Virol 60: 227–238

Shanley JD, Pesanti EL (1985) The relation of viral replication to interstitial pneumonitis in murine cytomegalovirus lung infection. J Infect Dis 151: 454–458

Shanley JD, Jordan MC, Stevens JG (1981) Modification by adoptive humoral immunity of murine cytomegalovirus infection. J Infect Dis 143: 231–237

Shanley JD, Pesanti EL, Nugent KM (1982) The pathogenesis of pneumonitis due to murine cytomegalovirus. J Infect Dis 146: 388–396

Shellam GR, Flexman JP, Farrell HE, Papadimitriou JM (1985) The genetic background modulates the effect of the beige gene on susceptibility to cytomegalovirus infection in mice. Scand J Immunol 22: 147–155

Skolnik PR, Kosloff BR, Hirsch MS (1988) Bidirectional interactions between human immunodeficiency virus type 1 and cytomegalovirus. J Infect Dis 157: 508–514

Spaete RR, Mocarski ES (1985) Regulation of cytomegalovirus gene expression: α and β promoters are trans activated by viral functions in permissive human fibroblasts. J Virol 56: 135–143

Spaete RR, Mocarski ES (1987) Insertion and deletion mutagenesis of the human cytomegalovirus genome. Proc Natl Acad Sci USA 84: 7213–7217

Spector DH, Spector SA (1984) The oncogenic potential of human cytomegalovirus. Prog Med Virol 29: 45–89

Stagno S, Reynolds DW, Huang ES, Thames SD, Smith RJ, Alford CA (1977) Congenital cytomegalovirus infection. N Engl J Med 296: 1254–1258

Stagno S, Reynolds DW, Pass RF, Alford CA (1980) Breast milk and the risk of cytomegalovirus infection. N Engl J Med 302: 1073–1076

Staprans SI, Rabert DK, Spector DH (1988) Identification of sequence requirements and trans-acting functions necessary for regulated expression of a human cytomegalovirus early gene. J Virol 62: 3463–3473

Starr SE, Allison AC (1977) Role of T lymphocytes in recovery from murine cytomegalovirus infection. Infect Immun 17: 458–462

Stenberg RM, Depto AS, Fortney J, Nelson JA (1989) Regulated expression of early and late RNAs and proteins from the human cytomegalovirus immediate early gene region. J Virol 63: 2699–2708

Stenberg RM, Stinski MF (1985) Autoregulation of the human cytomegalovirus major immediate-early gene. J Virol 56: 676–682

Stenberg RM, Thomsen DR, Stinski MF (1984) Structural analysis of the major immediate early gene of human cytomegalovirus. J Virol 49: 190–199

Stenberg RM, Witte PR, Stinski MF (1985) Multiple spliced and unspliced transcripts from human cytomegalovirus immediate-early region 2 and evidence for a common initiation site within immediate-early region 1. J Virol 56: 665–675

Stevens JG (1980) Herpetic latency and reactivation. In: Rapp F (ed) Oncogenic herpesviruses, vol 2. CRC, Boca Raton, pp 1–12

Stevens JG, Wagner EK, Devi Rao GB, Cook ML, Feldman LT (1987) RNA complementary to a herpesvirus α gene mRNA is prominent in latently infected neurons. Science 235: 1056–1059

Stinski MF (1977) Synthesis of proteins and glycoproteins in cells infected with human cytomegalovirus. J Virol 23: 751–767

Stinski MF (1978) Sequence of protein synthesis in cells infected by human cytomegalovirus: early and late virus-induced polypeptides. J Virol 26: 686–701

Stinski MF (1983) Molecular biology of cytomegalovirus. In: Roizman B (ed) The herpesviruses, vol 2. Plenum, New York, pp 67–114

Stinski MF, Roehr TJ (1985) Activation of the major immediate early gene of human cytomegalovirus by cis-acting elements in the promoter-regulatory sequence and by virus-specific trans-acting components. J Virol 55: 431–441

Stinski MF, Thomsen DR, Stenberg RM, Goldstein LC (1983) Organization and expression of the immediate early genes of human cytomegalovirus. J Virol 46: 1–14

Stroop WG, Rock DL, Fraser NW (1984) Localization of herpes simplex virus in the trigeminal and olfactory systems of the mouse central nervous system during acute and latent infections by in situ hybridization. Lab Invest 51: 27–38

Thomsen DR, Stenberg RM, Goins WF, Stinski MF (1984) Promoter-regulatory region of the major immediate early gene of human cytomegalovirus. Proc Natl Acad Sci USA 81: 659–663

Tocci MJ, St Jeor SC (1979) Susceptibility of lymphoblastoid cells to infection with human cytomegalovirus. Infect Immun 23: 418–423

Tumilowicz JJ, Gawlik ME, Powell BB, Trentin JJ (1985) Replication of cytomegalovirus in human arterial smooth muscle cells. J Virol 56: 839–845

Turtinen LW, Saltzman R, Jordan MC, Haase AT (1987) Interactions of human cytomegalovirus with leukocytes in vivo: analysis by in situ hybridization. Microb Pathog 3: 287–297

Volkmer H, Bertholet C, Jonjic S, Wittek R, Koszinowski UH (1987) Cytolytic T lymphocyte recognition of the murine cytomegalovirus nonstructural immediate-early protein pp89 expressed by recombinant vaccinia virus. J Exp Med 166: 668–677

Wathen MW, Stinski MF (1982) Temporal patterns of human cytomegalovirus transcription: mapping the viral RNAs synthesized at immediate early, early, and late times after infection. J Virol 41: 462–477

Weller TH (1971a) The cytomegalovirus: ubiquitous agents with protean clinical manifestations I. N Engl J Med 285: 203–214

Weller TH (1971b) The cytomegaloviruses: ubiquitous agents with protean clinical manifestations II. N Engl J Med 285: 267–274

Wilkinson GW, Akrigg A, Greenaway PJ (1984) Transcription of the immediate early genes of human cytomegalovirus strain AD169. Virus Res 1: 101–106

Winston DJ, Pollard RB, Ho WG, Gallagher JG, Rasmussen LE, Huang SN, Lin CH, et al. (1982) Cytomegalovirus immune plasma in bone marrow transplant recipients. Ann Intern Med 97: 11–18

Wroblewska Z, Wellish MC, Wolinsky JS, Gilden D (1981) Comparison of human cytomegalovirus growth in MRC-5 human fibroblasts, brain, and choroid plexus cells in vitro. J Med Virol 8: 245–256

Wu BC, Ho M (1979) Characteristics of infection of B and T lymphocytes from mice after inoculation with cytomegalovirus. Infect Immun 24: 856–864

Regulation and Tissue-Specific Expression of Human Cytomegalovirus

J. A. NELSON[1], J. W. GNANN, Jr.[2], and P. GHAZAL[1]

1   Introduction   75
2   Tissue-Specific Expression of HCMV   75
2.1 Peripheral Blood Mononuclear Cells   76
2.2 Kidney   79
3   Replication of HCMV in Teratocarcinoma Cells   82
4   Cellular and Viral Components Regulating HCMV Expression   84
4.1 Promoter   84
4.2 Enhancer   85
4.3 NF-1/CTF-Binding Domain   89
4.4 Modulator   90
5   IE Genes of Regions 1 and 2   91
6   Conclusion   96
References   97

1 Introduction

Human cytomegalovirus (HCMV) establishes a lifelong latent state after primary infection, as do the other members of the human herpesvirus family. The site of latency and the molecular mechanisms involved in the establishment and maintenance of latent virus in the cell are unknown for HCMV. In this chapter, we will discuss experimental approaches to identifying cell types naturally infected in the human host by HCMV. We will examine cell culture systems and transcription factor interactions in vitro which may identify HCMV-host cell interactions that regulate expression of the virus.

2 Tissue-Specific Expression of HCMV

Classically, HCMV-infected cells are identified histologically by specific nuclear and cytoplasmic inclusions. Examination of tissue from individuals acutely infected with HCMV for the presence of cytomegalic cells has identified the virus in a wide variety

[1] Department of Immunology, Scripps Clinic and Research Foundation, La Jolla, CA 92037, USA
[2] Division of Infectious Diseases, University of Alabama at Birmingham, Birmingham, AL 35294, USA

Current Topics in Microbiology and Immunology, Vol. 154
© Springer-Verlag Berlin · Heidelberg 1990

of organs (MYERSON et al. 1984; WILEY et al. 1986; HO 1982). Generally, infection has been restricted to cells of epithelial and endothelial origin. However, with the advent of more sensitive virus detection techniques such as immunocytochemistry and in situ hybridization, morphologically normal-appearing cells may be identified as potential reservoirs for HCMV. In this section, we will examine the expression of HCMV in two tissues, blood and kidney, that are well recognized for their ability to transmit virus to seronegative recipients.

2.1 Peripheral Blood Mononuclear Cells

Epidemiological studies have implicated transfused blood as an important source of HCMV infection (PRINCE et al. 1971; YEAGER 1974; BALLARD et al. 1979). Attempts to identify the blood cell types that are infected by HCMV have been hampered by the difficulty in detecting low levels of virus in a small percentage of cells. We (unpublished results) and others (BRAUN and REISER 1986) have been able to detect HCMV RNA in lymphocytes by northern blot hybridization. However, the signal is low, probably due to the small percentage of cells infected. We circumvented this sensitivity problem by applying the technique of in situ hybridization to detect viral nucleic acid in peripheral blood mononuclear (PBMN) cells using ^{35}S probes representing different regions of the HCMV genome. Our hypothesis was that a low copy number of HCMV genomic DNA templates are present in PBMN cells. Therefore, mRNA produced from regions of the HCMV genome that are heavily transcribed in nonpermissive or semipermissive cells should be better targets for in situ hybridization. In addition, utilizing fragments of the HCMV genome that are transcribed during different viral replication phases [i.e., immediate-early (IE), early, and late], we may be able to differentiate whether HCMV is permissively or nonpermissively infecting the cell. The knowledge that nonpermissively infected cells often express IE viral genes (RICE et al. 1984) led us to select the *Eco*RI J fragment of HCMV strain AD169 as our IE probe. This region of the viral genome encodes at least seven IE mRNAs and is abundantly transcribed during the IE phase of replication (DEMARCHI 1981; WATHEN and STINSKI 1982; JAHN et al. 1984; WILKINSON et al. 1984; STENBERG et al. 1985) (Fig. 1). Viral genes encoded in this region produce protein(s) that are capable of increasing transcription from heterologous promoters (DAVIS et al. 1987; HERMISTON et al. TEVETHIA et al. 1987; PIZZORNO et al. 1988). Late genes encode viral structural proteins and are transcribed after the onset of viral DNA replication (DEMARCHI 1981; WATHEN and STINSKI 1982). As our HCMV late gene probe, we used a 6.6-kb *Bam*HI R fragment derived from strain AD169. This fragment detects 4.0-kb and 1.9-kb late mRNAs coding for the 65-kDa phosphorylated matrix protein and a related 71-kDa phosphoprotein (NOWAK et al. 1984). The IE and late probes do not contain sequences homologous with human DNA and do not cross-hybridize (RÜGER et al. 1984).

We have examined blood from 20 asymptomatic HCMV-seropositive individuals over a period of time and find that approximately 0.01% of their PBMNCs hybridize to the IE probe (Fig. 2). This figure is somewhat lower than the percentage

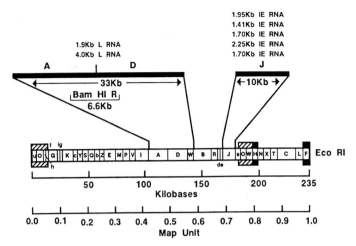

Probes used to detect different kinetic classes of HCMV transcripts

Fig. 1. A physical map for the *Eco*RI fragments of HCMV DNA, strain AD169, is shown with the relative positions of the viral DNA fragments used for in situ hybridization. The immediate-early (IE) probe is a 10-kb *Eco*RI J fragment which encodes the various IE mRNAs shown. The late probe is a 6.6-kb *Bam*HI R fragment which encodes the two late mRNAs shown.

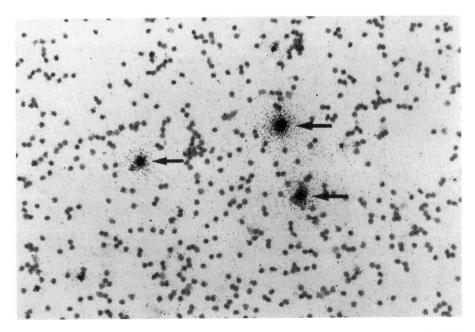

Fig. 2. In situ hybridization of PBMN cells using the *Eco*RI J fragment of AD169 as an IE probe. Cells hybridizing to the HCMV fragment (silver grains) are indicated by the *arrows*, x 200

previously reported, but frequencies of hybridizing cells can clearly vary in an individual due to factors not yet identified (SCHRIER et al. 1985). Not all HCMV-seropositive patients have PBMNCs that hybridize to HCMV probes, but the majority of patients do. The PBMNCs from most HCMV-seronegative individuals do not hybridize to HCMV probes. Fluctuations also occur in the frequency of hybridizing cells from an individual seen on serial samples. Generally, hybridization of PBMN cells from asymptomatic HCMV-seropositive persons with the late probe was negative, but a few individuals had some positive cells. (at a much lower frequency than with the IE probe). Further experiments indicate that the primary infected populations are monocytes (up to 5%) and OKT4$^+$ lymphocytes (up to 2.4%). A few OKT8-positive cells (0.8%) but no NK or B cells showed hybridization with the HCMV IE probe (SCHRIER et al. 1985). Culture of lymphocytes from hybridization-positive donors on permissive fibroblasts produced no cytopathic effects. These results are consistent with many observations that HCMV-infected lymphocytes produce little, if any, infectious virus under such circumstances. Therefore, we conclude that HCMV nucleic acid is present in a small number of circulating mononuclear cells, that certain cells are preferentially infected (monocytes, OKT4 cells), and that HCMV infection of mononuclear cells appears to be nonpermissive.

   The finding that HCMV RNA can be detected in circulating mononuclear cells harvested from some clinically healthy individuals has several implications. First, a population of cells capable of harboring HCMV has been identified. The detection of only HCMV RNA (and not DNA) indicates that virus replication is restricted. Whether PBMN cells serve as the major reservoir for this virus or whether HCMV is maintained elsewhere and is seeded either continuously or periodically into circulating mononuclear cells as they traffic is not yet clear. This restriction of viral replication in monocytes and lymphocytes may be lifted by immunosuppression (i.e., bone marrow transplantation, HIV infection) allowing productive infection of these cells. Therefore, to determine whether the immune status of the individual affects viral replication in PBMN cells, we studied HCMV expression in the peripheral blood of AIDS patients. By in situ hybridization, individuals representing the three different groups seropositive for HIV [seropositive asymptomatic, AIDS-related complex (ARC) and overt AIDS] were examined for the presence of HIV and HCMV. The results of the study are shown in Fig. 3. We found that HIV-infected patients in all groups as well as the HIV-uninfected homosexual group had approximately fivefold more cells hybridizing with the HCMV IE probe as compared with patients who were HIV seronegative. However, the greatest contrast was observed with the use of the HCMV late probe. PBMN cells from HIV-seronegative HCMV-seropositive individuals generally did not hybridize with the late probe. However, PBMNs from all the HIV-infected patients hybridized with the late probe and the IE probe with similar frequencies. The fact that IE gene expression is inactive late in infection suggests that a higher proportion of cells are infected by HCMV if you total cells positive for both the IE and late probes. These results, taken together with the ease of isolating infectious virus from PBMN cells of AIDS patients, suggest that HCMV can productively infect these blood cells (unpublished results). The removal of restriction of virus expression in PBMN cells

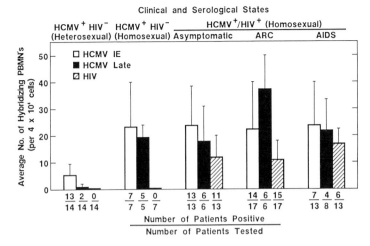

Fig. 3. Examination of PBMN cells for the presence of HCMV and HIV by in situ hybridization. PBMN cells from patients with varying clinical and serological status were purified by ficoll-hypaque gradients. Approximately 40 000 PBMN cells/spot were fixed and hybridized with either ^{35}S-labeled HIV or HCMV [AD169 *Eco*RI J (IE) or *Bam*R (late)] probes. After hybridization and washing, slides were dipped in photoemulsion (NTB-2) and developed with standard developer and fixative. Cells containing silver grains were counted as positive for hybridization. The average number of cells hybridizing to each probe in each clinical category with the range of hybridizing cells is shown. The number of patients positive for hybridization and the number of patients tested is shown below.

may be due either to decreased immune surveillance or a general activation of monocytes and T cells in AIDS patients. The latter scenario appears more likely since in vitro treatment of PBMN cells with mitogens (PHA) or antigens to which the donor is immune increases (10- to 20-fold) the number of cells hybridizing to HCMV probes (unpublished results). Therefore, the state of monocyte or T-cell activation may have profound effects on HCMV replication.

2.2 Kidney

HCMV is an extremely important cause of morbidity and mortality in renal transplant recipients (PETERSON et al. 1980; GLENN 1981; MARKER et'al. 1981; BETTS 1982). In this population, disease caused by HCMV can range from a syndrome of fever and malaise, to severe retinitis, to lethal pneumonia (BETTS et al. 1977; RUBIN et al. 1977; SUWANSIRIKUL et al. 1977). In addition, HCMV infection has an important but poorly understood impact on the rate of allograft survival (PASS et al. 1979). Potential sources of infection for HCMV-seronegative recipients include the graft and transfused blood. HCMV-seropositive transplant recipients may, in addition, reactivate their own latent virus. Epidemiological evidence to date has suggested that the donor kidney is the likliest source of HCMV (BETTS et al. 1975; CHOU 1986), although no laboratory has been able reproducibly to isolate the virus from healthy kidneys (NANKERVIS 1976; BALFOUR et al. 1977; NARAQI et al. 1978). In support of this hypothesis, work with a murine model has shown that murine cytomegalovirus (MCMV) can be transferred via kidney allografts (HAMILTON and SEAWORTH 1985; KLOTMAN et al. 1985; BRUNING et al. 1986).

In an effort to identify HCMV latently infected cells in human kidney, we attempted to detect viral nucleic acid sequences by in situ hybridization in tissue obtained from healthy donor kidneys prior to transplantation (GNANN et al. 1988). The seven transplant recipients studied were all HCMV seronegative before transplantation. One patient received a graft from an HCMV-seropositive living-related donor, and the remainder of the patients received cadaveric grafts. Five of the donors were HCMV seropositive, one was seronegative, and one was of unknown status. Only leukocyte-depleted packed red blood cells were used for transfusions, a practice that reduces the incidence of HCMV infection (LANG et al. 1977). All the transplant patients developed active HCMV infection within 10 weeks of trans-plantation. Using in situ hybridization with the HCMV IE and late probes described above, we examined biopsy specimens from these kidneys obtained throughout the transplant period. We detected no HCMV nucleic acids in the pretransplant biopsies from seven donor kidneys. In contrast, biopsies taken at later times when HCMV infection or graft rejection was clinically suspected showed prominent hybridization with the HCMV IE and late gene probes. Virtually all of the hybridization was with mononuclear inflammatory cells in the renal interstitial spaces. Very little hybridiz-ation with renal parenchymal cells was observed (Fig. 4). These experiments clearly demonstrate that mononuclear inflammatory cells are the predominant HCMV-infected cell in renal grafts. The observation that both IE and late HCMV probes hybridize to the infiltrating cells in the renal graft indicates that these cells may be permissively infected.

On the basis of these data at least two hypotheses can be proposed for the pathogenesis of primary HCMV infection in transplant patients. First, virus carried in a small number of cells in the graft may be reactivated by a combination of allogeneic stimulation (OLDING et al. 1985) and therapeutic immunosuppression (JORDAN et al. 1977) and begin to replicate. Activated host mononuclear cells infiltrating the kidney as part of the host-versus-graft response may then be infected by HCMV. These infected mononuclear cells could disseminate HCMV to distant target organs (e.g., retina, lung). Alternatively, a small number of HCMV-infected donor lymphocytes or monocytes carried into the graft may become activated and begin to express virus. These donor leukocytes could move into the bloodstream and infect circulating host PBMN cells that may later enter the graft as part of the rejection response (Fig. 5). Indeed, the two hypotheses are not mutually exclusive and both could be operative (Fig. 6).

The lack of HCMV hybridization in the pretransplant kidney does not support the hypothesis that HCMV is transmitted to the seronegative recipient in the organ. However, one possible explanation is that latently infected cells do not express sufficient amounts of IE mRNA to be detected by this system. An alternative and more likely explanation is that HCMV is present only in a small number of cells in the healthy donor kidney and may have gone undetected by sampling error with the small number of biopsies obtained.

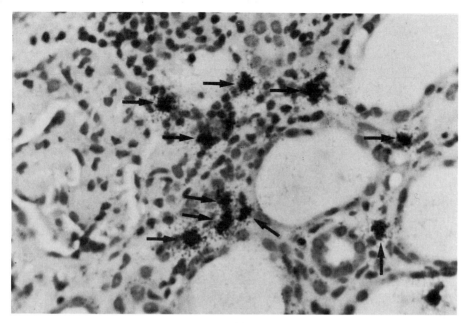

Fig. 4. In situ hybridization of a kidney biopsy (posttransplant) using the IE probe of HCMV. The majority of cells hybridizing to the probe (silver grains) are inflammatory cells as indicated by the *arrows*, x 600

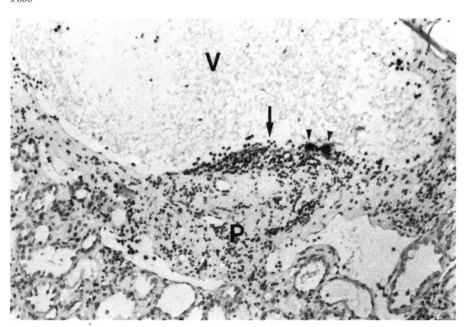

Fig. 5. In situ hybridization of a kidney biopsy (posttransplant) using the IE probe of HCMV. Infiltrating cells marginating on the vessel wall (*arrow*) are hybridizing to the IE probe (*arrowheads*). The vein (*V*) and the parenchyma (*P*) are shown, x 200

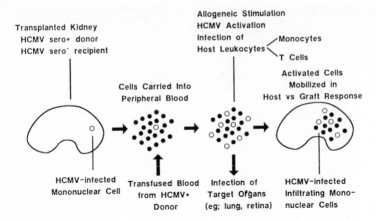

Fig. 6. Potential model for transmission of HCMV to seronegative renal transplant patients. In this model, HCMV can be introduced into a seronegative recipient either through a kidney from a seropositive donor (most probable source) or transfused blood (*open circles* represent HCMV-infected cells). Allogeneic activation of donor cells in peripheral blood would activate HCMV to replicate, resulting in spread of infection. Infected PBMN cells would act as a vector for disseminating virus throughout the body to target organs such as lung. Infiltrating cells in the kidney hybridizing to IE and late probes may represent cells mobilized to reject the kidney in the host-versus-graft response

Both the peripheral blood and kidney studies demonstrate that mononuclear cells are an important site of HCMV infection and may act as vectors for dissemination of the virus throughout the body. Replication of the virus may be naturally restricted in undifferentiated cells. However, mitogenic or allogeneic stimulation of these cells to differentiate may induce cellular factors necessary for HCMV replication. The next section will explore cell systems to define possible events leading to latency/reactivation.

3 Replication of HCMV in Teratocarcinoma Cells

Teratocarcinoma cell systems have provided a unique in vitro tool to dissect molecular events involved in the regulation of viral genes after cellular differentiation. These cells are derived from embryonal carcinomas which can be stimulated to differentiate into a wide variety of somatic cell types. HCMV was shown to replicate in a differentiated human teratocarcinoma cell line (Tera-2), but there was an unidentified block in viral replication in undifferentiated cells (GONZCOL et al. 1984). This cell line, therefore, provided a unique system to analyze the cellular events which occur when a cell is activated and allows HCMV replication.

The first genes of HCMV to be expressed are IE genes which encode transcriptional activator proteins. Our hypothesis was that the level of expression of these genes is an important determinant of permissiveness of HCMV in a cell. Therefore, we first studied regulation of expression of these IE genes in undifferentiated and differentiated Tera-2 cells. By comparison of steady-state RNA levels and in vitro run-on transcription of nuclei, we demonstrated that the major IE gene (region 1) is inactive in undifferentiated but active in differentiated Tera-2 cells. Thus, the block in HCMV replication in these cells is at the transcriptional level (NELSON and GROUDINE 1986).

A comparison of the structural features of chromatin on the promoter regulatory region with the active and inactive IE gene showed the presence of constitutive and inducible DNaseI sites. The majority of the constitutive sites existed at -175, -275, -375, -425, and -525 relative to the start of transcription (Fig. 7) (NELSON and GROUDINE 1986). This region was shown to have SV40 enhancer function (BOSHART et al. 1985). In contrast, the inducible DNaseI sites were located outside this region at -650, -775, -875, -975, and in an area within the first exon (NELSON and GROUDINE 1986) (Fig. 7). Since this 5'-flanking region regulates transcription of several important IE genes (regions 1 and 2) (STENBERG et al. 1985), the increased DNaseI hypersensitivity in the region 5' to the enhancer may reflect an unusual DNA conformation which allows transcription factors to bind easily. Conversely, the decreased hypersensitivity may indicate that negative regulatory factors are bound to the inducible region, protecting it from DNaseI digestion. The structure of this region was examined for non-B conformation with the chemical carcinogen chloracetaldehyde. A single site was detected when the gene was active (-836) in the inducible DNaseI-hypersensitive region (Fig. 7 (KOHWI-SHIGEMATSU and NELSON 1988)). No chloracetaldehyde sites were observed in the 5'-flanking sequence of the major IE gene while the gene was inactive. These results indicate that major conformational changes occur in the region 5' to the enhancer when the IE genes are active.

To test the significance of the upstream inducible DNaseI-hypersensitive sites, we have constructed plasmids which contain the chloramphenicol acetyl transferase (CAT) gene under the control of variously deleted portions of the HCMV IE promoter. We assayed for activity in transient transfection CAT assays using differentiated and undifferentiated Tera-2 cells. Our results indicated that removal

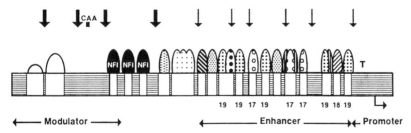

Fig. 7. Structure of the MIEP regulatory region. The *bar* represents the 5'-flanking sequences with the *blank areas* marking regions of in vitro DNaseI protection. The different-coded nodules positioned over these protected areas illustrate the distinctive nature and multiplicity of interacting nuclear proteins. The *numbers* refer to the repeat elements protected. *Slim vertical arrows* mark in vivo constitutive nuclease hypersensitive sites while the *bold vertical arrows* mark inducible hypersensitive sites. CAA marks the interaction point of the carcinogen chloroacetylaldehyde. *T*, TATA box; *NF1*, nuclear factor 1 protein

of a 395-bp portion of the HCMV IE regulatory region (-750 to -1145) resulted in a tenfold increase in activity in undifferentiated cells (NELSON et al. 1987). However, in permissive differentiated Tera-2 cells, human foreskin fibroblasts, or HeLa cells, removal of this regulatory region resulted in a decrease in activity. In addition, attachment of this HCMV upstream element onto the homologous or heterologous promoter increased activity three- to fivefold, depending on the premissive cell. No increase in CAT activity was observed in HCMV-superinfected, undifferentiated cells transiently transfected with these HCMV promoter constructions. A two- to threefold stimulation occurred with all constructions in the differentiated cells. These results indicate that a *cis*-regulatory element exists in the 5'-flanking sequence of the major IE gene of HCMV which negatively modulates expression in undifferentiated cells but positively influences expression in differentiated cells. The identification of a dual function *cis* regulatory region (modulator) 5' to the enhancer indicates that sequences in addition to those previously described (BOSHART et al. 1985; STINSKI and ROEHR 1985) are important in IE expression. Therefore, by utilizing this in vitro cell culture system we have shown that the state of the virus within the cell is dependent on the level of IE gene expression. In addition, the corresponding regulatory *cis*-acting regulatory elements of major IE promoter (MIEP) will be discussed in the next section.

4 Cellular and Viral Components Regulating HCMV Expression

Human cytomegalovirus has at least three different parts of the genome transcribed at IE times (JAHN et al. 1984; STENBERG et al. 1984; KOUZARIDES et al. 1988; WESTON 1988). The majority of the IE transcription originates from the MIEP located in the *Hind*III E fragment (strain AD169) of the long unique region of the genome (JAHN et al. 1986; STENBERG et al. 1984). This promoter directs the synthesis of RNA-containing multiple exons that are differentially spliced to produce a series of transcripts that result in the translation of multiple related and/or unrelated proteins (STENBERG et al. 1985, 1988). The expression of the IE proteins are by definition independent of prior viral gene expression and are therefore predominantly dependent on host-cell factors. The 5'-flanking region of MIEP consists of distinct functional units: promoter, enhancer, NFI/CTF cluster, and modulator sequences. The task of this section is to summarize what we know about the dependence of transcriptional control of the MIEP on host-cell factors and the possible interactions of viral components with the cellular regulatory network.

4.1 Promoter

The promoter of the major IE gene of HCMV utilizes the host's RNA polymerase II and associated factors for transcription. Generally, a eukaryotic RNA polymerase II promoter consists of at least two kinds of *cis*-acting DNA sequences. These motifs are upstream elements positioned at around -100 and TATA elements. TATA elements consist of a ubiquitous sequence of 7 bp, TATAWAW, located between 19 and 34 bp upstream of the initiation site of transcription (BREATHNACH and CHAMBON 1981). This *cis* element plays an important role in control of gene expression and appears to interact with a component(s) of the basic transcription machinery (VAN DYKE et al. 1988). The sequence between -29 and -23 of MIEP is identical to the 7 bp consensus TATA box sequence. Interestingly, the MIEP TATA box demonstrates ten of ten identities with that of the HIV-LTR TATA box. The significance of this homology is at present unknown; however, the MIEP TATA box is functional and directs RNA polymerase II transcription (THOMSON et al. 1984; GHAZAL et al. 1987, 1988a).

Immediately upstream of the MIEP TATA box between nucleotides -72 and -53 is a sequence that is similar to the 19-bp palindromic elements located within the enhancer region (see below, Fig.8). This redundant form of the 19-bp palindromic element binds a sequence-specific transcription factor that resembles or is identical to the 19-bp enhancer-binding factor(s) (GHAZAL et al. 1988a). The extent of this interaction is distinct from the interaction of the factors with the enhancer 19-bp elements, as shown by DNaseI protection analysis (GHAZAL et al. 1988a). Nevertheless, the sequence is important for transcription from MIEP and appears to be equivalently functional in a variety of different cell types (GHAZAL et al. 1988a; LUBON et al. 1988).

4.2 Enhancer

A remarkable array of short sequences ranging in size from 16/17 nucleotides to 21 nucleotides occur between -510 and -50 (AKRIGG et al. 1985; THOMSON et al. 1984; BOSHART et al. 1985). This region is an important regulatory region (STINSKI and ROEHR 1985) and possesses strong enhancer activity (BOSHART et al. 1985). These repetitive sequence motifs are thought to represent potential regulatory elements. A similar highly repetitive arrangement of short sequences also exists in the 5′-flanking sequence of the major IE genes of murine and simian CMV (DORSCH-HÄSLER et al. 1985; JEANG et al. 1987). Some of the mouse and simian CMV-repetitive elements are identical to repetitive sequences of HCMV.

The activity of MIEP enhancer has been reproduced partially in vitro using nuclear extracts (GHAZAL et al. 1987). In vitro transcription offers an experimentally amenable system to investigate the functional relevance of the relationship between MIEP regulatory elements and potential interacting cellular transcription factors. A competition assay was used to determine whether the stimulation of transcription by the enhancer sequences could be due to specific *trans*-acting factors. In vitro transcription of templates with or without enhancer sequences in the presence of various fragments from MIEP regulatory region has shown directly that enhancer activity is mediated by binding *trans*-acting factors (GHAZAL et al. 1987). Using the technique of in vitro DNaseI footprinting with transcriptionally active nuclear proteins, we have demonstrated the existence of multiple distinct cellular proteins that bind specifically to the various repeat sequences as well as to unique sequences

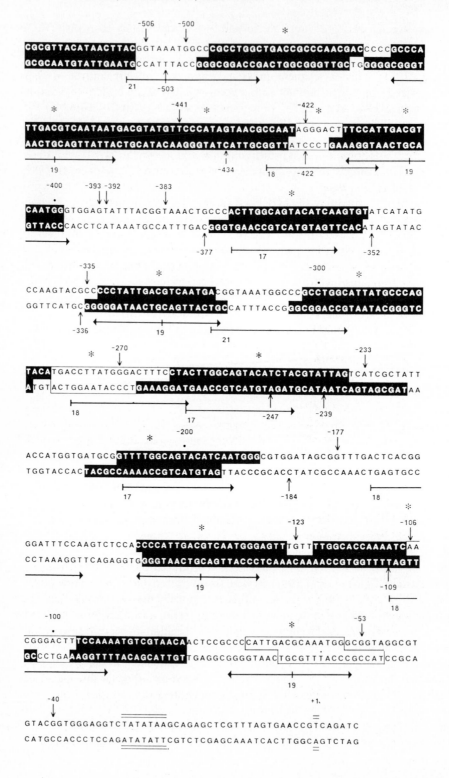

(GHAZAL et al. 1987, 1988a). Complete protection of all 19-bp and 17-bp repeat elements was observed while only partial and/or weak interactions were observed for the 18- and 21-bp repeats (see Fig. 8). In the case of the 21-bp repeats, protection extended from the 3′-end half of the repeat and sequences immediately adjacent. A comparison of these protected sequences revealed a common motif of TGGCN$_5$GCCCA (GHAZAL et al. 1987). In addition, unique sequences outside the repeat elements were also bound by nuclear proteins. A summary of the sequences contacted by sequence-specific nuclear proteins is depicted in Figs. 7 and 8.

The functionality of sequences bound by nuclear proteins was shown by developing an in vitro transcription oligonucleotide-competition assay (GHAZAL et al. 1988b). This technique involves the use of synthetic double-stranded oligonucleotides corresponding to the target sequences of the DNA-binding proteins in an in vitro transcription competition assay. These experiments clearly demonstrated the requirement for the 18-bp repeat, 19-bp repeat, and binding sites associated with the 21-bp repeat, as well as a unique sequence-binding site to provide enhancer function. The 17-bp repeat only marginally contributed to the action of the enhancer; however, it should be noted that the activities of different enhancer-binding proteins are unlikely to be equivalent under all circumstances. Importantly, this work suggests that the enhancer requires the coordinated action of several distinct elements, some of which are reiterated while others only occur once. Those binding sites so far shown to be functional are marked with an asterisk in Fig. 8. The extent of binding, as determined by the degree of protection, differs between the individual elements. For example, the 19-bp repeat at nucleotide position -70 binds to a lesser extent with factor(s) that interact strongly with the upstream 19-bp repeat elements (see promoter section above, GHAZAL et al. 1988a). Nevertheless, this type of interaction does not appear to be critical in determining the efficacy of these elements toward transcriptional regulation (GHAZAL et al. 1988a, b). This observation calls to question the existence of weakly interacting binding sites that may not be detected, but are critical for regulating transcription. Intriguingly, the 5′-end halves of many of the binding sites thus far determined for MIEP have a common sequence motif, (T)TG(G/A)C. This homology may suggest a particular class of nuclear factor(s) associated with this sequence, while the 3′-end half of the binding site may associate with distinct factors (GHAZAL et al. 1988a).

Many of the sequence-specific transcription factor-binding sites are also represented within the simian and murine MIEP 5′-flanking sequences (Table 1), such as the 19-bp repeat and the 21-bp repeat associated binding site, TGGCN$_5$GCCCA. However, some sequence motifs are absent, such as the 18-bp repeat (including the 10-bp core GGGACTTTCC) in the simian MIEP and the 17-

Fig. 8. Sites of protein-DNA interaction on the MIEP regulatory region. *Numbers* represent the distance in base pairs located upstream of the transcription start site (+ 1). Sequences protected from DNaseI cleavage are marked by *reverse printing* (strong protection) or a *box* (weak protection). *Vertical arrows* denote positions of enhanced protein-induced DNaseI cleavage in vitro. Repeated sequence elements are designated by *horizontal arrows* with the respective repeat size indicated below. Those binding sites shown to be functional (see text) are marked with an *asterisk*

Table 1. Summary of nuclear protein-binding sites in HCMV and related sequences in the simian and murine CMV MIEP region

Repeat	HCMV		SCMV		MCMV	
17/16	-373	ACTTGGCAGTACATCAA	-253	ACTTGGCAGTACATCAA	NDI	
	-260	ACTTGGCAGTACATCTA	-220	ACTTGGCAAGTACATTAC		
	-209	TTTTGGCAGTACATCAA	-203	TATTGGCAAGTACGCCAA		
	-122	(TTTTGGCACCAAAATCAA)				
18	-428	CCAATAGGGACTTTCCAT	NDI		-767	TCAATAGGGACTTTCCAT
	-277	CCTTATGGGACTTTCCTA			-674	TCAATAGGGACTTTCCAT
	-109	ATCAACGGGACTTTCCAA			-581	TCAATAGGGACTTTCCAA
					-488	TCATTAGGGACTTTCCAA
					-396	TCAATAGGGACTTTCCAT
19	-469	GCCCATTGACGTCAATAAT	-488	CCCCATTGACGTCAATGGT	-236	CACCATTGACGTCAATGGG
	-416	TTCCATTGACGTCAATGGG	-453	TCCTATTGACGTCATATGG		
	-333	CCCTATTGACGTCAATGGC	-430	TCCTATTGACGTCATATGGC		
	-147	CCCCATTGACGCAAATGGG	-406	CCCCATTGACGTCAATTAC		
	-73	CCCCATTGACAAATGGG	-303	GCCCATTGACGTCAATAGG		
			-338	CACCATTGACGTCAATGGG		
			-284	CCTCATTGACGTCAATGAC		
			-167	TCCCATTGACGTCAATGGC		
			-113	CCCCATTGACGTCAATGGG		
			-91	GGGCAATGACGCAAATGGG		
			-70	TTCCATTGACGTAAATGGC		
(21)	-495	GCCTGGCTGACCGCCCA	-417	ATATGGCGCCTCCCCCA	-515(Rev)	CATTGGCTTACCACCCA
	-302	GCCTGGCATTA t GCCCA	(21)-375	GCCTGGCTCAATGCCCA		
			-321	GGATGGCTCATTGCCCA		
u	-440	CCCATAGTAACGCCA	NDI		NDI	
	-239	TTAGTCATCGCT	NDI		NDI	
	-93	AAAATGTCGTAA	NDI		NDI	

u, unique sequence-binding sites; (21), 21-bp repeat element associated binding site consensus TGGGCN$_5$GCCCA; (Rev), reverse sequence; NDI, no detectable identity

bp repeat in the murine MIEP. Differences in the modular arrangement and combinations of sequence elements between species-specific strains of CMV may confer unique programs of cell-type or tissue-specific regulation.

An important aspect that should not be overlooked is the similarity of regulatory sequences of cellular and other viral genes to sequences within the HCMV MIEP. For example, the core of the 19-bp palindromic sequence, TGACGTCA, occurs within cAMP-regulated genes (MONTMINY et al. 1986). This sequence motif serves as an important *cis*-acting sequence that also confers responsiveness to cAMP (MONTMINY et al. 1986; HURST and JONES 1987). A nuclear protein family, ATF/CREB (43–47 kDa), binds to this sequence (HAI et al. 1988; HURST and JONES 1987; MONTMINY and BILEZSIKJIAN 1987) following cAMP treatment (mediated by protein kinase A), and ATF/CREB is phosphorylated and dimerizes (YAMAMOTO et al. 1988). The dimerization of ATF/CREB is thought to be important for increasing the transcriptional efficacy of the factor. The fact that the 19-bp repeat confers cAMP responsiveness to MIEP (FLECKENSTEIN and STINSKI, personal communication) suggests that ATF is a potential factor(s) binding to the HCMV enhancer. Moreover, ATF/CREB has been implicated in mediating the *trans*-activation of the adenovirus early E2 promoter in combination with the E1A protein (LIN and GREEN 1988). This observation may be of some significance since the HCMV IE genes can complement *trans*-activation functions of adenovirus E1A-defective mutants (TEVETHIA et al. 1987).

Another example of a sequence motif conserved between HCMV MIEP and other regulatory elements is the sequence bound by the NF-κB factor (55–62 kDa) (LENARDO et al. 1988). This protein binds a sequence identical to the 10-bp core sequence of the 18-bp repeat (GGGACTTTCC) present in cellular (immunoglobulin and interleukin-2 receptor genes) and viral (HIV and SV40 regulatory sequences) genes. The NF-κB-binding element confers phorbol ester inducibility, as well as B-cell preference for expression (SEN and BALTIMORE 1986, 1987). In most cells, with the exception of the mature B-cell, NF-κB forms a reversible heterodimer with IκB (60–70 kDa), an inhibitory molecule in the cytosol (BAEUERLE and BALTIMORE 1988). Phorbol esters that are mediated by protein kinase C are thought to activate a dissociation event leading to the nuclear translocation of the factor and activation of transcription (BAEUERLE and BALTIMORE 1988). However, other ubiquitously available nuclear proteins also bind functionally to this sequence (BALDWIN and SHARP 1987). These sequence homologies exemplify the subtle dynamic relationship between virus and host cell.

4.3 NF-1/CTF-Binding Domain

Sequence analysis of the MIEP demonstrates the presence of four consensus nuclear factor 1 (NF-1) sequences (TGGA/CN$_5$GCCAA) that bind NF-1 (HENNIGHAUSEN and FLECKENSTEIN 1988; JEANG et al. 1987). NF-1 belongs to a family of proteins involved in replication and transcription (CTF) (JONES et al. 1987). These NF-1 sequences exist between the enhancer and modulator element described above. Simian CMV (SCMV), which constitutively expresses a homologous IE gene in undifferentiated Tera-2 cells (LaFemina and Hayward 1986, 1988), contains a region in the regulatory sequence 5' to the enhancer that is composed of 23 NF-1-binding sites (Jeang et al. 1987), compared with four in HCMV. The presence of 19 more NF-1 sites in SCMV relative to HCMV suggests that the protein may have a role in activation. Jeang et al. have argued that the large cluster of NF-1 sites in SCMV may act by overcoming the effects of repressors. However, there are perhaps many more functionally relevant differences. For example, the HCMV MIEP 18-bp repeat or the unique sequence elements are absent in the SCMV regulatory region (above and Table 1). In addition, the presence of the HCMV modulator sequence that is absent in SCMV may also contribute to the differences in viral expression in Tera-2 cells. The functional significance of the NF-1-binding sites is unknown. However, the coincidence of two inducible in vivo DNaseI-hypersensitive sites near these sequences (Fig. 7) suggests the NF-1/CTF protein may be involved in regulation of MIEP.

4.4 Modulator

The modulator region was shown above to affect MIEP function negatively in undifferentiated nonpermissive Tera-2 cells while positively influencing transcription from MIEP in the differentiated cells. We have examined whether the modulator sequences 5' to the enhancer (described above) confer cell specificity for expression in other types of cells (Lubon et al. 1989). Several different cell types (epithelial, T cells, B cells) were transiently transfected with plasmids containing the CAT gene under the control of the HCMV MIEP with and without the modulator region. The effect of the modulator sequence on CAT activity differed depending on the cell type. A negative effect (two- to fourfold) was observed in H-9 and SW480 cells, but expression in Jurkat, 293, Raji, Namalwa, and U937 cells was unaffected by the presence of the modulator sequence. These results indicate that the HCMV modulator sequence can influence MIEP activity in cell types other than teratocarcinoma cells. In particular, the modulator negatively affects expression in cell types that are important during natural infection—T cells and epithelial cells (see above).

In order to identify cellular factors that may mediate the modulation of the HCMV MIEP, we established a library of transcriptionally active nuclear extracts from a variety of different cell types (Jurkat, CEM, H9, U937, Raji, B cells, T47D, Hela, and 293 cells) (Lubon et al. 1989). We analyzed transcriptional activities of the MIEP with and without the modulator sequence in these extracts. Transcriptional activity from the modulator-containing template was significantly reduced in nuclear extracts from CEM, U937, and Raji cells. Slightly lower levels of repression were detected in HeLa and H-9 cells, whereas extracts from Jurkat, B cells, and 293 and T47D cells exerted only a marginal effect. Therefore, we are able partially to mimic the regulatory activity of the modulator sequence in transcriptionally active nuclear extracts.

To determine whether protein-DNA complexes in the modulator region correlated with transcriptional activity, the nuclear extracts described above were utilized in mobility shift assays. Similar migrating nuclear protein-DNA complexes formed between the modulator region and the various nuclear extracts. A simple correlation was not observed between transcriptional activity and a specific migrating nucleoprotein complex (LUBON et al. 1989). Nucleoproteins from these extracts were found to interact with distinct regions of the modulator. A major complex mapped to sequences containing a large dyad symmetry (Fig. 9, unpublished). The above studies demonstrate that the modulator sequence exerts differential activities in a variety of cells. We suggest that the unequal pattern of activity of the modulator sequence may be an important determinant toward viral latency and reactivation.

Summing our current knowledge of the MIEP region, we conclude that the 5'-flanking sequence of the major IE gene is highly complex and appears to be composed of several distinct elements. The known regulatory domains and protein-DNA interactions of the HCMV MIEP are summarized in Fig. 7. The elements appear to be acting coordinately to contribute to DNA conformations important for accessibility to transcription factors and subsequent gene expression. We think that the overall activity of the negative and positive domains of the HCMV MIEP within any given cell determines the final level of IE expression.

5 IE Genes of Regions 1 and 2

The major IE promoter regulates transcription of several different transcripts in two distinct regions of the HCMV genome designated IE regions 1 and 2 (IE-1, IE-2) (Fig. 10) (STENBERG et al. 1985). We (unpublished) as well as others (DAVIS et al. 1987; HERMISTON et al. 1987; TEVETHIA et al. 1987; PIZZORNO et al. 1988; STAPRANS et al. 1988) have shown that viral protein products from these regions are capable of increasing PolII transcription from heterologous promoters. Figure 11 demonstrates the ability of IE-1 and IE-2 to increase the level of expression from the HIV LTR in H-9 and HeLa cells. Levels of these transcriptional activation proteins may be critical in determining HCMV permissiveness in a cell.

Structural analysis of IE-1 indicates that a 2.6-kb nuclear transcript containing four exons is spliced into a 1.95-kb cytoplasmic RNA which codes for the 72-kDa major IE phosphoprotein (STENBERG et al. 1984; AKRIGG et al. 1985). This transcript is not detectable at late times during infection possibly due to autoregulation (STENBERG et al. 1984; STENBERG and STINSKI 1985). However, levels of this protein remain constant throughout the HCMV replication cycle (Fig. 10) (STENBERG et al. 1989). IE-2 codes for a series of transcripts that share exons from IE-1 (Fig. 10). A common feature of the IE-1 and IE-2 mRNAs is that all the transcripts contain the 5'

-962 G*ATATCGC*CATTTTTCCAAAAGTTGATTTTTGGGCATAC*GCGATAT*C

Fig. 9. Major dyad symmetry within the modulator region of HCMV strain AD169

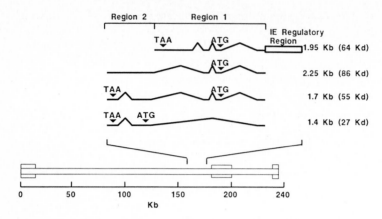

Fig. 10. HCMV IE transcription in regions 1 and 2 showing the splicing pattern and IE proteins encoded by these mRNAs (STENBERG et al. 1985, 1989)

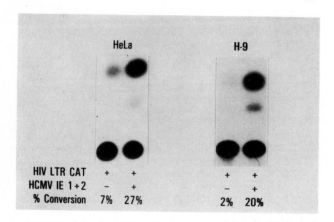

Fig. 11. Transactivation of the HIV LTR attached to CAT gene with HCMV regions 1 and 2 in HeLa and H9 cells. Subconfluent monolayers of HeLa or logarithmically growing H9 cells were translated with the HIV LTR with (+) and without (−) the HCMV AD169 *Eco*RI J fragment containing IE regions 1 and 2. Cells were harvested and lysed 48h after transfection and protein extracts assayed for (200 µg/assay) CAT activity. The percentage conversion of chloramphenicol to acetylated products is shown

leader exon of IE-1. Predicted IE products encoded by IE-1/IE-2 transcripts include 86-, 55-kDa, and 27-kDa proteins (STENBERG et al. 1985, 1989).

In an effort to understand the functions of IE-1 and IE-2 gene products, we have generated a variety of antibodies to synthetic peptides derived from predicted amino acid sequences in exons from IE-1 and IE-2. The position of the peptide sequences utilized for antibody production in relationship to the 72-kDa and 86-kDa proteins are shown in Fig. 12. Multiple levels of regulation occur with expression of IE proteins from IE-1 and IE-2 including transcriptional and posttranscriptional

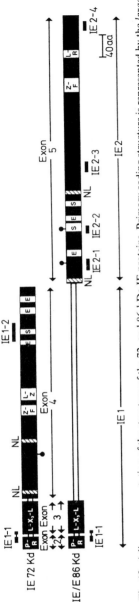

Fig. 12. A linear representation of the structure of the 72- and 86-kDa IE proteins. Primary coding structure is represented by the *large black boxes* while intergenic regions (not to scale) are shown by the *interconnecting bars*. The *horizontal arrows* delineate the exons of the IE-1 and 2 region. The location of the peptide antibodies IE1-1, -2 and IE2-1, -2, -3, -4 are shown by the *small black boxes*. The scale indicates amino acid number. Structural features of interest are marked within the coding sequences. *P-R*, proline-rich region; *L-X₃*, leucine repeat unit; L NL, nuclear localization sequence; L Z-F, putative zinc finger motif; L L-L L Z, putative leucine leucine-zipper motif; L L-R, leucine-rich region; L E, polyglutamic acid segment; L S, polyserine segment; (●), potential N-linked glycosylation sites

events (STENBERG et al. 1989). In cycloheximide reversal experiments in which IE
RNA is accumulated to high levels in the presence of cycloheximide, IE antibodies
generated above detect predicted HCMV proteins (STENBERG et al. 1989). However,
using antipeptide antibody to the amino terminus (IE1-1 or 8528) or antipeptide
antibody to the carboxy terminus in IE-2 (IE2-4 or 1218), kinetic analysis of IE
proteins produced during a synchronized infection indicate that the predominant
proteins at the IE phase are the 72-kDa and 86-kDa proteins (Fig. 13). These IE
proteins appear to be produced in equal molar amounts throughout infection. The
other IE proteins produced in IE-1 and IE-2 do not appear until late in the viral
replication cycle, suggesting regulation of these proteins at the posttranscriptional
level. Therefore, the 72-kDa and 86-kDa proteins are the predominant HCMV
proteins from this region at IE times and may play a vital role in subsequent gene
activation necessary for viral replication.

Examination of the primary sequence structure of the 72-kDa and 86-kDa
proteins demonstrates several interesting features characteristic of nuclear proteins
and transcription factors (Fig. 12). Both proteins share a repeated motif of proline-
N_{1-5}-proline at the N terminus which is characteristic of other transcription factors
including CTF/NF-1, C/EBP, AP-1, c-Fos, Fral, AP-2, and *tat* (ARYA et al. 1985;

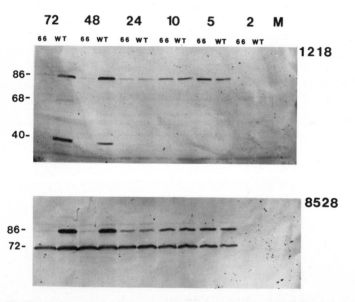

Fig. 13. Kinetic analysis of steady-state levels of region 1 and 2 proteins. Human fibroblast cells were
infected with wild-type (WT) HCMV and an early temperature-sensitive mutant (*ts66*). The *ts* mutant was
grown at the restrictive temperature (39.5°C). Infected cells were harvested at the indicated times and
protein extracts were electrophoresed on a 15% SDS-polyacrylamide gel. Western blots of these gels with
IE antibodies to the NH$_2$ terminal of region 1 (8528 or IE1-1) or the COOH terminus of region 2 (1218 or
IE2-4) (see Fig. 10) revealed the presence of two predominant proteins (86 kDa and 72 kDa) at IE times
postinfection. Other HCMV proteins sharing common epitopes with these IE proteins predicted from
HCMV proteins sharing common epitopes with these IE proteins predicted from S-1 mapping (STENBERG
et al. 1985, 1989) are seen later in infection. Mock infected cells (*M*) did not react with these antibodies
(STENBERG et al. 1989)

BOHMANN et al. 1987; LANDSCHULTZ et al. 1988a; COHEN and CURREN 1988; SANTORO et al. 1988). In the case of CTF/NF-1 this proline-rich stretch maps to a domain of the protein which is important for transcriptional activation (WILLIAMS et al. 1988).

Another amino acid sequence motif found in transcription factors is the "zinc finger." This DNA-binding motif was orginally discovered in *Xenopus laevis* transcription factor TFIIIA (MILLER et al. 1985), an RNA polymerase III transcriptional factor, and later in a variety of factors that influence polymerase II transcription (RHODES and KLUG 1988). At least two classes of these protein motifs exist and are characterized according to the number and position of the cysteine and histidine residues available for zinc coordination (BERG 1986). The first class (C_2H_2), typified by TFIIIA, comprises pairs of cysteines and histidines separated by a loop of 12 amino acids. Generally proteins with the C_2H_2 motif have the zinc finger tandemly repeated a minimum of two times with a seven- to eight-amino-acid linker. The other classes of metal-binding proteins have a variable number of conserved cysteines available for metal chelation. For example, the steroid receptors contain two unrelated fingers encoded by separate exons with four to five conserved cysteines (HUCKABY et al. 1987). The HCMV 72-kDa and 86-kDa IE proteins each contain a distinct single putative zinc finger motif shown in Fig. 14. The significance of the single zinc finger motif in the separate IE proteins is unknown. However, these structures may facilitate interactions of the IE proteins with viral nucleic acids.

Another sequence motif present in the 72-kDa protein of HCMV that is present in other proven or suspected gene regulatory proteins is a structure called the "leucine zipper" (LANDSCHULTZ et al. 1988b). Leucine side chains of this structure are proposed to interdigitate with those of another to hold two proteins together. This interaction would facilitate DNA-binding domains of two proteins to attach to DNA at specific sites. The 72-kDa protein contains a heptad repeat of leucine residues (a putative leucine zipper) in the fourth exon adjacent to the zinc finger (Fig. 12). The leucine zipper is not present in the 86-kDa protein, but this protein does contain a leucine-rich region adjacent to the zinc finger.

An additional similarity of the 72-kDa and 86-kDa sequence motifs to other DNA-binding proteins and transcription factors is the presence of polyglutamic acid and polyserine stretches. Similar stretches of these amino acids are found in the transcription factor ACE-1 (FÜRST et al. 1988), Sp1 (KADONGA et al. 1987), AP-2

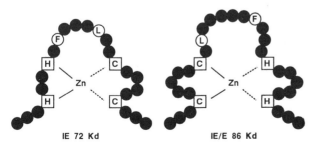

IE 72 Kd   **IE/E 86 Kd**

Fig. 14. Two-dimensional folding scheme for a linear arrangement of putative "zinc fingers" of the 72- and 86-kDa IE proteins. Labeled amino acids indicate conserved residues including the Cys and His zinc ligands

(WILLIAMS et al. 1988), and heat shock transcription factor (HSTF) (WIEDERRECHT et al. 1988). Finally, both proteins contain at least two potential nuclear localization sequences that are characterized by the clustering of four to six basic residues (DINGWALL and LASKY 1986). Another feature of these two proteins is the leucine-X_3-leucine repeat unit in exon 3. Finally, these proteins contain asparagine-X-threonine/serine motifs that are potential sites of N-linked glycosylation (MARSHALL 1972). No other major amino acid sequence similarities of the IE-1 and -2 proteins were detected in a comparative analysis with the Doolittle protein data bank (DOOLITTLE, personal communication).

Comparative analysis of amino acid sequence similarities only infers potential functions of these IE proteins. However, these homologies may indicate that several distinct and shared modular units exist in these proteins that enable these factors to interact with cellular and viral components to modulate HCMV gene expression.

6 Conclusion

In this chapter we have described the importance of the PBMN cells and their state of differentiation in the biology of HCMV. Model tissue culture systems that were utilized to study how the differentiation state may regulate viral gene expression strongly indicate the importance of cellular elements influencing transcription of IE genes and subsequent viral state. The interactions of cellular transcription factors with the MIEP region, encompassing promoter, enhancer, NF-1/CTF cluster, and modulator sequences have been investigated using a functional in vitro biochemical approach. This work has revealed a highly complex arrangement of distinct sequence-specific transcription factor interactions with each region that appear to act in a coordinated manner to control the level of IE gene expression. The products of this major IE region regulate (in *trans*) transcription of heterologous cellular and viral promoters and may constitute the earliest event directing the viral replication cycle. Therefore, identification of *cis* and *trans* regulatory factors controlling the expression of these IE genes is expected to be pivotal in determining the mechanisms of latency and reactivation.

Acknowledgments. This is publication Number 5815-IMM from the Department of Immunology, Scripps Clinic and Research Foundation, La Jolla, CA 92037. This work was supported by United States Public Health Service grant AI-21640 and AI-24178 from the National Institute of Allergy and Infectious Diseases and a grant from the Universitywide Task Force on AIDS. JAN is a recipient of a Faculty Award from the American Cancer Society. We thank Catherine Reynolds-Kohler, Richard Landes, and Emi Giulietti for valuable technical assistance and Drs. Richard Stenberg, Henry Lubon, Clayton Wiley, Janet Lathey, and Rachel Schrier for valuable discussions. We also wish to thank Dr. Michael B.A. Oldstone for his support and encouragement; and Gay Schilling for preparation of the manuscript.

References

Akrigg A, Wilkinson GWG, Oram JD (1985) The structure of the major immediate-early gene of human cytomegalovirus strain AD169. Virus Res 2: 107–121

Arya SK, Guo C, Joseph SF, Wong-Staal F (1985) Transactivator gene of human T lymphotropic virus type III (HTLV-III). Science 229: 69–73

Baeuerle PA, Baltimore D (1988) IκB: a specific inhibitor of the NF-κB transcription factor. Science 242: 540–546

Baldwin AS, Sharp PA (1987) Binding of a nuclear factor to a regulatory sequence in the promoter of the mouse H-2K^b class I major histocompatibility gene. Mol Cell Biol 7: 305–313

Balfour HH, Slade MS, Kalis JM, Howard RJ, Simons RL, Najarian JS (1977) Viral infections in renal transplant donors and their recipients: a prospective study. Surgery 81: 487–492

Ballard RA, Drew WL, Hufnagle KG, Riedel PA (1979) Acquired cytomegalovirus infection in preterm infants. Am J Dis Child 133: 482–485

Berg J (1986) Potential metal-binding domains in nucleic acid binding proteins. Science 232: 485–487

Betts RF (1982) Cytomegalovirus infection in transplant patients. Prog Med Virol 28: 44–64

Betts RF, Freeman RB, Douglas RG Jr, Talley TE, Rundell B (1975) Transmission of cytomegalovirus infection with renal allograft. Kidney Int 8: 387–394

Betts RF, Freeman RB, Douglas RG, Talley TE (1977) Clinical manifestations of renal allograft derived primary cytomegalovirus infection. Am J Dis Child 131: 759–763

Bohmann DT, Bos TJ, Adman A, Nishimura T, Vogt PK, Tjian R (1987) Human proto-oncogene c-jun encodes a DNA binding protein with structural and functional properties of transcription factor AP1. Science 238: 1386–1392

Boshart M, Weber F, Jahn G, Dorsch-Häsler K, Fleckenstein B, Schaffner W (1985) A very strong enhancer is located upstream of an immediate-early gene of human cytomegalovirus. Cell 41: 521–530

Braun RW, Reiser HC (1986) Replication of human cytomegalovirus in human peripheral blood T cells. J Virol 60: 29–36

Breathnach R, Chambon p (1981) Organization and expression of eukaryotic split genes coding for protein. Annu Rev Biochem 50: 349–383

Bruning JH, Bruggeman CA, van Boven CPA, van Breda Vriesman PJC (1986) Passive transfer of cytomegalovirus by cardiac and renal organ transplants in a rat model. Transplantation 41: 695–698

Chou S (1986) Acquisition of donor strains of cytomegalovirus by renal transplant recipients. N Engl J Med 314: 1418–1423

Cohen DR, Curran T (1988) Fra1: a serum-inducible, cellular immediate-early gene that encodes a Fos-related antigen. Mol Cell Biol 8: 2063–2069

Davis MG, Kenney SC, Kamine J, Pagano JS, Huang E-S (1987) Immediate-early gene region of human cytomegalovirus trans-activates the promoter of human immunodeficiency virus. Proc Natl Acad Sci USA 84: 8642–8646

DeMarchi JM (1981) Human cytomegalovirus DNA: restriction enzyme cleavage maps and map locations for immediate-early, early, and late RNAs. Virology 114: 23–38

Dingwall C, Laskey RA (1986) Protein import into the cell nucleus. Annu Rev Cell Biol 2: 367–390

Dorsch-Häsler K, Keil GM, Weber F, Jasin M, Schaffner W, Koszinowski UH (1985) A long and complex enhancer activates transcription of the gene coding for the highly abundant immediate-early mRNA in murine cytomegalovirus. Proc Natl Acad Sci USA 82: 8325–8329

Fürst P, Hu S, Hackett R, Hamer D (1988) Copper activates metallothionein gene transcription by altering the conformation of a specific DNA binding protein. Cell 55: 705–717

Geelen JLMC, Boom R, Klaver GPM, Minnaar RP, Feltkamp MCW, van Milligen FJ, Sol CJA, van der Noordaa J (1987) Transcriptional activation of the major immediate-early transcription unit of human cytomegalovirus by heat-shock, arsenite and protein synthesis inhibitors. J Gen Virol 68: 2925–2931

Ghazal P, Lubon H, Fleckenstein B, Hennighausen L (1987) Binding of transcription factors and creation of a large nucleoprotein complex on the human cytomegalovirus enhancer. Proc Natl Acad Sci USA 84: 3658–3662

Ghazal P, Lubon H, Hennighausen L (1988a) Specific interactions between transcription factors and the promoter-regulatory region of the human cytomegalovirus major immediate-early gene. J Virol 62: 1076–1079

Ghazal P, Lubon H, Hennighausen L (1988b) Multiple sequence-specific transcription factors modulate cytomegalovirus enhancer activity in vitro. Mol Cell Biol 8: 1809–1811

Glenn J (1981) Cytomegalovirus infections following renal transplantation. Rev Infect Dis 3: 1151–1178

Gnann JW, Ahlmen J, Svalander C, Olding L, Oldstone MBA, Nelson JA (1988) Inflammatory cells in transplanted kidneys are infected by human cytomegalovirus. Am J Pathol 132: 239–248

Gonczol E, Andrews PW, Plotkin SA (1984) Cytomegalovirus replicates in differentiated but not undifferentiated human embryonal carcinoma cells. Science 224: 159–161

Hai T, Liu F, Allegretto EA, Kanin M, Green MR (1988) A family of immunologically related transcription factors that includes multiple forms of ATF and AP-1. Genes Dev 2: 1216–1226

Hamilton JD, Seaworth BJ (1985) Transmission of latent cytomegalovirus in a murine kidney tissue transplantation model. Transplantation 39: 290–296

Hennighausen L, Fleckenstein B (1986) Nuclear factor 1 interacts with five DNA elements in the promoter region of the human cytomegalovirus major immediate-early gene. EMBO J 5: 1367–1371

Hermiston T, Malone C, Witte P, Stinski M (1987) Identification and characterization of the human cytomegalovirus immediate-early region 2 gene that stimulates gene expression from an inducible promoter. J Virol 61: 3214–3221

Ho M (1982) Cytomegalovirus biology and infection. Plenum, New York, pp 119–129

Huckaby CS, Conneely OM, Beattie WG, Dabron AW, Tsai MJ, O'Malley BW (1987) Structure of the chromosomal chicken progesterone receptor gene. Proc Natl Acad Sci USA 84: 8380–8384

Hurst HC, Jones N (1987) Identification of factors that interact with the E1a-inducible adenovirus E3 promoter. Genes Dev 1: 1132–1146

Jahn G, Knust E, Schmolla H, Sarre T, Nelson JA, McDougall JK, Fleckenstein B (1984) Predominant immediate-early transcripts of human cytomegalovirus AD169. J Virol 49: 363–370

Jeang K, Rawlins DR, Rosenfeld PJ, Shero JH, Kelly TJ, Hayward GS (1987) Multiple tandemly repeated binding sites for cellular nuclear factor 1 that surround the major immediate-early promoters of simian and human cytomegalovirus. J Virol 61: 1559–1570

Jones KA, Kadonaga JT, Rosenfeld PJ, Kelly JJ, Tjian R (1987) A cellular DNA binding protein that activates eukaryotic transcription and DNA replication. Cell 48: 79–89

Jordan MC, Shanley JD, Stevens JG (1977) Immunosuppression reactivates and disseminates latent murine cytomegalovirus. J Gen Virol 37: 419–423

Kadonaga JT, Cavner KR, Masiarz FR, Tjian R (1987) Isolation of cDNA encoding transcription factor Spl and functional analysis of the DNA binding domain. Cell 51: 1079–1090

Klotman ME, Starnes D, Hamilton JD (1985) The source of murine cytomegalovirus in mice receiving kidney allografts. J Infect Dis 152: 1192–1196

Kohwi-Shigematsu T, Nelson JA (1988) The chemical carcinogen, chloracetaldehyde, modifies a specific site within the regulatory sequence of human cytomegalovirus major immediate gene in vivo. Mol Carcinog 1: 20–25

Kouzarides T, Bankier AT, Satchwell SC, Preddy E, Barrell BG (1988) An immediate-early gene of human cytomegalovirus encodes a potential membrane glycoprotein. Virology 165: 151–164

LaFemina R, Hayward GS (1986) Constitutive and retinoic acid-inducible expression of cytomegalovirus immediate-early genes in human teratocarcinoma cells. J Virol 58: 434–440

LaFemina R, Hayward GS (1988) Differences in cell type-specific blocks to immediate-early gene expression and DNA replication of human, simian and murine cytomegalovirus. J Gen Virol 69: 355–374

Landschulz WH, Johnson PF, Adashi EY, Graves BJ, McKnight SM (1988a) Isolation of a recombinant copy of the gene encoding C/EMP. Genes Dev 2: 786–800

Landschulz WH, Johnson PF, McKnight SL (1988b) The leucine zipper: a hypothetical structure common to a new class of DNA binding proteins. Science 240: 1759–1764

Lang DJ, Ebert PA, Rodgers BM, Boggess HP, Rixse RS (1977) Reduction of post perfusion CMV infections following the use of leukocyte depleted blood. Transplantation 17: 391–395

Lenardo MJ, Kuang A, Gifford A, Baltimore D (1988) NF-kB protein purification from bovine spleen: nucleotide stimulation and binding site specificity. Proc Natl Acad Sci USA 85: 8825–8829

Lin YS, Green MR (1988) Interaction of a common transcription factor, ATF, with regulatory elements in both E1a and cyclic AMP-inducible promoters. Proc Natl Acad Sci USA 85: 3396–3400

Lubon H, Ghazal P, Nelson JA, Hennighausen L (1988) Cell-specific activity of the human immunodeficiency virus enhancer repeat in vitro. AIDS Res Hum Retro Viruses 4: 381–391

Lubon H, Ghazal P, Hennighausen L, Reynolds-Kohler C, Lockshin C, Nelson JA (1989) Cell-specific activity of the modulator region in the human cytomegalovirus major immediate-early gene. Mol Cell Biol 9: 1342–1345

Marker SC, Howard RJ, Simmons RL, Kalis JM, Connelly DP, Najarian JS, Balfour HH (1981) Cytomegalovirus infection: a quantitative prospective study of three hundred and twenty consecutive renal transplants. Surgery 89: 660–671

Marshall RD (1972) Glycoproteins. Annu Rev Biochem 41: 673–701

Miller J, McLachlan AD, Klug A (1985) Repetitive zinc-binding domains in the protein transcription factor IIIA from *Xenopus* oocytes. EMBO J 4: 1609–1614

Montminy MR, Bilezsikjian LM (1987) Binding of a nuclear protein to the cyclic AMP response element of the somatostatin gene. Nature 328: 175–178

Montminy MR, Sevarino KA, Wagner JA, Mandel G, Goodman RH (1986) Identification of a cyclic-AMP-responsive element within the rat somatostatin gene. Proc Natl Acad Sci USA 83: 6682–6686

Myerson D, Hackman RC, Nelson JA, Ward DC, McDougall JK (1984) Widespread presence of histologically occult cytomegalovirus. Hum Pathol 15: 430–439

Nankervis GA (1976) Comments on CMV infections in renal transplant patients. Yale J Biol Med 49: 27–28

Naraqi S, Jackson GG, Jonasson O, Rubenis M (1978) Search for latent cytomegalovirus in renal allografts. Infect Immun 19: 699–703

Nelson JA, Groudine M (1986) Transcriptional regulation of the human cytomegalovirus major immeditate-early gene is associated with induction of DNaseI hypersensitive sites. Mol Cell Biol 6: 452–461

Nelson JA, Reynolds-Kohler C, Smith B (1987) Negative and positive regulation by a short segment in the 5′-flanking region of the human cytomegalovirus major immediate-early gene. Mol Cell Biol 7: 4125–4129

Nowak B, Gmeiner A, Sarnow P, Levine AJ, Fleckenstein B (1984) Physical mapping of human cytomegalovirus genes: identification of DNA sequences coding for a virion phosphoprotein of 71 kDa and a viral 65-kDa polypeptide. Virology 134: 91–102

Olding LB, Jenson FC, Oldstone MBA (1975) Pathogenesis of cytomegalovirus infection. I. Activation of virus from bone marrow-derived lymphocytes by in vitro allogenic reaction. J Exp Med 141: 561–572

Pass RF, Whitley RJ, Diethelm AG, Whelchel JD, Reynolds DW, Alford CA Jr (1979) Outcome of renal transplantation in patients with primary cytomegalovirus infection. Transplant Proc 11: 1288–1290

Peterson PK, Balfour HH, Marker SC, Fryd DS, Howard RJ, Simmon RL (1980) Cytomegalovirus disease in renal allograft recipients: a prospective study of the clinical features, risk factors and impact on renal transplantation. Medicine (Baltimore) 59: 283–300

Pizzorno MC, O'Hare P, Sha L, LaFemina RL, Hayward GS (1988) Transactivation and autoregulation of gene expression by the immediate-early region 2 gene products of human cytomegalovirus. J Virol 62: 1167–1179

Prince AM, Szmuness W, Millian SJ, David DS (1971) A serologic study of cytomegalovirus infections associated with blood transfusions. N Engl J Med 284: 1125–1131

Rhodes D, Klug A (1988) "Zinc fingers": a novel motif for nucleic acid binding. Nucleic Acids Mol Biol 2: 149–166

Rice GPA, Schrier RD, Oldstone MBA (1984) Cytomegalovirus infects human lymphocytes and monocytes: virus expression is restricted to immediate-early gene products. Proc Natl Acad Sci USA 81: 6134–6138

Rubin RH, Cogimi AB, Tolkoff-Rubin NE, Russell PS, Hirsch MS (1977) Infectious disease syndromes attributable to cytomegalovirus and their significance among renal transplant recipients. Transplantation 24: 458–464

Rüger R, Bornkamon GW, Fleckenstein B (1984) Human cytomegalovirus DNA sequences with homologies to the cellular genome. J Gen Virol 65: 1351–1364

Santoro CN, Mermod N, Andrews PC, Tjian R (1988) A family of human CCAAT box-binding proteins active in transcription and DNA replication: cloning and expression of multiple cDNAs. Nature 334: 218–224

Schrier RD, Nelson JA, Oldstone MBA (1985) Detection of human cytomegalovirus in peripheral blood lymphocytes in a natural infection. Science 230: 1048–1051

Sen R, Baltimore D (1986) Multiple nuclear factors interact with the immunoglobulin enhancer sequences. Cell 46: 705–716

Sen R, Baltimore D (1987) Inducibility of k immunoglobulin enhancer-binding protein NF-kB by a post-translational mechanism. Cell 47: 921–928

Spaete R, Mocarski E (1985) Regulation of cytomegalovirus gene expression: alpha and beta promoters are transactivated by viral functions in permissive human fibroblasts. J Virol 56: 135–143

Staprans SI, Rabert DK, Spector DH (1988) Identification of sequence requirements and *trans*-acting functions necessary for regulated expression of a human cytomegalovirus early gene. J Virol 62: 3463–3473

Stenberg RM, Stinski MF (1985) Autoregulation of the human cytomegalovirus major immediate-early gene. J Virol 56: 676–682

Stenberg RM, Thomsen DR, Stinski MF (1984) Structural analysis of the major immediate-early gene of human cytomegalovirus. J Virol 49: 190–199

Stenberg RM, Witte PR, Stinski MF (1985) Multiple spliced and unspliced transcripts from human cytomegalovirus immediate-early region two and evidence for a common initiation site within immediate-early region. J Virol 56: 665–675

Stenberg RM, Depto AS, Fortney J, Nelson JA (1989) Regulated expression of early and late RNA and protein from the human cytomegalovirus immediate-early gene region. J Virol (in press)

Stinski MF, Roehr TS (1985) Activation of the major immediate-early gene of human cytomegalovirus by cis-acting elements in the promoter-regulatory sequence and by virus-specific trans-acting components. J Virol 55: 431–441

Stinski MF, Thomson DR, Stenberg RM, Goldstein LC (1983) Organization and expression of the immediate-early genes of human cytomegalovirus. J Virol 46: 1–14

Suwansirikul S, Rao N, Dowling JN, Ho M (1977) Primary and secondary cytomegalovirus infection: clinical manifestations after renal transplantation. Arch Intern Med 137: 1026–1030

Tevethia MJ, Spector DJ, Leisure KM, Stinski MF (1987) Participation of two human cytomegalovirus immediate-early gene regions in transcriptional activation of adenovirus promoters. Virology 161: 276–285

Thomson DR, Stenberg RM, Goins WF, Stinski MF (1984) Promoter-regulatory region of the major immediate-early gene of human cytomegalovirus. Proc Natl Acad Sci USA 81: 659–663

Van Dyke MW, Roeder RG, Sawadogo M (1988) Physical analysis of transcription preinitiation complex assembly in a class II gene promoter. Science 241: 1335–1338

Wathen MW, Stinski MF (1982) Temporal patterns of human cytomegalovirus transcription: mapping the viral RNAs synthesized at immediate-early, early, and late times after infection. J Virol 41: 462–477

Weston K (1988) An enhancer element in the short unique region of human cytomegalovirus regulates the production of a group of abundant immediate-early transcripts. Virology 162: 406–416

Wiederrecht G, Seto D, Parker CS (1988) Isolation of the gene encoding the S. cereviside heat shock transcription factor. Cell 54: 841–853

Wiley CA, Schrier RD, Denaro FJ, Nelson JA, Lampert PW, Oldstone MBA (1986) Localization of cytomegalovirus proteins and genome during fulminant central nervous system infection in an AIDS patient. J Neuropathol Exp Neurol 45: 127–139

Wilkinson GWG, Akrigg A, Greenaway PJ (1984) Transcription of the immediate-early genes of human cytomegalovirus strain AD169. Virus Res 1: 101–116

Williams T, Admon A, Lüscher B, Tjian R (1988) Cloning and expression of AP-2, a cell-type-specific transcription factor that activates inducible enhancer elements. Genes Dev 2: 1557–1569

Yamamoto KK, Gonzalez GA, Biggs WH, Montminy MR (1988) Phosphorylation-induced binding and transcriptional efficacy of nuclear factor CREB. Nature 334: 494–498

Yeager AS (1974) Transfusion-acquired cytomegalovirus infection in newborn infants. Am J Dis Child 128: 478–483

Guinea Pig Cytomegalovirus Gene Expression

H. C. Isom and C. Y. Yin

1   Introduction   101
2   Expression of GPCMV in Specific Organs and Cell Types   102
2.1 Salivary Gland   102
2.2 Brain   104
2.3 Ear   105
2.4 Placenta   107
2.5 Hematopoietic and Lymphoid Tissues and Cells   108
2.6 Other Organs and Cell Types   109
3   Molecular Analyses of GPCMV Gene Expression   110
3.1 Characterization of GPCMV DNA   110
3.2 GPCMV Gene Expression at the RNA Level   113
3.3 GPCMV Gene Expression at the Protein Level   117
4   Conclusions   118
References   119

1 Introduction

Human cytomegalovirus (HCMV) is a significant human pathogen and its clinical importance has recently become more predominantly recognized because of the severity of HCMV infections in immunocompromised hosts, transplant recipients, and individuals with AIDS. Since HCMV is species specific, it is important to have an appropriate animal model to help understand the pathogenicity of this virus. Guinea pig cytomegalovirus (GPCMV) infection of the guinea pig is species specific, produces many of the same clinical syndromes that occur during HCMV infection of the human, and has been shown in numerous studies to be an excellent model for studying the pathogenicity of HCMV. One approach that has been taken to understand the replication and pathogenicity of viruses has been to characterize gene expression by these viruses and to study the regulation of virus gene expression.

In this chapter we will use the term "gene expression" simply to mean expression of the virus genome. We will not limit our discussion to gene expression at a molecular level but will also include classical methods of measuring virus gene expression including detection of infectious virus by biological methods, detection of virus particles by electron microscopy, and detection of virus antigens by

Department of Microbiology and Immunology, The Pennsylvania State University College of Medicine, Hershey, Pennsylvania 17033, USA

immunofluorescence or immunohistochemistry. Since a long-range goal at least of the research ongoing in our laboratory on GPCMV is to understand how GPCMV genes are expressed amid the background of cellular gene expression that occurs in the infected cell, we will examine GPCMV gene expression in particular organs and in specific cell types within those organs. We will ask questions such as: In what tissues can virus be found during an acute infection? In what tissues does virus infection persist? What are the effects of virus infection at the cellular level in different cell types?

In the latter part of the chapter, we will discuss the molecular biology of GPCMV and review what is known about virus gene expression of GPCMV-permissive infection in vitro at the level of GPCMV RNA and protein synthesis. At this time, very few molecular studies to analyze GPCMV gene expression in vivo have been carried out. The goal of this chapter is to describe what is currently known about (a) GPCMV gene expression in different tissues and cell types in GPCMV-infected guinea pigs and (b) GPCMV gene expression during productive infection of cells in culture. In the future, the correct fusion of these two bodies of knowledge may make it possible to understand how GPCMV (a) interacts with different cell types to produce acute infection or to persist in vitro and in vivo, (b) elicits the immune response, and (c) causes the pathogenicity that is observed during in vivo infection.

2 Expression of GPCMV in Specific Organs and Cell Types

During acute and persistent GPCMV infection, GPCMV gene expression can be detected in many organs and in specific cell types within these organs. In the following sections we will review what is known about GPCMV infection in vivo and in vitro with regard to cell type. We will discuss in detail only the most recent studies since the pathogenicity of GPCMV has been reviewed previously (Hsiung et al. 1980; Bia et al. 1983; Isom and Gao 1988).

2.1 Salivary Gland

GPCMV infection was first recognized in the salivary gland duct cells of naturally infected animals (Jackson 1920). The salivary gland is a primary site of GPCMV infection during acute and persistent infection (Tenser and Hsiung 1976) and the salivary gland duct cells contain typical inclusions that can be easily recognized and enumerated (Fong et al. 1980). The ultrastructural effects of GPCMV infection of the salivary gland, which were first reported by Middlekamp in 1967 (Middlekamp et al. 1967), showed that GPCMV infects primarily the duct cell epithelium of the guinea pig salivary gland. Mononuclear infiltrates were seen surrounding the ducts of the gland. The infected epithelial cells were enlarged and protruded into the lumen of the duct, containing large acidophilic intranuclear Cowdry type A inclusions and smaller cytoplasmic granules. When weanling Hartley guinea pigs were infected intracerebrally or subcutaneously with GPCMV, the titer of virus from salivary gland was sufficiently high by 24 days postinfection (p.i.) that infectious virus could be measured directly from tissue homogenates and did not require cocultivation (CONNOR and JOHNSON 1976). When adult Hartley guinea pigs were infected, infectious virus was first isolated from the salivary gland at 5 days p.i. (HSIUNG et al. 1978). GPCMV inclusions in the salivary gland were first detected 2 weeks after virus inoculation, increased to a maximum number at 3–4 weeks, and were no longer detectable by 8 weeks. Virus infectivity titers increased in parallel and peaked at 4 weeks postinoculation, but infectious virus could still be detected by 30 weeks p.i. even though inclusions were not detected beyond 8 weeks (FONG et al. 1980). GPCMV does not persist in all organs but it does persist in salivary gland.

Electron microscopic examination of salivary gland duct cells from guinea pigs at 4 weeks p.i. showed aggregated dense matrix with a lattice-like structure in the central portion of the nucleus, nucleocapsids scattered throughout the nucleus, and mature virions enclosed in cytoplasmic vacuoles in the cytoplasm (FONG et al. 1980). The electron-dense matrix in the nucleus was composed of hollow fibrillar structures and the nucleocapsids contained cores at different stages of assembly. The GPCMV nucleocapsids acquired an outer envelope from the cell inner nuclear membrane. Vacuoles containing small numbers of virions fused to form larger vacuoles. Tubular structures that are seen in GPCMV-infected guinea pig embryo fibroblast cells (MIDDLEKAMP et al. 1967; FONG et al. 1979) were not seen in salivary gland duct cells. At the cell surface, which was adjacent to the duct lumen, it was possible to observe breaks in the cytoplasmic vacuoles which allowed virions to be released into the duct lumen. Release of mature virions appeared to result from fusion of the vacuoles with the plasma membrane. Free virus particles were observed in the duct lumen. In disseminated GPCMV infection in strain 2 inbred guinea pigs the ultrastructural development of GPCMV was the same for infection of outbred Hartley animals. The development of GPCMV in the salivary gland as measured ultrastructurally closely resembles that of HCMV (KAWANISHI et al. 1967).

When the techniques of light and electron microscopy were used to study GPCMV infection of the salivary glands from GPCMV-infected animals it was concluded that GPCMV infection was present only in the duct cells. In a more recent study (GRIFFITH et al., unpublished data), these results were confirmed when salivary gland tissue was examined histologically for intranuclear inclusions or immunocytochemically for GPCMV antigens. However, when the technique of in situ hybridization to detect GPCMV nucleic acids was used, GPCMV nucleic acids were detected not only in duct cells but also in salivary gland cells outside of the duct. Nucleic acids were detected primarily in duct cells that also had intranuclear inclusions but GPCMV nucleic acids were also detected in duct cells that did not contain intranuclear inclusions. Intranuclear inclusions were detected in salivary glands from 11 of 33 animals, GPCMV antigens were detected in 13 of 33 animals, and GPCMV nucleic acids were detected in 15 of 33 animals. It is clear from this study that the ability to detect GPCMV infection and gene expression is dependent upon the sensitivity of the technique used in examining the infected tissue. Further studies will have to be carried out using specific molecular probes and antibodies, when they become available and characterized, to determine which GPCMV genes are expressed in nonduct salivary gland cells.

2.2 Brain

Although MARKHAM and HUDSON showed in 1935 that intracerebral inoculation of guinea pigs with GPCMV led to meningoencephalitis, studies on GPCMV infection of the brain have not been pursued and studied in more detail until recently. In 1982, GPCMV infection of the brain was observed in neonatal guinea pigs that had been infected with the virus congenitally (GRIFFITH et al. 1982). The microscopic lesions that were seen in the brains of the neonatal animals were characterized as glial nodule encephalitis and reported to be similar to lesions seen in human babies infected congenitally with HCMV. In 1986, it was demonstrated that GPCMV can replicate in guinea pig fetal primary brain cell cultures with susceptibility to virus infection varying with the age of the fetus (KARI and GEHRZ 1986). GPCMV replicated to higher levels in 31- and 37-day gestation cultures than in 25-day gestation cultures. This difference was most likely attributable to the fact that cultures from older fetuses contained more differentiated cells. In 37-day gestation cultures, cells which stained for both GPCMV antigens and glial fibrillary acid protein, a marker for astrocytes, were found but cells which stained for GPCMV antigens and neuron-specific enolase or acetylcholinesterase, markers for neurons, were not found, indicating that GPCMV productively infects astrocytes but not neurons in these cultures. Since neurons could only be detected in 37-day gestation cultures, it was not possible to make this comparison in cultures from younger fetuses. These studies demonstrate that GPCMV replication and gene expression as detected by immunofluorescence staining for GPCMV antigens using virus-specific antiserum can be observed in fetal brain cells.

More recently, Booss et al. (1988) have examined GPCMV gene expression in vivo in brain cells of young guinea pigs. When young guinea pigs were inoculated intracerebrally with GPCMV, virus was recovered from the brain and peak titers were obtained at 3–4 days p.i. Virus was cleared from the brain between 15 and 23 days p.i. Appearance of circulating neutralizing antibody at 3–4 weeks p.i. correlated with the loss of recoverable virus from the brain. During the 1st week p.i. the predominant histopathological change in the brain was the development of leptomeningitis; mononuclear cell infiltrates and intranuclear inclusion-bearing cells were observed in the leptomeninges and a low to moderate number of reactive monocytes were occasionally observed in the molecular layer of the cortex. Encephalitis and ependymitis were first observed toward the end of the 1st week of infection and peaked at day 10. Parenchymal changes included perivascular infiltrates and diffuse inflammatory changes but the most characteristic finding was focal microglial nodules. The nodules consisted of swirled and elongated cells that were sometimes in association with intranuclear inclusion-bearing cells. The nodules consisted of rod cells and macrophages. The local host defense responses included activation of astrocytes and glial nodule formation. Systemic host defense responses also contributed to the pathological changes. Characterization of the circulating immune cells that invaded the CNS showed that monocytes, and not T cells, predominated in the leptomeninges and in parenchymal foci (Booss et al. 1989). It is interesting to note that the finding of glial nodules in the parenchyma has also been seen in HCMV encephalitis. These findings suggest that the GPCMV-guinea pig model may be an excellent system for studying HCMV encephalitis and the host defense response to HCMV infection of the brain. Having such a model to study HCMV encephalitis is important since HCMV encephalitis is seen in AIDS (MORGELLO et al. 1987) and immunologically compromised allograft (SCHNECK 1965) patients, and the pathogenesis of HCMV infection in the CNS is poorly understood.

2.3 Ear

One major consequence of HCMV infections is sensorineural hearing loss. HCMV is the leading infectious cause of congenital sensorineural hearing loss (STAGNO et al. 1977). Deafness has also been associated with primary HCMV infections in adults and the hearing loss and central auditory dysfunction found in a large percentage of AIDS patients may also be associated with HCMV infection. In line with the general problem of the species-specific nature of HCMV it has been difficult to study the pathogenicity of HCMV deafness. Few human temporal bones have been available for study. Autopsies of infants who have died of generalized HCMV infection have shown labyrinthitis that involved predominantly the endolymphatic compartment of both the auditory and vestibular systems (MYERS and STOOL 1968; DAVIS et al. 1977, 1981). A model for HCMV labyrinthitis has been established by infecting GPCMV-seronegative guinea pigs with GPCMV via the intracochlear or intrathecal routes (HARRIS et al. 1984). Control studies using inactivated virus showed that the procedure of injecting virus into the perilymphatic compartment had no effects on cochlear morphology, did not cause inflammation, and did not affect function as measured by cochlear electrophysiological recordings. When animals were inoculated with GPCMV there was a precipitous decline in cochlear electrophysiological recordings at 8 days p.i. Examination of the temporal bones at 8 days p.i. showed marked inflammation and hemorrhage in the scala tympani. Guinea pigs which had developed antibody to GPCMV as a result of footpad inoculation with the virus showed no signs of morphological damage or hearing loss when they were subsequently inoculated in the inner ear with GPCMV. In the guinea pigs, perilymphatic involvement predominated while in the inner ears of human infants who have died of cytomegalic inclusion disease HCMV was mainly confined to the endolymphatic structures. In this study virus gene expression was not directly measured except for the observation that typical cytomegalic cells lined the scala tympani. It is assumed that the degeneration in the spiral ganglion cells was caused by virus gene expression and virus replication and that the damage due to inflammation was caused by the ability of virus gene expression to trigger the immune response.

In an independent study in which guinea pigs were inoculated directly into the scala tympani through the round window membrane, GPCMV inclusion-body-bearing cells were seen in the labyrinth between the limbus and the tectorial membrane and in some cases the endolymphatic sac contained cell debris and fluid (NOMURA et al. 1988). The endolymphatic sac appears to be the site of host defense within the inner ear. When GPCMV was inoculated into the endolymphatic sac, infection was accompanied by loss of cochlear function and GPCMV antigens were detected in endolymphatic epithelial cells, infiltrative cells, giant cells in the perisaccular connective tissue, mesothelial and inflammatory cells in the scala tympani, and spiral ganglion cells (FUKUDA et al. 1988). Seropositive animals were protected against the damage caused by viral replication and did not demonstrate loss of cochlear function, but inflammation in the endolymphatic sac was observed. Prophylactic treatment of guinea pigs with ganciclovir 1 day prior to inoculation with GPCMV prevented the cochlear histopathological changes and hearing loss that are seen during experimental GPCMV labyrinthitis (WOOLF et al. 1988). These studies suggest that damage to the inner ear that accompanies GPCMV infection appears to result from the direct cytopathic effects of virus gene expression and also from the indirect effects of the response of the immune system to virus gene expression.

It also has recently been demonstrated that a female guinea pig which had been inoculated with GPCMV in the round window membrane shortly before becoming pregnant gave birth to a guinea pig which had an abnormal cochlea (NOMURA et al. 1988). This latter study indicates that infection is not limited to that which can be introduced experimentally by direct inoculation of the inner ear of animals with virus but shows that infection of the inner ear by GPCMV can occur by a more "natural" route.

In a recent more detailed study, GPCMV gene expression in GPCMV labyrinthitis was monitored with time after inoculation of the scala tympani with GPCMV using IgG from seropositive animals (KEITHLEY et al. 1988). The first cells to express GPCMV antigens were the tympanic lamellar cells, the mesothelial cells lining the scala tympani. At 3 days p.i., GPCMV antigens were detected in the inflammatory cells in the scala tympani and by 4 days p.i. the infection had spread and GPCMV antigens were detected in the osseous spiral lamina, mesothelial cells of Reissner's membrane, and the spiral ganglion cells. Eventually virus antigens were also detected in the inflammatory cells in the modiolus, in mesothelial cells in the scala vestibuli, and in Scarpa's ganglion cells. Virus antigens were detected more frequently in mesothelial and inflammatory cells than in other cell types. Infection spread toward the brain and it is possible that GPCMV particles are carried within infected inflammatory cells. Typical GPCMV inclusions were seen in some of the cells expressing GPCMV antigens but not in all, indicating that in some cells virus gene expression may be occurring but may be limited such that virus replication and the production of typical inclusions is not occurring. These studies clearly show that the interaction of GPCMV with specific host cell types is important in determining pathogenicity. These studies, which are limited by the fact that they were carried out with antiserum obtained from guinea pigs inoculated with virus, one of the few reagents available at this time for carrying out studies of this nature, clearly demonstrate why molecular reagents and specific, characterized antibodies are needed so that more precise information can be obtained about tissue-specific expression of GPCMV.

2.4 Placenta

The most frequent cause of congenital viral infection in humans is HCMV (Ho 1982). Congenital HCMV infections are thought to be acquired via the placenta but the mechanisms of transplacental transmission are not known. Although there are several reports describing HCMV infection of the placenta at the histological level and isolation of HCMV from the human placenta (FELDMAN 1969; HAYES and GIBAS 1971; FRENCH et al. 1977), these studies have been quite limited. Transplacental transmission of GPCMV to the guinea pig fetus does occur and it has been demonstrated in several reports that the GPCMV model is an excellent system for analyzing HCMV congenital infection (CHOI and HSIUNG 1978; KUMAR and NANKERVIS 1978; JOHNSON and CONNOR 1979; GRIFFITH and HSIUNG 1980; KUMAR and PROKAY 1982; BIA et al. 1984; GRIFFITH et al. 1986). GPCMV gene expression and replication in the placenta and its role in transplacental transmission can be studied more thoroughly in the animal model because of the availability of tissue and the ability to manipulate the system. In the animal model, it is possible to (a) examine placentas at various times during the course of a pregnancy, (b) localize the site(s) of GPCMV infection and/or GPCMV gene expression within the placenta, (c) establish whether the timing of primary infection during gestation effects when placental infection occurs and the severity of placental infection, and (d) determine the relationship between placental infection and fetal infection.

GPCMV infection of the placenta has been studied in guinea pigs infected at midgestation (GRIFFITH et al. 1985) or during the first trimester (GOFF et al. 1987). In the first study, pregnant Hartley guinea pigs were inoculated at midgestation with virus and studied at 8, 14, 21, and 28 days postinoculation. Since the gestation for guinea pigs is 68–70 days, the last time point was close to term. These studies demonstrated that (a) GPCMV virus was present in the placenta long after the virus was cleared from the blood stream, (b) GPCMV was present in the placenta and not in maternal blood that was filling placental blood spaces, (c) virus could be isolated from the placenta at times when significant levels of circulating GPCMV-neutralizing antibody were present in the maternal circulation, (d) there was a delay between establishment of infection of the placenta and infection of the fetus, and (e) virus infectivity titers were the highest at 21 and 28 days p.i., which coincided with late gestation. Since infection in these animals was initiated at midgestation, it was not possible to determine whether the peak of infection occurred at 28 days p.i. because of the time course of the infection or because infection is maximal at late gestation. To address this issue, pregnant guinea pigs were infected during the first trimester of pregnancy at 17 days gestation and infection of the placenta was measured through 48 days p.i., which was late in gestation and close to term (GOFF et al. 1987). The initial viremia was cleared by 2–3 weeks p.i. but returned during the last 2 weeks of gestation. The secondary viremia could have resulted from virus coming from leukocytes, the salivary gland, the spleen, or the placenta. GPCMV infection in the placentas of these animals was biphasic, with the first peak occurring during the 2nd week of infection and the second equal or even greater peak occurring during the last 2–3 weeks of gestation. These studies show that GPCMV infection of the placenta is maximal during late gestation whether infection is initiated during the first or second trimesters and that GPCMV can persist in the placenta and serve as a continuing source of virus throughout the pregnancy. The rise in GPCMV titer in the placenta near the end of pregnancy may be due to changes in placental structure and function that take place late in gestation or to hormonal changes that occur. The data also suggest that increased virus replication in late gestation may cause an increase in the incidence of fetal infection.

Placentas from guinea pigs infected at midgestation were examined histologically for GPCMV infection and tissues were also stained by the immunoperoxidase method for detection of GPCMV antigens using guinea pig serum containing neutralizing antibodies to GPCMV (GRIFFITH et al. 1985). Histopathology typical of an HCMV infection was seen in placentas from animals killed at 21 and 28 days postinoculation and typical GPCMV intranuclear cytomegalic inclusions were only observed in placentas at 28 days p.i. GPCMV-induced lesions detected histologically and with specific antiserum were localized at the transitional layer between the capillarized labyrinth and the noncapillarized interlobium. Electron microscopic examination revealed that intranuclear inclusions were seen in trophoblastic cells, virions and dense bodies were found in extracellular spaces surrounding the infected cells, and viral nucleocapsids not associated with typical intranuclear inclusions were also seen in the nuclei of nontrophoblastic cells.

2.5 Hematopoietic and Lymphoid Tissues and Cells

In HCMV infections, a series of hematological abnormalities have been described. In HCMV mononucleosis, there are atypical circulating lymphocytes, lymphadenopathy, and splenomegaly. When the effects of experimentally induced acute GPCMV infection of guinea pigs were studied, virus-induced changes in the hematopoietic and lymphoid tissues were observed and many of these changes were similar to what had been seen for HCMV (GRIFFITH et al. 1981). Young nonpregnant guinea pigs were used in these studies and they were inoculated with a dose of virus that caused a nonlethal, self-limiting infection. Anemia was evident from day 5 to 12 p.i., leukocyte counts dropped during the 1st week p.i. and returned to normal by 3 weeks p.i., and lymphocytosis with atypical lymphocytes was also seen. GPCMV was isolated from the granulocyte-erythrocyte fraction of the blood from day 1 to 11 p.i. but was no longer present at day 13–16 p.i. GPCMV persisted in the mononuclear fraction of the blood and was detected from day 1 to at least day 16. GPCMV was also isolated from the bone marrow and thymus but no virus inclusions were seen in either tissue. GPCMV infection of the lymphoid tissues differs from infection of the salivary gland in that GPCMV intranuclear inclusions were rarely seen in lymphoid tissue.

Splenomegaly was apparent from day 7 to 15 p.i. and infectious GPCMV was isolated from the spleen from 3 to 30 days p.i. with the highest titers found on day 7. GPCMV was recovered from the B- and T-cell fractions at 3 days p.i. By day 13,

GPCMV infectivity titers were no longer detectable in the macrophage fraction and by day 16, virus was no longer isolated from the T-cell fraction. GPCMV persisted in the B-cell fraction through day 60. Distinct virus-induced inclusions were not seen in the spleen. Stimulation in both the B- and T-cell areas of the spleen was observed consistent with the concept that both B-cell and T-cell immune responses accompany a GPCMV infection.

The lymphadenopathy that was observed during acute GPCMV infection was also studied (Lucia et al. 1985). GPCMV was isolated from the mesenteric and axillary lymph nodes during the first 2–4 weeks p.i. and from the cervical nodes through at least 8 weeks p.i. Although inclusion-bearing cells were rarely observed in the lymph nodes during GPCMV infection, GPCMV antigens were detected in the nuclei of noncervical lymph node cells from day 3 through 14 after inoculation. Examination of lymph node tissue with sensitive molecular probes may reveal GPCMV gene expression in even more noninclusion-bearing cells than was seen using antiserum to detect GPCMV antigens.

In a recent study, congenitally infected guinea pigs were analyzed for changes in immune function and for alterations produced by GPCMV in tissues associated with immune functions (Zheng et al. 1987). GPCMV-infected neonatal guinea pigs develop splenomegaly, thymic hypoplasia, and immunodepression. GPCMV was recovered from both the spleen and the thymus of congenitally-infected neonates but higher titers of infectious virus were recovered from the spleen than from the thymus. The number of T, B, and inflammatory cells increased in the spleens and T cells were depleted from the thymus. There was no evidence of virus-induced thymic cell lysis and it is possible that T-cell depletion occurred as a result of T-cell migration to another site, perhaps to the spleen. Both B- and T-cell functions were impaired in the infected neonatal animals as had been seen previously in GPCMV-infected adult guinea pigs (Griffith et al. 1984); both adult and congenitally infected guinea pigs had reduced proliferative responses to the T-cell mitogen, conconavalin A, and the B-cell mitogen, lipopolysaccharide. The response to T-cell mitogens was more severely altered in congenitally infected neonates than in infected adult guinea pigs and the T-cell immune depression lasted longer in the neonates. It is not known which spleen and thymus cell types become infected in GPCMV congenital infection. It is important to realize that the spleen and the thymus in these animals were undergoing differentiation and development at the time when they were infected. To understand how thymic hypoplasia and splenomegaly develop, it will be necessary to analyze the state of differentiation of infected cells in these tissues, determine which cell types in the spleen and the thymus express GPCMV genes, and establish which GPCMV genes are expressed.

2.6 Other Organs and Cell Types

GPCMV can also infect many organs and cell types not listed in the above paragraphs. Which cell types and tissues become infected and the severity of infection depends upon many variables including the amount of virus inoculated, the route of inoculation, the strain of the animal, and whether the animal is pregnant.

For example, the severity of GPCMV infection is enhanced in pregnant compared with nonpregnant animals (GRIFFITH et al. 1983) and in inbred strain 2 guinea pigs compared with random-bred Hartley animals (FONG et al. 1983). In the studies described above, inclusions were not seen in lymphoid tissues; however, if the animals were inoculated with larger doses of infectious virus, the animals became severely ill and inclusions were found in the spleen, lymph nodes, and bone marrow (GRIFFITH et al. 1981). When inbred strain 2 guinea pigs are inoculated with salivary gland-passaged GPCMV, the animals develop severe disseminated disease (FONG et al. 1983). Under these conditions, infectious GPCMV was isolated from spleen, lungs, liver, pancreas, heart, adrenals, kidneys, and salivary glands and intranuclear virus inclusions were present in many cell types in these organs.

3 Molecular Analyses of GPCMV Gene Expression

Although expression of the GPCMV genome can be studied by measuring infectious virus, by histological detection of virus particles, and by detection of antigens with virus-specific antisera, these techniques cannot be used to detect low levels of gene expression or to identify which portions of the genome are expressed during limited gene expression. To understand GPCMV gene expression in more detail during acute and persistent infections, it is necessary to characterize the virus at the molecular level and develop reagents that can be used to identify expression of specific RNA species and proteins in tissue and at the individual cellular level.

3.1 Characterization of GPCMV DNA

Molecular characterization of GPCMV was initiated by examining the DNA of this virus (ISOM et al. 1984) and preparing recombinant DNA plasmids containing GPCMV DNA fragments spanning the genome (GAO and ISOM 1984). A procedure was developed for the purification of GPCMV DNA (ISOM et al. 1984) and the molecular cloning of approximately 97% of the GPCMV genome was accomplished (GAO and ISOM 1984). The cloning of GPCMV DNA has made it possible to determine the structure of the GPCMV genome (GAO and ISOM 1984), generate restriction endonuclease maps of the DNA (GAO and ISOM 1984), identify regions of DNA sequence homology with HCMV (ISOM and GAO 1988), begin to analyze GPCMV transcription (ISOM and GAO 1988), and detect GPCMV infection in cultured cells (SHA et al. 1987) and in salivary gland (GRIFFITH et al., unpublished data) by in situ hybridization.

The *Hind*III, *Eco*RI, and *Xba*I restriction endonuclease cleavage sites of the GPCMV genome were mapped by hybridizing ^{32}P-labeled fragments to Southern blot transfers of total GPCMV DNA cleaved with the three different enzymes (GAO and ISOM 1984). No cross-hybridization between any internal fragments was seen. Cross-hybridization to multiple bands in each of the other two digests made it possible to position many of the fragments on the genome. The GPCMV genome has three terminal fragments and two populations of GPCMV molecules exist. The predominant form (70% of the population) consists of molecules in which both terminal fragments contain repeat sequences of a maximum of 0.7×10^6 daltons. The minor population (about 30%) consists of molecules in which one terminal fragment is identical to that in the predominant structural form, whereas the remaining terminal fragment is identical except it is missing the 0.7×10^6-dalton repeat sequence. The data originally obtained from hybridization with cloned, gel-isolated internal and terminal fragments and from double digestions allowed linear arrangement of all the GPCMV HindIII DNA fragments and all but four of the EcoRI DNA fragments, EcoRI e, O, H, and i (GAO and ISOM 1984). In recent studies, several regions of the GPCMV genome have been mapped in more detail and the map positions for EcoRI e and O were determined (YIN and ISOM, unpublished data; Fig. 1). In addition, it was established in this analysis that the EcoRI-a fragment was originally incorrectly mapped to the right of the region of uncertainty for EcoRI e and O and that the correct alignment is EcoRI a, e, O. The XbaI restriction endonuclease cleavage map was previously generated and three regions of uncertainty still exist for this map. Two important conclusions were obtained from the molecular cloning and physical mapping of the GPCMV genome: (a) the size of GPCMV DNA is 239 kilobases (kb), corresponding to a molecular weight of 158 $\times 10^6$; and (b) the GPCMV genome consists of a long unique sequence with terminal repeat sequences but without internal repeat regions.

DNA sequence homology has been observed between GPCMV and HCMV DNAs (ISOM et al. 1984; ISOM and GAO 1988). It is of interest to note that the HCMV Ad169 HindIII E fragment, a region which contains the major IE HCMV genes (JAHN et al. 1984) and sequences associated with HCMV transformation (NELSON et al. 1984), contains sequences homologous to GPCMV DNA. Hybridization of HCMV Ad169 HindIII E fragment DNA with the GPCMV HindIII D fragment

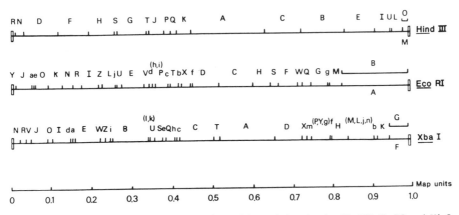

Fig. 1. Schematic diagram of the GPCMV genome with restriction sites for HindIII, EcoRI, and XbaI. *Parentheses* indicate that the order of fragments in this region is unknown. *Open rectangles* at the termini indicate regions containing sequence homology. This figure is a modification of the original GPCMV restriction endonuclease map (GAO and ISOM 1984)

has been observed. It is of interest to note that sequences within the GPCMV *Hind*III D fragment code for three size classes of mRNA that are expressed during GPCMV IE infection (see below). When hybridization between HCMV *Hind*III E and GPCMV *Hind*III D DNA fragments was carried out in the presence of a DNA with high G + C content (*Micrococcus luteus*) DNA, no decrease in hybridization intensity was observed, suggesting that the hybridization is not simply due to high G + C content regions binding to each other, but rather to authentic base homology. The GPCMV *Hind*III D DNA fragment is 21.3 kb and contains within it the *Xba*I J DNA fragment, which is only 7.9 kb. Further analysis demonstrated that homology with the HCMV Ad169 *Hind*III E fragment was restricted to the *Xba*I J DNA fragment. Southern blot hybridization was then carried out to map in more detail the region of sequence homology within the HCMV *Hind*III E fragment (Fig. 2). HCMV DNA fragments from subclones of the HCMV *Hind*III E fragment were cleaved with the appropriate restriction endonucleases, purified from vector, electrophoretically separated, and transferred to nitrocellulose filters. The *Xba*I J DNA fragment was purified, radioactively labeled, and used as probe. No hybridization was detected to the pCM4000 subclone, which contains the DNA sequences that have transforming capabilities (NELSON et al. 1984), and no hybridization was detected to the sequences that encode the 1.9-kb major IE transcript (JAHN et al. 1984). Strong hybridization was detected between the GPCMV *Xba*I J DNA fragment and the HCMV pGJ3 subclone.

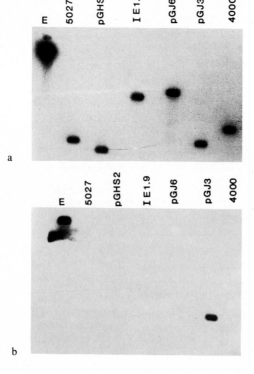

Fig. 2a, b. Southern blot hybridization between GPCMV *Xba*I-J DNA fragment and HCMV *Hind*III-E(E) fragment. HCMV DNA from subclones of the HCMV *Hind*III-E fragment (pCM5027, 1.9IE, pGJ6, pGH52, pGJ3, and pCM4000) were cleaved with the appropriate restriction endonucleases, purified from vector, electrophoretically separated, and transferred to nitrocellulose filters. Hybridization was carried out to purified **a** HCMV *Hind*III E to localize the HCMV DNA fragments and to **b** GPCMV *Xba*I-J DNA fragment to detect DNA sequence homology. Subclones of the HCMV *Hind*III-E fragment were kindly provided by Drs. B. Fleckenstein and J. Nelson

A comparison of GPCMV and HCMV DNAs reveals similarities and differences. GPCMV and HCMV DNAs are similar in size (158×10^6 Da for GPCMV DNA compared with 150×10^6 Da for HCMV DNA) and similar in G + C content (54% for GPCMV DNA compared with 57% for HCMV DNA). Indeed, there is some DNA sequence homology between the two virus DNAs. In contrast, the structural organization of the GPCMV genome does not contain isomers and is considerably less complex than that of HCMV.

3.2 GPCMV Gene Expression at the RNA Level

In the herpesviruses including the cytomegaloviruses, virus gene expression is divided into three phases: (a) the immediate early (IE) phase observed in the absence of protein synthesis; (b) the early phase which occurs before the onset of virus DNA synthesis; and (c) the late phase which occurs after the onset of virus DNA replication. The availability of cloned GPCMV DNA fragments and the restriction endonuclease physical maps made it possible to begin to examine transcription of GPCMV during productive infection of guinea pig cells in culture. GPCMV IE RNA was defined experimentally as the RNA isolated from GPCMV-infected cells treated with cycloheximide for 1 h prior to infection and for 4 h p.i.; GPCMV early RNA was defined experimentally as the RNA isolated from cells treated with phosphonoacetic acid during infection and harvested at 20–24 h p.i., and GPCMV late RNA was defined experimentally as the RNA isolated from cells at 48–72 h p.i. GPCMV IE, early and late transcription was analyzed initially using large HindIII and EcoRI GPCMV fragments in order roughly to determine the regions of the genome that encode the IE, early, and late transcripts. cDNA probes were synthesized from IE, early, and late poly A^+ RNAs and hybridized to cloned GPCMV HindIII and EcoRI DNA fragments that spanned the GPCMV genome (GAO and ISOM 1984). The autoradiograms were scanned and the values for the hybridization intensities were used to determine the percentage of transcription from various portions of the genome. More than 70% of the IE transcripts were derived from sequences contained within the HindIII-D, HindIII-G (EcoRI-E), and HindIII-B fragments. These three portions of the genome containing sequences that hybridize to IE RNA were designated regions I, II, and III respectively. Early RNAs were transcribed from 16 out of 18 cloned fragments but 35% of the early RNAs were derived from the HindIII-N and -L fragments. Late RNAs were transcribed from recombinant DNAs, representing 99% of the virus genome. Different patterns of percentage hybridization occur at IE, early, and late times after infection, indicating that GPCMV transcription is temporally regulated (ISOM and GAO 1988). Temporal regulation of transcription has been observed for other cytomegaloviruses and is a general property of herpesviruses.

In a more recent study, a detailed analysis of transcription from regions I, II, and III has been carried out (YIN and ISOM, unpublished data). Northern blot hybridization was used to determine the size classes of RNAs encoded by the DNA sequences from these three regions of the genome. Total poly A^+ and poly A^- IE RNA from GPCMV-infected or uninfected cells was fractionated according to size by electrophoresis in agarose gels and transferred to nitrocellulose filters. RNA was hybridized to ^{32}P-labeled HindIII-D (region I), EcoRI-E (region II), and HindIII-B (region III) DNA fragments. The results of the northern blot hybridizations showed that region I encodes three size classes of IE RNAs (3.9, 3.3, and 2.0 kb), region II encodes two size classes of IE RNAs (3.8 and 2.0 kb) and region III encodes four size classes of IE RNAs (3.6, 2.9, 2.7, and 1.9 kb) or a total of nine RNA species. In order to map these transcripts within the three regions, detailed restriction endonuclease maps of these three regions were generated and subclones containing smaller GPCMV DNA fragments were prepared. The smaller DNA fragments were subcloned into pGEM vectors containing Sp6 and T7 promoters so that strand-specific RNA probes could be generated to determine the direction of transcription.

The HindIII, XbaI, EcoRI, BamHI, and PstI restriction endonuclease sites for region I were determined. The poly A$^+$ fraction of cytoplasmic IE RNA extracted from GPCMV-infected cells was fractionated by electrophoresis in agarose gels, transferred to nitrocellulose filters and hybridized to ^{32}P-labeled cRNA riboprobes transcribed from GPCMV DNA fragments inserted into pGEM-1 or pGEM-2 vectors. Only DNA sequences from the right end of the HindIII-D fragment, i.e., from the EcoRI-O and -K fragments, encode IE RNA. The three transcripts are transcribed in the same direction and are overlapping. All three initiate near the right end of EcoRI K and the 3.9- and 2.0-kb transcripts are spliced. It appears that the multiple overlapping transcripts may have the same promoter and that different-sized transcripts are generated by differential splicing, but mapping in even greater detail is necessary before this conclusion can be reached. The results of nothern blot hybridization indicate that the three transcripts are expressed at reasonably equal levels.

To map IE transcription from region II, the SacI, SalI, and PstI restriction endonuclease sites within the EcoRI-E fragment were determined. The results of northern blot hybridization using subclones from region II showed that the 3.8-kb transcript is transcribed from the left half of the fragment while the 2.0-kb transcript is transcribed from the right half and they do not overlap. The transcripts are transcribed in the same direction. The 2.0-kb transcript is present in significantly higher levels than the 3.8-kb transcript. In fact, of all the GPCMV IE transcripts, the region II 2.0-kb transcript is one of the most abundantly expressed. The significance of the 2.0-kb transcript will be discussed in more detail below.

The existence of overlapping transcripts observed for region I was also seen when IE transcription from region III was analyzed. Transcription from the large HindIII-B fragment is restricted to the EcoRI-G and EcoRI-M DNA fragments. The HindIII, EcoRI, BamHI, PstI, and SalI restriction endonuclease sites for region III were determined. Three of the four IE transcripts from region III, the 3.6-, 2.7-, and 1.9-kb transcripts are transcribed in the same direction and are overlapping. All three appear to initiate near the right end of the HindIII-B fragment and at least one, the 1.9-kb fragment, is spliced. The fourth IE transcript, the 2.9-kb fragment, is encoded by sequences contained within the left end of the EcoRI-G fragment. The three overlapping transcripts are transcribed from one strand of DNA and the 2.9-kb transcript is transcribed from the other. Of the four region III transcripts, the 2.7- and 2.9-kb transcripts are the most abundantly transcribed.

We were interested in determining whether the same GPCMV genes that were transcribed in the presence of cycloheximide were also transcribed at early times during the course of a natural productive in vitro infection. To carry out these studies, we chose to use the dot blot procedure to hybridize in vivo-labeled RNA to cloned GPCMV DNA fragments. To test the validity of the procedure, we first carried out the in vivo labeling in the presence of cycloheximide and compared the results obtained from the dot blots with those obtained from northern blot analysis using radioactively labeled DNA as probe. Guinea pig cells were treated with cycloheximide for 1 h prior to infection and 4 h p.i. with GPCMV. [^{32}P] Orthophosphate was added to the infected cells from 1 to 4 h p.i. Cytoplasmic RNA was extracted from the [^{32}P] orthophosphate-labeled infected cells and hybridized to cloned EcoRI DNA fragments immobilized on a nitrocellulose filter. Strong hybridization was detected to EcoRI-O, -K (region I), EcoRI-E (region II), and EcoRI-G, -M (region III) DNA fragments. These results paralleled what had been observed when (a) radioactively labeled cDNA was used in Southern blot analysis or (b) nick-translated DNA was used as probe in northern blot analysis. In addition, strong hybridization was also observed to EcoRI-N and EcoRI-I fragments that are located adjacent to region I on the GPCMV genome and HindIII-E and HindIII-I fragments to the right of region III on the GPCMV genome. Hybridization had been previously detected to these sequences when cDNA was used as probe (Isom and Gao 1988). In the northern blot analyses described above, hybridization to these sequences was not examined. The results of the in vivo labeling studies using RNA extracted from cycloheximide-treated cells demonstrate that GPCMV IE RNA is transcribed from several different regions of the GPCMV genome and from the same regions identified by other techniques.

We then used in vivo labeling to examine GPCMV IE transcription at early times during the course of a natural productive infection. When ^{32}P-labeled RNA was extracted from guinea pig cells infected with GPCMV for short intervals (1 or 2 h) in the absence of cycloheximide and hybridized to GPCMV DNA from the large HindIII and EcoRI DNA fragments and also DNA from the recombinant subclones, hybridization of RNA isolated from cells infected for 1 h to GPCMV DNA fragments containing the DNA sequences for the region II 2.0-kb transcript was significantly stronger than hybridization to any of the other fragments. When RNA isolated from cells infected for 2 h was used, the DNA fragments encoding the 2.0-kb species continued to hybridize intensely and strong hybridization dots were also observed for sequences encoding the region I 3.9-, 3.3-, and 2.0-kb transcripts and the region III 2.9- and 2.7-kb transcripts. Sequences encoding the region II 3.8-kb and the region III 1.9-kb transcripts demonstrated hybridization but the intensity was weaker. Hybridization was also observed to the HindIII-E, HindIII-I, EcoRI N, and EcoRI I DNA fragments. Northern blot hybridization was subsequently carried out using nick-translated HindIII-E, HindIII-I, EcoRI-N, and EcoRI-I DNA fragments as probe. At least eight additional transcripts were identified from these regions and two of them are expressed at reasonably high levels but the 2.0-kb transcript from region II still appears to be the most abundant IE transcript.

Subclones that contain small GPCMV DNA fragments that were generated because they encode sequences for GPCMV IE RNA were used in northern analyses to determine whether these fragments are IE specific or also encode sequences for GPCMV early or late transcripts. RNA from uninfected cells, and IE, early and late GPCMV RNAs were fractionated by size in agarose gels, transferred to nitro-cellulose filters and hybridized to GPCMV DNA probes that identify regions I, II and III. None of the IE transcripts continued to be expressed strongly at early times but some were expressed weakly. Two probes hybridized strongly and many of the probes hybridized weakly to late RNAs of different size classes, indicating that the sequences contained in these probes also encode portions of specific late transcripts. The probe which hybridizes to the 2.0-kb transcript from region II was particularly IE specific and did not hybridize to early or late RNA.

We conclude that there are at least 17 GPCMV IE transcripts as defined by the cycloheximide block. The steady-state level for some of these transcripts is higher than for others and the region II 2.0-kb transcript appears to be the most abundant transcript during a cycloheximide block and during a natural infection. The 2.0-kb transcript can be detected by 1 h p.i. in the absence of cycloheximide but by 2 h p.i. almost all of the other transcripts are also detected.

Comparison of what we know to date about GPCMV IE transcription with what is known about HCMV and MCMV IE transcription indicates certain differences and some similarities. HCMV (STINSKI et al. 1983; STENBERG et al. 1984, 1985; JAHN et al. 1984; WESTON 1988) and MCMV (KEIL et al. 1984, 1985, 1987a, b) IE transcription have been characterized extensively. The major IE transcript of HCMV is 1.95 kb, is encoded by sequences located at 0.739–0.755 map units (IE1), and encodes a 72-kDa phosphoprotein. Sequences just to the left of this region are also transcribed IE (the IE2 gene). At least six overlapping spliced IE RNAs can be transcribed from the IE1 and IE2 genes. Four differentially spliced IE transcripts are also encoded by sequences located in the short unique region of the HCMV genome. Initially, studies of HCMV IE transcription concentrated on the IE1 1.95-kb transcript. Recently, interest has centered on the IE2 gene because the products of this region appear to act alone or in combination with other HCMV IE proteins to regulate heterologous promoters (HERMISTON et al. 1987; PIZZORNO et al. 1988). The major IE transcript of MCMV is 2.75 kb, is encoded by sequences located at 0.769–0.815 map units, and encodes an 89-kDa phosphoprotein. The MCMV major IE transcript is generated by splicing and originates from four exons in the gene. Five minor IE transcripts are also encoded by the same region (DORSCH-HASLER et al. 1985) and low levels of IE transcription have also been detected from both termini of the genome. The MCMV major IE gene product can activate transcription (KOSZINOWSKI et al. 1986). One strong similarity between GPCMV, HCMV, and MCMV IE transcription is the existence of overlapping differentially spliced IE transcripts. Although there is only one major IE transcript for MCMV and HCMV, both viruses transcribe a reasonably large number of IE RNAs. The number of GPCMV IE transcripts that we have identified is greater than the number reported for the other two viruses and GPCMV IE transcription is derived from a larger number of regions of the genome than HCMV.

At this time it is not possible to identify which of the GPCMV transcripts will be the most interesting functionally. Some of these transcripts may not even be translated into proteins. The most abundant transcript may or may not be the most significant. The most significant transcript for regulation of productive infection in one cell type may not be the most important for regulating maintenance of latency in a different cell type. These questions remain to be answered not only for GPCMV but also for HCMV and MCMV. We have provided the foundation for understanding GPCMV IE transcription and have generated a series of probes that selectively hybridize to one or at most two of the transcripts. These probes can be used in in situ hybridization to examine GPCMV gene expression in vitro and in vivo. The subclones can be used to identify IE proteins encoded by the sequences and can be sequenced to identify regulatory and coding sequences. Availability of well-characterized cloned small GPCMV DNA fragments will enable us to begin to study regulation of IE transcription and how GPCMV IE products function to regulate GPCMV gene expression.

3.3 GPCMV Gene Expression at the Protein Level

Little is known about the GPCMV proteins, which is unusual in light of the fact that the identity of the virion and infected cell proteins for many of the herpesviruses was known long before their DNA or RNA were well characterized. To our knowledge, only two papers have been published on GPCMV proteins and both are from the same laboratory (Tsutsui et al. 1986; Nogomi-Satake and Tsutsui 1988). To begin to characterize GPCMV proteins, Tsutsui et al. (1986) generated hybridomas producing monoclonal antibodies to GPCMV-infected cells. Three groups of monoclonal antibodies were prepared. The first group immunoprecipitated a 50-kDa polypeptide which is located in nuclear inclusions and is most likely a late nonstructural protein. These antibodies reacted predominantly with filamentous structures in nuclear inclusions and occasionally stained nucleocapsids but did not react with intracytoplasmic or extracellular virions. In a subsequent study, it was determined that the 50-kDa protein is phosphorylated and is a protein which binds single- and double-stranded cell and virus DNA in an in vitro assay (Nogomi-Satake and Tsutsui 1988). Synthesis of the 50-kDa protein began to increase at approximately 12 h after GPCMV infection and paralleled GPCMV DNA synthesis. The increase in synthesis of the 50-kDa protein was not seen when phosphonoacetic acid was present in the culture medium. The second group of antibodies reacted with a 76-kDa polypeptide, which is found in cytoplasmic inclusions and extracellular dense virions, and the third group of antibodies reacted with a 78-kDa core protein. None of the ten antibodies generated detected IE virus antigens.

We have recently initiated studies to identify GPCMV IE protein synthesis. Guinea pig cells were treated with cycloheximide for 1 h prior to infection and 9 h p.i. Cells were washed free of cycloheximide and radioactively labeled with [^{35}S] methionine. Cells that had not been infected were also labeled as a control. By 30 min of labeling, five major (approximately 102, 68, 52, 42, and 12 kDa) and seven less prominent IE GPCMV protein bands that were not seen in the control cells were detected (Fig. 3). Comparison of the transcriptional analyses with the protein synthesis data suggest that many of the IE RNA species are most likely translated.

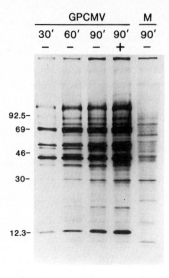

Fig. 3. GPCMV IE proteins. Guinea pig cells were infected with GPCMV at a multiplicity of infection of 20 plaque-forming units/cell. Guinea pig cells were treated with cycloheximide for 1 h prior to infection and 9 h p.i. Cells were washed free of cycloheximide and radioactively labeled with [^{35}S] methionine for 30, 60, or 90 min in the absence of actinomycin D or 90 min in the presence of actinomycin D. Cells that had not been infected were also labeled as a control (*M*). Cells were lysed, and radioactively labeled cell extracts were subjected to polyacrylamide gel electrophoresis and autoradiography. Molecular weight markers are indicated

Further characterization of GPCMV IE gene expression will require identifying which GPCMV genes encode the proteins detected. These studies indicate that GPCMV IE expression during productive infection is complex and involves expression of several genes from various different regions of the genome.

4 Conclusions

The species specificity of HCMV prevents the study of HCMV in animals and necessitates finding an appropriate animal model. A variety of animals, including the guinea pig, become infected with their own species-specific cytomegaloviruses. The similarities in the pathogenicity of GPCMV and HCMV in their respective hosts are impressive. In both HCMV and GPCMV infections, acute infection is followed by chronic persistent infection and virus is isolated from many of the same tissues and organs. HCMV and GPCMV can cross the placenta, causing congenital infection, and can be transmitted by blood transfusion.

It is readily apparent from some of the studies on GPCMV infection that we have described above that an animal model for HCMV makes it possible to study the infection in detail; it is possible to examine numerous body tissues and fluids for virus gene expression and the samples can be obtained at specified time points. In addition, the intensity of the infection can be manipulated. Using the guinea pig, it is possible to study specific HCMV infections such as encephalitis, labyrinthitis, mononucleosis, and infection of the placenta, and it is also possible to study disseminated disease. It is clear from the many excellent biological and histological analyses of GPCMV-infected guinea pigs that the virus selectively infects specific tissues and cell types and that the age and state of differentiation of the cell may influence the outcome of infection. The data obtained using antisera also suggest that limited virus gene expression may occur in some cell types without production of virus. It is equally apparent that the immune response to GPCMV plays an important role systemically and locally in the pathogenicity of this virus.

Studies on the pathogenicity of GPCMV in the animal, in particular with regard to long-term persistence of the virus and virus genome in the tissues of the infected guinea pig, cannot progress without molecular reagents. We conclude from the molecular studies described above that GPCMV gene expression is beginning to be understood in productive infection in vitro in one cell type and reagents that can be used to study GPCMV gene expression in detail are beginning to be prepared. However, no information is currently available about regulation of GPCMV expression even at the in vitro level. In order to understand any aspect of CMV-induced pathogenicity, it will be necessary to determine which cell types within a tissue or organ become productively infected, what genes are expressed in specific cell types, what genes need to be expressed to elicit immune responses, and how expression of the virus genes is differentially regulated in various cell types. In future experiments, it will be necessary to use nucleic acid probes for GPCMV coding and regulatory sequences as well as characterized polyclonal and monoclonal antibodies to examine GPCMV expression in vivo. The GPCMV-infected guinea pig models to study many different aspects of CMV infection are well described and are awaiting further characterization at the molecular level.

Acknowledgments. These studies were supported in part by grant CA27503 awarded by the National Cancer Institute.

References

Bia FJ, Griffith BP, Fong CKY, Hsiung GD (1983) Cytomegalovirus infections in the guinea pig: experimental models for human disease. Rev Infect Dis 5: 177–195

Bia FJ, Miller SA, Davidson KH (1984) The guinea pig cytomegalovirus model of congenital human cytomegalovirus infection. Birth Defects 20: 233–241

Booss J, Dann PR, Griffith BP, Kim JH (1988) Glial nodule encephalitis in the guinea pig: serial observations following cytomegalovirus infection. Acta Neuropathol (Berl) 75: 465–473

Booss J, Dann PR, Griffith BP, Kim JH (1989) Host defense response to cytomegalovirus in the central nervous system. Am J Pathol 134: 71–78

Choi YC, Hsiung GD (1978) Cytomegalovirus infection in guinea pigs. II. Transplacental and horizontal transmission. J Infect Dis 138: 197–202

Connor WS, Johnson KP (1976) Cytomegalovirus infection in weanling guinea pigs. J Infect Dis 134: 442–449

Davis GL, Spector GJ, Strauss M, MiddleCamp JN (1977) Cytomegalovirus endolabyrinthitis. Arch Pathol Lab Med 101: 118–121

Davis LE, Johnsson L-G, Kornfield M (1981) Cytomegalovirus labyrinthitis in an infant: morphological, virological, and immunofluorescent studies. J Neuropathol Exp Neurol 40: 9–19

Dorsch-Hasler K, Keil GM, Weber F, Jasin M, Schaffner W, Koszinowski UH (1985) A long and complex enhancer activates transcription of the gene coding for the highly abundant immediate early mRNA in murine cytomegalovirus. Proc Natl Acad Sci USA 82: 8325–8329

Feldman RA (1969) Cytomegalovirus during pregnancy (a prospective study and report of 6 cases). Am J Dis Child 117: 517–521

Fong CKY, Bia FJ, Hsiung GD, Madore P, Chang PW (1979) Ultrastructural development of guinea pig cytomegalovirus in cultured guinea pig embryo cells. J Gen Virol 42: 127–140

Fong CKY, Bia FJ, Hsiung GD (1980) Ultrastructural development and persistence of guinea pig cytomegalovirus in duct cells of guinea pig submaxillary gland. Arch Virol 64: 97–108

Fong CKY, Lucia H, Bia FJ, Hsiung GD (1983) Histopathologic and ultrastructural studies of disseminated cytomegalovirus infection in strain 2 guinea pigs. Lab invest 49: 183–194

French ML, Thompson JF, White A (1977) Cytomegalovirus viremia with transmission from mother to fetus. Ann Intern Med 86: 748–749

Fukuda S, Keithley E, Harris JP (1988) The development of endolymphatic hydrops following CMV inoculation of the endolymphatic sac. Laryngoscope 98: 439–443

Gao M, Isom HC (1984) Characterization of the guinea pig cytomegalovirus genome by molecular cloning and physical mapping. J Virol 52: 436–447

Goff E, Griffith BP, Booss J (1987) Delayed amplification of cytomegalovirus infection in the placenta and maternal tissues during late gestation. Am J Obstet Gynecol 156: 1265–1270

Griffith BP, Hsiung GD (1980) Cytomegalovirus infection in guinea pigs. IV. Maternal infection at different stages of gestation. J Infect Dis 141: 787–793

Griffith BP, Lucia HL, Bia FJ, Hsiung GD (1981) Cytomegalovirus-induced mononucleosis in guinea pigs. Infect Immun 32: 857–863

Griffith BP, Lucia HL, Hsiung GD (1982) Brain and visceral involvement during congenital cytomegalovirus infection of guinea pigs. Pediatr Res 16: 455–459

Griffith BP, Lucia HL, Tillbrook JL, Hsiung GD (1983) Enhancement of cytomegalovirus infection during pregnancy in guinea pigs. J Infect Dis 147: 990–998

Griffith BP, Lavallee JT, Booss J, Hsiung GD (1984) Asynchronous depression of response to T- and B-cell mitogens during acute infection with cytomegalovirus in the guinea pig. Cell Immunol 87: 727–733

Griffith BP, McCormick SR, Fong CKY, Lavallee JT, Luica HL, Goff E (1985) The placenta as a site of cytomegalovirus infection in guinea pigs. J Virol 55: 402–409

Griffith BP, McCormick SR, Booss J, Hsiung GD (1986) Inbred guinea pig model of intrauterine infection with cytomegalovirus. Am J Pathol 122: 112–119

Harris JP, Woolf NK, Ryan AF, Butler DM, Richman DD (1984) Immunologic and electrophysiologic response to cytomegaloviral infection in the guinea pig. J Infect Dis 150: 523–530

Hayes K, Gibas H (1971) Placental cytomegalovirus infection without fetal involvement following primary infection in pregnancy. J Pediatr 79: 401–402

Hermiston TW, Malone CL, Witte PR, Stinski MF (1987) Identification and characterization of the human cytomegalovirus immediate-early region 2 gene that stimulates gene expression from an inducible promoter. J Virol 61: 3214–3221

Ho M (1982) Cytomegalovirus: biology and infection. In: Greeough WB III, Merrigan TC (eds) Current topics in infectious diseases. Plenum, New York, pp 131–151

Hsiung GD, Choi YC, Bia FJ (1978) Cytomegalovirus infection in guinea pigs. I. Viremia during acute primary and chronic persistent infection. J Infect Dis 138: 191–196

Hsiung GD, Bia FJ, Fong CKY (1980) Viruses of guinea pigs: considerations for biomedical research. Microbiol Rev 44: 468–490

Isom HC, Gao M (1988) The pathogenicity and molecular biology of guinea pig cytomegalovirus. In: Viruses diseases in laboratory and captive animals. Nijhoff, Boston

Isom HC, Gao M, Wigdahl B (1984) Characterization of guinea pig cytomegalovirus DNA. J Virol 49: 426–436

Jackson L (1920) An intracellular protozoan parasite of the ducts of the salivary glands of the guinea pig. J Infect Dis 26: 347–350

Jahn G, Knust E, Schmolla H, Sarre T, Nelson JA, McDougall JK, Fleckenstein B (1984) Predominant immediate-early transcripts of human cytomegalovirus AD 169. J Virol 49: 363–370

Johnson KP, Connor WS (1979) Guinea pig cytomegalovirus: transplacental transmission. Arch Virol 59: 263–267

Kari B, Gehrz R (1986) Susceptibility of fetal guinea pig brain cell cultures to replicating guinea pig cytomegalovirus infection is increased with increasing fetal age: infection of astrocytes. J Virol 58: 960–962

Kawanishi H, Takeda T, Matsumoto M (1967) Human cytomegalovirus infection: electron and light microscope observations of the parotid glands of an autopsy case. Acta Pathol Jpn 17: 171–189

Keil GM, Ebeling-Keil A, Koszinowski UH (1984) Temporal regulation of murine cytomegalovirus transcription and mapping of viral RNA synthesized at immediate early times after infection. J Virol 50: 784–795

Keil GM, Fibi MR, Koszinowski NK (1985) Characterization of the major immediate early polypeptides encoded by murine cytomegalovirus. J Virol 54: 422–428

Keil GM, Ebeling-Keil A, Koszinowski UH (1987a) Immediate early genes of murine cytomegalovirus: location, transcripts, and translation products. J Virol 61: 526–533

Keil GM, Ebeling-Keil A, Koszinowski UH (1987b) Sequence and structural organization of murine cytomegalovirus immediate-early gene 1. J Virol 61: 1901–1908

Keithley EM, Sharp P, Woolf NK, Harris JP (1988) Temporal sequence of viral antigen expression in the cochlea induced by cytomegalovirus. Acta Otolaryngol (Stockh) 106: 46–54

Koszinowski UH, Keil GM, Volkmer H, Fibi MR, Ebeling-Keil A, Munch K (1986) The 89,000-Mr murine cytomegalovirus immediate-early protein activates gene transcription. J Virol 58: 59–66

Kumar ML, Nankervis GA (1978) Experimental congenital infection with cytomegalovirus: a guinea pig model. J Infect Dis 138: 650–654

Kumar ML, Prokay SL (1983) Experimental primary cytomegalovirus infection in pregnancy: timing and fetal outcome. Am J Obstet Gynecol 145: 56–60

Lucia HL, Griffith BP, Hsiung GD (1985) Lymphadenopathy during cytomegalovirus-induced mononucleosis in guinea pigs. Arch Pathol Lab Med 109: 1019–1023

Markham FS, Hudson NP (1935) Susceptibility of the guinea pig fetus to the submaxillary gland virus of guinea pigs. Am J Pathol 12: 175–182

Middlekamp JN, Patrizi G, Reed CA (1967) Light and electron microscope studies of the guinea pig cytomegalovirus. J Ultrastruct Res 18: 85–101

Morgello S, Cho ES, Nielson S, Devinsky O, Petito CK (1987) Cytomegalovirus encephalitis in patients with acquired immune deficiency syndrome: an autopsy study of 30 cases and a review of the literature. Hum Pathol 18: 289–297

Myers EN, Stool S (1968) Cytomegalovirus inclusion disease of the inner ear. Laryngoscope 78: 1904–1915

Nelson JA, Fleckenstein B, Jahn G, Galloway DA, McDougall JK (1984) Structure of the transforming region of human cytomegalovirus Ad169. J Virol 49: 109–115

Nogomi-Satake T, Tsutsui Y (1988) Identification and characterization of a 50K DNA-binding protein of guinea pig cytomegalovirus. J Gen Virol 69: 2267–2276

Nomura Y, Harada T, Hara M (1988) Viral infection and the inner ear. ORL J Otorhinolaryngol Relat Spec 50: 201–211

Pizzorno MC, O'Hare P, Sha L, LaFeminaRL, Hayward GS (1988) trans-Activation and autoregulation of gene expression by the immediate-early region 2 gene products of human cytomegalovirus. J Virol 62: 1167–1179

Schneck SA (1965) Neuropathological features of human organ transplantation. I. Probable cytomegalovirus infection. J Neuropathol Exp Neurol 24: 415–429

Sha M, Griffith BP, Raveh D, Isom HC, Ward DC, Hsiung GD (1987) Detection of guinea pig cytomegalovirus nucleic acids in cultured cell with biotin-labelled hybridization probes. Virus Res 6: 317–329

Stagno S, Reynolds DW, Amos CS, Dahle AJ, McCollister FP, Mohindra I, Ermocilla R, Alford CA (1977) Auditory and visual defects resulting from symptomatic and subclinical congenital cytomegaloviral and Toxoplasma infections. Pediatrics 59: 669–678

Stenberg RM, Thomsen DR, Stinski MF (1984) Structural analysis of the major immediate early gene of human cytomegalovirus. J Virol 49: 190–199

Stenberg RM, Witte PR, Stinski MF (1985) Multiple spliced and unspliced transcripts from cytomegalovirus immediate-early region 2 and evidence for a common initiation site within immediate-early region 1. J Virol 56: 665–675

Stinski MF, Thomsen DR, Stenberg RM, Goldstein LC (1983) Organization and expression of the immediate early genes of human cytomegalovirus. J Virol 46: 1–14

Tenser RB, Hsiung GD (1976) Comparison of guinea pig cytomegalovirus and guinea pig herpes-like virus; pathogenesis and persistence in experimentally infected animals. Infect Immun 13: 934–940

Tsutsui Y, Yamazaki Y, Kashiwai A, Mizutani A, Furukawa T (1986) Monoclonal antibodies to guinea pig cytomegalovirus: an immunoelectron microscopic study. J Gen Virol 67: 107–118

Weston K (1988) An enhancer in the short unique region of human cytomegalovirus regulates the production of a group of abundant immediate early transcripts. Virology 162: 406–416

Woolf NK, Ochi JW, Silva EJ, Sharp PA, Harris JP, Richman DD (1988) Ganciclovir prophylaxis for cochlear pathophysiology during experimental guinea pig cytomegalovirus Labyrinthitis. Antimicrob Agents Chemother 32: 865–872

Zheng Z, Lavallee JT, Bia FJ, Griffith BP (1987) Thymic hypoplasia, splenomegaly and immune depression in guinea pigs with neonatal cytomegalovirus infection. Dev Comp Immunol 11: 407–418

Protein Coding

Analysis of the Protein-Coding Content of the Sequence of Human Cytomegalovirus Strain AD169

M. S. Chee, A. T. Bankier, S. Beck, R. Bohni, C. M. Brown, R. Cerny,
T. Horsnell, C. A. Hutchison III, T. Kouzarides, J. A. Martignetti,
E. Preddie, S. C. Satchwell, P. Tomlinson, K. M. Weston, and
B. G. Barrell

1	Introduction	126
2	Sequence Analysis	126
3	Prediction of Reading Frames	135
3.1	Criteria for Selection	135
3.2	Codon Bias	136
3.3	HCMV Map	136
4	Identification of Homologs	141
5	IE Genes	143
5.1	MIE Early Gene Region	143
5.2	HCMV US3 IE Gene	144
5.3	UL37 IE Gene	145
6	Early and Late Genes	145
6.1	Major Early Transcripts	145
6.2	Enzymes of Nucleotide and DNA Metabolism	147
6.2.1	Nucleotide Metabolism	147
6.2.2	DNA Replication	148
6.2.3	DNA Repair	148
6.2.4	Deoxyribonuclease	149
6.3	Phosphotransferase	149
6.4	Early Phosphoprotein genes	149
6.5	Late DNA-Binding Proteins	150
6.6	Capsid Proteins	150
6.7	Structural Phosphoprotein Genes	151
6.8	Surface Glycoproteins	154
6.8.1	Glycoproteins B and H	155
6.8.2	HLA Homolog	155
6.8.3	T-Cell Receptor Homology	156
7	Gene Families	157
7.1	RL11 Family	157
7.2	The US6 Family	158
7.3	The US22 Family	158
7.4	The G-Protein Coupled Receptor (GCR) Family	159
8	Relationship to α and γ-Herpesvirus Genomes	160
9	Perspectives	162
References		163

MRC Laboratory of Molecular Biology, Hills Road, Cambridge CB2 2QH, UK

Current Topics in Microbiology and Immunology, Vol. 154
© Springer-Verlag Berlin · Heidelberg 1990

1 Introduction

Large-scale sequence analysis of the AD169 strain of human cytomegalovirus (HCMV) began in this laboratory in 1984 when very little was known about the sequence or location of genetic information in the viral genome. At that time sequence analysis was confined to the major immediate-early gene (STENBERG et al. 1984), a region of the Colburn strain that contained CA tracts (JEANG and HAYWARD 1983), the L-S junction region (TAMASHIRO et al. 1984), and what has been termed the transforming region (KOUZARIDES et al. 1983). This chapter is being written in March 1989 when the sequence is complete except for some remaining polishing of certain areas which is still going on (manuscript in preparation). As far as we know there are no major discrepancies in the data which might lead to the sequence changing although of course this cannot be ruled out. We present a preliminary analysis of the HCMV genome and limit ourselves mainly to the potential protein-coding content of over 200 reading frames.

2 Sequence Analysis

The sequence has been determined by M13 shotgun cloning and chain termination sequencing. In this random approach each base is sequenced many times on average so that the consensus produced should be highly accurate. The sequencing strategy involved applying this random procedure to each HindIII fragment of the viral genome (ORAM et al. 1982). However, the high G + C content caused severe problems as manifested in the many compressions encountered on the sequencing gels. This entailed resequencing many clones substituting dITP or 7-deazaGTP for dGTP in the reactions to minimize the effect. All sequences have been determined on both strands. Detailed accounts of the methods used are published elsewhere (BANKIER et al. 1987; BANKIER and BARRELL 1989). The sequences at the ends of the genome which were not generated in the HindIII library were obtained from the HindIII junction fragments C (equivalent to I andQ) and G (equivalent to K and Q) which were sequenced in their entirety, and from a portion of the HindIII B (K and H) junction fragment from the HindIII W/H end to the EcoRI site 21.2 kb downstream (WESTON and BARRELL 1986) (Fig. 1). Sequences were also obtained across all the HindIII sites. Double-stranded sequencing on appropriate overlapping cosmid and plasmid clones (FLECKENSTEIN et al. 1982) confirmed that the sequence was contiguous except for an extra 393-bp fragment which was found between HindIII T and E, and which we have named HindIII d. The final map in the prototypical orientation of the viral genome with the HindIII fragments predicted from the sequence is shown in Fig. 1. As the precise ends of the molecule are not known, we have chosen to number the sequence from the start of the direct repeat (DR1) found by TAMASHIRO et al. (1984). By analogy with the "a" sequence of other herpesviruses, this is the closest feature to the end of the genome (MOCARSKI and

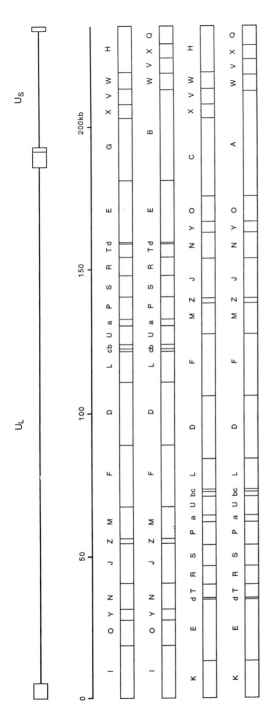

Fig. 1. HindIII restriction maps of the four HCMV strain AD169 isomers and their relationships to the genome structure (ORAM et al. 1982). The restriction map of the prototype isomer is *topmost* of the four. Individual *Hind*III fragments are named alphabetically by size Above the restriction maps a scale is given in kilobase pairs (*kb*). The *uppermost line* shows the genome structure with *UL* (long unique region) and *US* (short unique region) marked; each of these is flanked by their respective repeat sequences shown as blocks

Table 1. A compilation of reading frames of HCMV strain AD169. The orientations, coordinates, and theoretical sizes are tabulated, together with the locations of predicted Kozak consensus ATG codons. For spliced genes exon coordinates represent open reading frame coordinates; donor and acceptor positions are not shown. Lengths are shown in amino acids. References to previous publications in which a HindIII fragment-based nomenclature is used are as follows: 1 (WESTON and BARRELL 1986); 2 (BECK and BARRELL 1988); 3 (KOUZARIDES et al. 1988); 4 (KOUZARIDES et al. 1987b); 5 (CHEE et al. 1989b); and 6 (CHEE et al. 1989a). References given in the comments section are minimal. Asterisked citations refer to assignments based on other herpesviruses, in particular HSV-1

Frame	Strand	Start	K-ATG	Stop	Length	MW	Old Name	(ref)	Family	Comments
HCMVJ1L	C	3		929	309	33176		1		Overlaps J1I & J1S
HCMVTRL1		934	970	1902	311	34822	HKLF1	1		= HCMVIRL1
HCMVTRL2		1893		2237	115	12324				= HCMVIRL2
HCMVTRL3		3141	3192	3533	114	13252				= HCMVIRL3. Glycoprotein?
HCMVTRL4	C	3785		4435	217	24929				= HCMVIRL4. ORF in major early transcript (GREENAWAY and WILKINSON 1987)
HCMVTRL5		4185	4266	4607	114	12835				= HCMVIRL5
HCMVTRL6	C	5615	5947	6010	111	12286				= HCMVIRL6
HCMVTRL7	C	6598	6843	6921	82	9718				= HCMVIRL7
HCMVTRL8		7227	7284	7670	129	14302				= HCMVIRL8
HCMVTRL9		7501		7929	143	15909				= HCMVIRL9
HCMVTRL10		8101	8182	8694	171	19035				= HCMVIRL10; D at position 38 is N in IRL10. Glycoprotein
HCMVTRL11		8648	8726	9427	234	26661			RL11 family	= HCMVIRL11. Glycoprotein
HCMVTRL12		9431	9434	10681	416	47417			RL11 family	= HCMVIRL12. Glycoprotein
HCMVTRL13		10778	10796	11236	147	15888				= HCMVIRL13. Glycoprotein exon?
HCMVTRL14		11140	11143	11700	186	21827			RL11 family	First 35 amino acids identical in IRL14. Glycoprotein exon?
HCMVUL1		11771	11810	12481	224	25578			RL11 family	Glycoprotein
HCMVUL2	C	12868	13047	13131	60	6763				Glycoprotein exon?
HCMVUL3	C	13010	13324	13330	105	12307				
HCMVUL4		13434	13464	13919	152	17751			RL11 family	Glycoprotein exon?
HCMVUL5		13986	14013	14510	166	18861			RL11 family	Glycoprotein exon?
HCMVUL6		14522	14612	15463	284	31447			RL11 family	Glycoprotein exon?
HCMVUL7		15523	15526	16191	222	24354			RL11 family	Glycoprotein exon?
HCMVUL8		16198	16234	16599	122	13787			RL11 family	Glycoprotein exon?
HCMVUL9		16606	16612	17295	228	26889			RL11 family	Glycoprotein
HCMVUL10		17222		18199	326	37366			RL11 family	Glycoprotein exon?
HCMVUL11		18268	18295	19119	275	31382			RL11 family	Glycoprotein
HCMVUL12	C	19103	19321	19351	73	8250				Glycoprotein exon?
HCMVUL13		19143	19320	20738	473	54614				Glycoprotein exon?
HCMVUL14		20798	20843	21871	343	38567				Glycoprotein

Gene	Strand				Residues	MW	Name		Family	Comments
HCMVUL15	C	21 639		22 604	322	35 338				Glycoprotein
HCMVUL16		22 342	22 414	23 103	230	26 148				
HCMVUL17		23 151	23 214	23 525	104	12 672				
HCMVUL18		23 631	23 637	24 740	368	41 736	H3OI	2		Glycoprotein homologous to class 1 HLA (BECK and BARRELL 1988)
HCMVUL19	C	24 701	24 740	25 033	98	11 281				
HCMVUL20	C	25 233	25 299	26 318	340	38 703				Glycoprotein. Homologous to TCR-γ?
HCMVUL21	C	26 500	27 024	27 039	175	19 940				
HCMVUL22		27 263		27 646	128	14 132				Hydrophobic
HCMVUL23	C	27 866		28 891	342	39 341			US22 family	
HCMVUL24	C	28 936	30 009	30 171	358	40 187			US22 family	
HCMVUL25		30 030	30 057	32 024	656	73 541			UL25 family	
HCMVUL26		32 212	32 775	32 994	188	21 156				
HCMVUL27		32 834	34 657	34 723	608	69 222				
HCMVUL28	C	34 757	37 005	35 893	379	42 739			US22 family	
HCMVUL29	C	35 926	37 500	37 092	360	40 779			US22 family	
HCMVUL30	C	37 138		37 533	121	14 047				
HCMVUL31	C	37 682		39 763	694	76 061				
HCMVUL32	C	39 850	42 993	43 050	1048	112 689				Large structural phosphoprotein (pp150) (JAHN et al. 1987)
HCMVUL33	C	43 128	43 251	44 420	390	43 806			GCR family	Multiply hydrophobic. Homology to G-protein-coupled receptors
HCMVUL34	C	44 500		46 011	504	56 185	HJLF4	3	UL25 family	
HCMVUL35	C	46 042	46 093	48 012	640	72 531	HILF3	3	US22 family	
HCMVUL36EX2	C	48 246		49 751	408.7	47 518	HJLF2	3	US22 family	
HCMVUL36EX1	C	49 354	49 776	49 863	67.3	7 483	HJLF1	3		
HCMVUL37EX3	C	49 913	52 123	50 842	310	35 476	HZLF3	3		IE glycoprotein exon 3
HCMVUL37EX2	C	50 893		51 015	14.3	1 561	HZLF2	3		IE glycoprotein exon 2
HCMVUL38	C	51 131	52 706	52 138	331	36 738				
HCMVUL37EX1	C	52 218		52 763	162.7	19 116				IE glycoprotein exon 1
HCMVUL39		53 024		53 395	124	13 533				Glycoprotein
HCMVUL40	C	53 216	53 878	53 893	221	24 368				
HCMVUL41	C	53 936		54 358	141	16 767				Glycoprotein exon?
HCMVUL42	C	54 384		54 854	157	17 066				
HCMVUL43	C	54 604	55 164	55 245	187	20 993			US22 family	
HCMVUL44	C	55 214	56 512	56 668	433	46 234				Encodes ICP36 protein family (LEACH and MOCARSKI 1989)
HCMVUL45	C	56 656		59 400	915	101 670				Homology to large subunit of ribonucleotide reductase (NIKAS et al. 1986)*

(*Continued*)

Table 1. (*Continued*)

Frame	Strand	Start	K-ATG	Stop	Length	MW	Old Name	(ref)	Family	Comments
HCMVUL46	C	59 519	60 388	60 562	290	33 028				Capsid assembly? PERTUISET et al. (1989)*
HCMVUL47		60 282	60 390	63 335	982	109 962				Virion protein? (BATTERSON et al. 1983*; McGEOCH et al. 1988a)*
HCMVUL48		62 921	63 335	70 057	2241	253 227	HFRF0	4		
HCMVUL49	C	70 403	72 112	72 334	570	63 852	HFLF5	4		Glycoprotein?
HCMVUL50	C	72 072	73 262	73 283	397	42 902	HFLF4	4		
HCMVUL51	C	73 287	73 757	73 910	157	16 968	HFLF3	4		
HCMVUL52		73 748	73 796	75 799	668	74 122	HFRF1	4		
HCMVUL53		75 789	75 795	76 922	376	42 314	HFRF2	4		
HCMVUL54	C	76 906	80 631	80 655	1242	137 104	HFLF2	4		DNA Polymerase (KOUZARIDES et al. 1987a)
HCMVUL55	C	80 775	83 492	83 654	906	102 005	HFLF1	4		gB (CRANAGE et al. 1986)
HCMVUL56	C	83 458	86 007	86 019	850	95 870	HFLF0	4		
HCMVUL57	C	86 577	90 281	90 326	1235	133 880				Major DNA-binding protein (ANDERS and GIBSON 1988)
HCMVUL58	C	90 864		91 235	124	14 418				
HCMVUL59	C	91 205	91 573	91 597	123	13 945				
HCMVUL60	C	92 336		92 815	160	18 241				
HCMVUL61	C	92 847		94 139	431	44 310				
HCMVUL62	C	94 114		94 764	217	23 686				
HCMVUL63		95 331		95 717	129	14 792				
HCMVUL64	C	95 904		96 203	100	11 245				
HCMVUL65	C	96 315		96 620	102	11 525				Segments in frame with 67-kDa phosphoprotein sequence of DAVIS and HUANG (1985)
HCMVUL66	C	96 475		96 816	114	13 921				
HCMVUL67	C	97 098	97 436	97 451	113	13 218				Glycoprotein exon?
HCMVUL68	C	97 750	98 079	98 100	110	12 728				
HCMVUL69	C	98 202	100 433	100 532	744	82 679				Transactivator? (McGEOCH et al. 1988a)*
HCMVUL70	C	100 536		103 721	1062	120 928				DNA replication? (McGEOCH et al. 1988b)*
HCMVUL71		103 239		104 471	411	45 728				dUTPase? (PRESTON and FISHER 1984)*
HCMVUL72	C	104 558	105 721	105 751	388	43 576				Glycoprotein
HCMVUL73		105 629	105 737	106 150	138	14 868				Glycoprotein exon?
HCMVUL74	C	106 128	107 525	107 585	466	54 236				
HCMVUL75	C	107 904	110 132	110 153	743	84 453				gH (CRANAGE et al. 1988)
HCMVUL76	C	110 324	110 327	111 301	325	36 070				

Gene	Strand				aa	MW	Name	No.	Family	Notes
HCMVUL77		110787	110907	112832	642	71188				Virion protein? (ADDISON et al. 1984*; McGEOCH et al. 1988a)*
HCMVUL78		112864	112924	114216	431	47358				
HCMVUL79	C	114277	115161	115779	295	33846				
HCMVUL80		115084	115198	117321	708	73853				Assembly protein read from internal start (ROBSON and GIBSON 1989)
HCMVUL81	C	117311		117658	116	12796				
HCMVUL82	C	117489	119165	119189	559	61950			UL82 family	pp71 (RUGER et al. 1987)
HCMVUL83	C	119355	121037	121094	561	62900			UL82 family	pp65 (RUGER et al. 1987)
HCMVUL84	C	121312	123069	123306	586	65430				
HCMVUL85	C	123104	124021	124090	306	34596				
HCMVUL86	C	124186	128295	128415	1370	153875	HaLF1	5		Major capsid protein (CHEE et al. 1989b)
HCMVUL87		128265	128355	131177	941	104805				
HCMVUL88		131144	131177	132463	429	47691				
HCMVUL89EX2	C	132466		133629	378	42776				Conserved herpesvirus spliced gene (COSTA et al. 1985)*
HCMVUL90	C	133639	133836	133920	66	7445				
HCMVUL91		133784	133835	134167	111	12028				
HCMVUL92		134020	134140	134742	201	22512				
HCMVUL93		134693	134711	136492	594	68464				
HCMVUL94		136008	136353	137387	345	38382				
HCMVUL89EX1	C	137382	138389	138803	296	34323				Conserved herpesvirus spliced gene (COSTA et al. 1985)*
HCMVUL95		138352	138388	139980	531	57214				
HCMVUL96		139821	140016	140360	115	13108				
HCMVUL97		140373	140484	142604	707	78234	HSRF3	6		Phosphotransferase? (CHEE et al. 1989a)
HCMVUL98		142626	142701	144452	584	65273				DNase (McGEOCH et al. 1986)*
HCMVUL99		144311	144392	144961	190	20924				Phosphoprotein pp28 (MEYER et al. 1988)
HCMVUL100	C	145229	146344	146413	372	42862				Multiply hydrophobic DNA replication? Position only (McGEOCH et al. 1988b)*
HCMVUL101		146353		146697	115	12184				DNA replication? Position only (McGEOCH et al. 1988b)*
HCMVUL102		146747		149140	798	85615				
HCMVUL103	C	149311	150057	150108	249	28637				Virion protein? (WELLER et al. 1983*; McGEOCH et al. 1988a)*
HCMVUL104	C	150008	152098	152167	697	78508				

(Continued)

Table 1. (*Continued*)

Frame	Strand	Start	K-ATG	Stop	Length	MW	Old Name (ref)	Family	Comments
HCMVUL105		151 806	151 926	154 793	956	106 501			Helicase (MARTIGNETTI 1987; CRUTE et al. 1989)*
HCMVUL106	C	154 950	155 324	155 330	125	14 500			
HCMVUL107	C	155 420		155 869	150	17 374			
HCMVUL108		156 016		156 384	123	14 501			
HCMVUL109	C	157 517	157 810	157 816	98	11 709			
HCMVUL110	C	157 896		158 276	127	14 224			
HCMVUL111	C	159 479		159 799	107	11 565			
HCMVUL111A	C	159 615	159 678	159 911	78	8 582			ORF in transforming region (RAZZAQUE et al. 1988)
HCMVUL112		160 484	160 589	161 392	252.3	26 415			Common N-terminus of four phosphoproteins (WRIGHT et al. 1988)
HCMVUL113		161 301		162 797	499	51 105			Probably spliced to UL112; internal splicing? (WRIGHT et al. 1988)
HCMVUL114	C	162 973	163 722	163 758	250	28 354			Uracil-DNA glycosylase (WORRAD and CARADONNA 1988)*
HCMVUL115	C	163 697		164 614	306	34 110			Glycoprotein exon?
HCMVUL116	C	164 533		165 564	344	37 519			
HCMVUL117	C	165 474	166 745	166 757	424	45 464			Glycoprotein exon?
HCMVUL118	C	166 861		167 487	209	24 599			Glycoprotein exon?
HCMVUL119	C	167 558	167 983	168 037	142	14 729			Glycoprotein exon?
HCMVUL120	C	168 041	168 643	168 700	201	22 768			Glycoprotein
HCMVUL121	C	168 697	169 236	169 269	180	20 138			Glycoprotein
HCMVUL122	C	169 367		170 878	494.7	51 084			IE2A. Spliced to IE1 EX4. Also KATG at 170599 (STENBERG et al. 1985)
HCMVUL123EX4	C	171 009		172 274	405.7	45 622			IE1 gene exon 4 (STENBERG et al. 1984; AKRIGG et al. 1985)
HCMVUL123EX3	C	172 301		172 654	61.7	6 865			IE1 gene exon 3 (STENBERG et al. 1984; AKRIGG et al. 1985)
HCMVUL123EX2	C	172 659	172 765	172 873	23.7	2 658			IE1 gene exon 2 (first coding exon) (STENBERG et al. 1984; AKRIGG et al. 1985)
HCMVUL124		172 783	172 798	173 253	152	15 887			Glycoprotein
HCMVUL125	C	173 114		173 419	102	11 000			
HCMVUL126	C	173 508		173 909	134	15 910			

Gene	Strand	Position			Amino acids	MW	Name	Copy	Family	Notes
HCMVUL127	C	174453	174495	174887	131	15248				Glycoprotein exon?
HCMVUL128	C	174868		175284	139	16036				Glycoprotein exon?
HCMVUL129	C	175357		175704	116	13288				
HCMVUL130	C	175665	176306	176438	214	24653				Glycoprotein
HCMVUL131	C	176644	176871	177042	76	8243				First 35 amino acids identical in TRL14
HCMVUL132	C	176934	177743	177845	270	29973				
HCMVIRL14	C	177776	178324	178327	183	20750				= HCMVTRL13. Glycoprotein
HCMVIRL13	C	178231	178671	178689	147	15888				exon?
HCMVIRL12	C	178786	180033	180036	416	47417			RL11 family	= HCMVTRL12. Glycoprotein
HCMVIRL11	C	180040	180741	180819	234	26661			RL11 family	= HCMVTRL11. Glycoprotein
HCMVIRL10	C	180773	181285	181366	171	19034				= HCMVTRL10; N at position 38 is D in TRL10. Glycoprotein
HCMVIRL9	C	181538	182183	181966	143	15909				= HCMVTRL9
HCMVIRL8	C	181797		182240	129	14302				= HCMVTRL8
HCMVIRL7		182546	182624	182869	82	9718				= HCMVTRL7
HCMVIRL6		183457	183520	183852	111	12286				= HCMVTRL6. Glycoprotein
HCMVIRL5	C	184860	185201	185282	114	12835				= HCMVTRL5
HCMVIRL4		185032		185682	217	24929				= HCMVTRL4. ORF in major early transcript (GREENAWAY and WILKINSON 1987)
HCMVIRL3	C	185934	186275	186326	114	13252				= HCMVTRL3. Glycoprotein?
HCMVIRL2	C	187230		187574	115	12324				= HCMVTRL2
HCMVIRL1	C	187565	188497	188533	311	34822				= HCMVTRL1
HCMVJ1I		188538		189560	341	36544	HKLF1	1		Positions 1 to 309 overlap J1L; 118 to 341 overlap J1S
HCMVIRS1		189702	189765	192302	846	91050	HQRF1	1	US22 family	V at position 190 is L in TRS1. Sequences diverge after position 549
HCMVUS1	C	192332	193715	192967	212	23481	HQLF3	1	US1 family	
HCMVUS2	C	193119		193850	199	23112	HQLF2	1	US2 family	Glycoprotein
HCMVUS3	C	194133	194690	194924	186	21575	HQLF1	1	US2 family	Spliced IE glycoprotein (WESTON 1988)
HCMVUS4		194832	195230	195188	119	13089				
HCMVUS5		195203		195607	126	14451				
HCMVUS6	C	195403	195951	195975	183	20640	HXLF6	1	US6 family	Glycoprotein
HCMVUS7	C	196377	197051	197069	225	26271	HXLF5	1	US6 family	Glycoprotein

(Continued)

Table 1. (*Continued*)

Frame	Strand	Start	K-ATG	Stop	Length	MW	Old Name	(ref)	Family	Comments
HCMVUS8	C	197256	197936	197960	227	26634	HXLF4	1	US6 family	Glycoprotein
HCMVUS9	C	197954	198694	198772	247	28054	HXLF3	1	US6 family	Glycoprotein
HCMVUS10	C	199083	199637	199646	185	20772	HXLF2	1	US6 family	Glycoprotein
HCMVUS11	C	199716	200360	200366	215	25265	HXLF1	1	US6 family	Glycoprotein
HCMVUS12	C	200549	201391	201562	281	32470	HVLF6	1	US12 family	Multiply hydrophobic
HCMVUS13	C	201474	202256	202307	261	29461	HVLF5	1	US12 family	Multiply hydrophobic
HCMVUS14	C	202328	203257	203311	310	34198	HVLF4	1	US12 family	Multiply hydrophobic
HCMVUS15	C	203305		204756	484	53049	HVLF3	1	US12 family	Multiply hydrophobic
HCMVUS16	C	204153	205079	205091	309	34718	HVLF2	1	US12 family	Multiply hydrophobic
HCMVUS17	C	205227	206105	206144	293	31910	HVLF1	1	US12 family	Multiply hydrophobic
HCMVUS18	C	206376	207197	207266	274	30195	HWLF5	1	US12 family	Multiply hydrophobic
HCMVUS19	C	207338	208057	208132	240	26424	HWLF4	1	US12 family	Multiply hydrophobic
HCMVUS20	C	208107		209177	357	39890	HWLF3	1	US12 family	Multiply hydrophobic
HCMVUS21	C	208978	209694	209793	239	26586	HWLF2	1	US12 family	Multiply hydrophobic
HCMVUS22	C	209874		211652	593	66971	HWLF1	1	US22 family	Early nuclear protein (MOCARSKI et al. 1988)
HCMVUS23	C	211717	213492	213510	592	68886	HHLF7	1	US22 family	
HCMVUS24	C	213591	215090	215105	500	57928	HHLF6	1	US22 family	
HCMVUS25		215097		215633	179	19655				
HCMVUS26	C	215730	217538	217574	603	70022	HHLF5	1	US22 family	Multiply hydrophobic. Homology to G-protein-coupled receptors
HCMVUS27		217859	217904	218989	362	41996	HHRF2	1	GCR family	
HCMVUS28		219083	219200	220168	323	37189	HHRF3	1	GCR family	Multiply hydrophobic. Homology to G-protein-coupled receptors
HCMVUS29		220420	220426	221811	462	51068	HHRF4	1		
HCMVUS30		221537	221618	222664	349	39115	HHRF5	1		
HCMVUS31		222674		223264	197	22936	HHRF6	1	US1 family	
HCMVUS32		223325	223385	223933	183	22058	HHRF7	1	US1 family	
HCMVUS33	C	224075		224485	137	15775	HHLF3	1		
HCMVUS34		224408	224480	224968	163	17767	HHRF8	1		Glycoprotein exon?
HCMVUS35	C	225212		225538	109	12966	HHLF2	1		
HCMVUS36	C	225429		225758	110	12352	HHLF1	1		
HCMVTRS1	C	226115	228478	228541	788	83983	HHLF1	1	US22 family	L at position 190 is V in IRS1. Sequences diverge after position 549
HCMVJ1S	C	228683		229354	224	23797				Overlaps J1L & J1I

ROIZMAN 1982; TAMASHIRO et al. 1984; SPAETE and MOCARSKI 1985b). Our sequence is numbered from base 2352 of TAMASHIRO et al. (1984) but reading backward on the complementary strand. It contains a single copy of a DR1-flanked 578-bp sequence at each end and at the junction of the internal repeats. The sequence we have determined consists of 229 354 base pairs. The long unique region (*UL*) is 166 972 bp and the surrounding repeats (IRL and TRL) are 11 247 bp each. The short unique region (*US*) is 35 418 bp and is flanked by 2524-bp repeats (*IRS* and *TRS*). In the sizes given above, *IRL* and *IRS* are considered as overlapping by one copy of the DR1-flanked repeat unit. The long repeats are identical except for two base changes: a C at position 5288 and a G at position 8293 are both substituted by As in the equivalent *IRL* positions. The former change does not affect any predicted coding sequences, while the latter affects *TRL/IRL10* (Table 1). Two differences were also found in the short repeats: in *IRS*, an A at position 189 887 and a G at position 190 332 are substituted by C and T respectively in *TRS*. The former difference is silent while the latter changes a valine residue in HCMV-IRS1 to a leucine in HCMV-TRS1.

3 Prediction of Reading Frames

Very little of the genome has been mapped in terms of its transcription or its expression. In order to analyze the protein-coding content of the sequence we need to define the criteria for the selection of the reading frames we think are most likely to be coding. A description of the procedures we have applied is given below.

3.1 Criteria for Selection

Analysis of other herpesvirus genomes shows that in most regions the reading frame that is coding is the longest and that such reading frames are arranged end to end on either strand with very little noncoding sequence in between. Very few overlapping genes have been found although there are sometimes small overlaps at the beginnings and ends of genes. Thus the strategy we have adopted has been to screen the sequence for reading frames that are over a certain length and then to filter out any smaller frames that overlap larger ones by a certain amount. The cutoffs that we have chosen are a minimum length of 300 bp (i.e., a coding potential of 100 amino acids) and a maximum allowable overlap of a larger reading frame of 60%. This latter figure allows for the fact that a reading frame may be open upstream of the actual initiation codon and that this may lie under the preceding gene. There are 778 reading frames over 300 bp of which 581 are screened out on the grounds that they are overlapped extensively by larger frames, leaving 197 candidate protein-coding genes. The sequence is then examined for reading frames of less than 300 bp that may lie in the gaps that are left. Likely frames are selected by experience using criteria such as logical combinations of potential transcription signals with the reading frame and any potential translational start; homology to other reading frames or known genes; and the presence of protein structural or functional motifs in the amino acid sequence. Codon bias can also be used as described below. The whole procedure will not work where genes are spliced and the exons are small. In those regions of the genome where the genes are highly spliced or in regions which are noncoding, small background noncoding reading frames will have been included which would otherwise have been screened out if larger coding reading frames were present. We think that this is particularly true in and bordering the repeat sequences and in certain regions of the HindIII D and E fragments. In a few cases we have substituted a smaller frame for a larger overlapping frame where we have found compelling reasons to choose the former.

3.2 Codon Bias

Patterns of codon usage that could conceivably be generated only through the genetic code are, in the absence of any other criteria, the best indication that a sequence is coding for protein. The high G + C content of HCMV (57.2%) leads to an accumulation of G and C in the third, degenerative, position of the codons. This is because in an average amino acid sequence the excess G and C cannot be accommodated in the first and second positions without biasing the sequence to amino acids encoded by GC-rich codons. Figure 2 shows a G + C plot across the entire sequence. As can be seen there is considerable variation in the G + C content across the genome, particularly in the repeat areas, the regions bordering the repeats, and the HindIII D fragment. Because of this variability we have not yet been able to find a single formula that we could apply equally to all areas of the genome to justify further our selection of reading frames on the basis of size and position. However, codon bias does serve as a useful check in those areas with a high G + C content.

3.3 HCMV Map

The preliminary map of 208 reading frames deduced from the sequence using the criteria discussed above is shown in Fig. 3. Details are given in the figure legend of individual frames that we have omitted from the original set of 197 (Sect. 3.1) and the criteria for inclusion of replacement frames. Although some of the frames shown are unlikely to be coding (for example, UL126 which overlaps the (noncoding) exon 1 of the major immediate-early gene and part of the enhancer) we preferred to include all frames meeting our minimal criteria unless a more plausible alternative candidate could be identified.

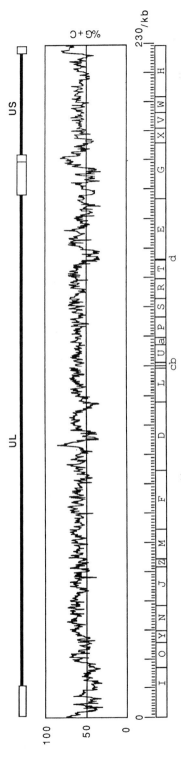

Fig. 2. Nucleotide composition of the HCMV strain AD169 genome. The % (G + C) content was plotted over the length of the genome using option 24 (plot base composition) of ANALYSEQ (STADEN 1986) with both span length and plot interval set at 201. The genome structure is shown above the plot, and a scale below. The orientation is that of the prototype isomer as indicated by the restriction map below the scale. The HCMV genome is relatively G + C rich (57.2% overall, 57.9% in UL, 55.7% in US, 49.9% in RL, 73.1% in RS). Within UL, marked variations in nucleotide composition are seen at either end in the HindIII fragments I, O, and E, and also in HindIIID. (see HONESS et al. 1989 for an analysis of dinucleotide frequencies)

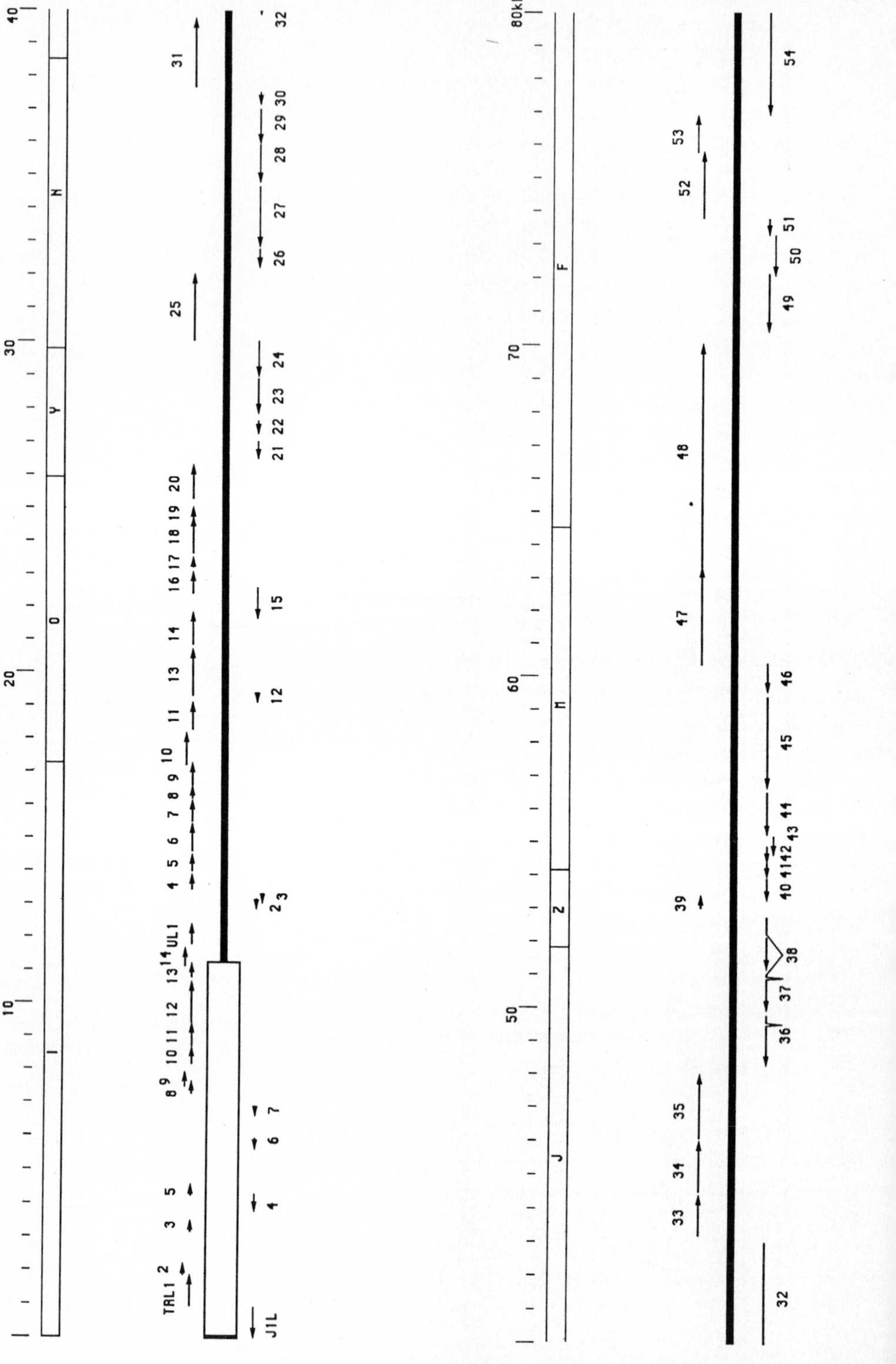

TRL1
UL1
J1L
10
20
30
40
50
60
70
80kb

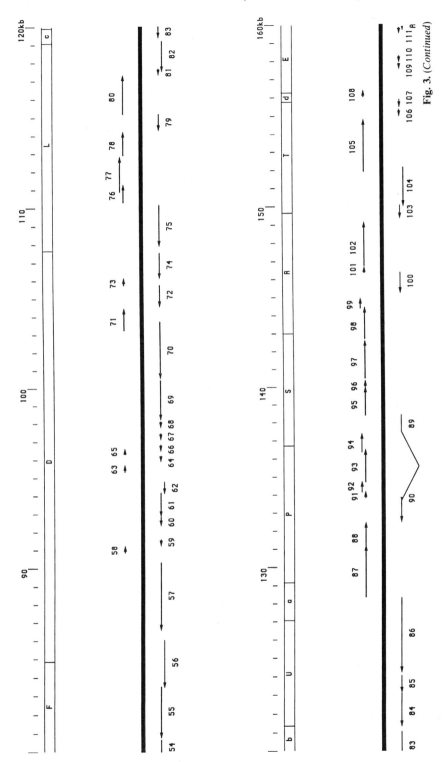

Fig. 3. (Continued)

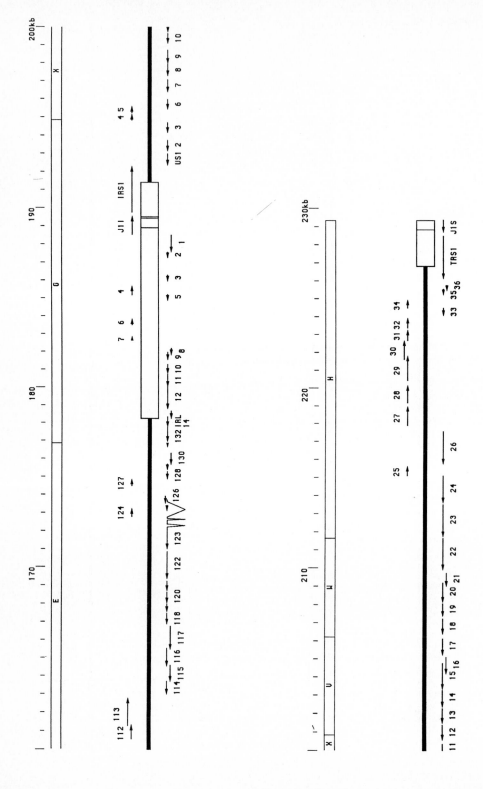

4 Identification of Homologs

The HCMV protein sequences were screened against the PIR (release 19.0; GEORGE et al. 1986), and SWISSPORT (release 8.0; BAIROCH 1988) libraries using the FastA program of PEARSON and LIPMAN (1988). Searches were also performed against a herpesvirus protein library including HSV-1, VZV, and EBV sequences. In these library comparisons alignments were examined when optimized FastA scores of 90 or greater were obtained, although in some cases lower-scoring matches were also scrutinized. Some of the HCMV sequences match numerous reading frames as a result of compositional bias, which may be general throughout the sequence or localized. For example, glycine-rich stretches occur in a number of reading frames, including HCMV-UL44, 56, 102, 112, and TRS/IRS1. In most cases highly biased matches have been excluded. Sometimes, however, these similarities are likely to reflect functional similarities, if not homology. For example, HCMV-UL122, which encodes an immediate-early transactivator, is similar to HSV-IE110, also an immediate-early transactivator. The results of overall homology searches, motif searches (STADEN 1988), and comparisons of gene layout with EBV, VZV, and HSV-1 have been amalgamated in the compilation of human herpesvirus and cellular homologs. Functions ascribed to HCMV genes or their homologs are noted in Table 1. Homologies detected to the sequenced herpesviruses are shown in Table 2. A

Fig. 3. A map of predicted open reading frames in HCMV strain AD169. Two hundred and eight individual frames are recognized, some of which are known to be spliced. The reading frame map is drawn in the prototype orientation below the *Hind*III restriction map. The diagram is scaled in kilobase pairs. Open reading frames which overlap on the same strand are displaced in the figure. Frames are numbered separately except for three genes for which splice sites have been precisely located (HCMV-UL36, UL37, and UL123) (KOUZARIDES et al. 1988; STENBERG et al. 1984, 1985), and one gene for which the splice sites are probably conserved with other herpesviruses (HCMV-UL89) (COSTA et al. 1985). Genes which may be spliced to upstream frames, but which are also capable of being initiated at a proximal ATG, are numbered separately (HCMV-UL36, UL38, UL122). Frames are designated TRL, IRL, UL, TRS, IRS, or US according to the region of the genome in which their 5' ends are located, and each of these six sets is numbered from *1*. A frame which spans the DR1 repeats (Sect. 2) and hence is capable of crossing the genomic termini has been designated *J* (junction) *1*. Three manifestations of this frame which differ in their 5' and 3' termini occur, and are shown as *J1L, J1S,* and *J1I* (where *L, S,* and *I* denote long, short and internal respectively; see also Table 1). The "a" sequence is shown as a *thin vertical line* located within the repeats. The following frames have been included in place of longer overlapping frames; the names of the latter (not shown) are given *in brackets*, together with reasons for the substitution; the orientations of the substituted frames are indicated by the direction of numbering : *1*, J1L, and TRL1 (TRL1X, positions 291–1361; these frames occupy the region more completely, with minimal overlap. TRL1 has a proximal TATA box and a Kozak consensus ATG). [NB. J1L completely overlaps a frame equivalent to HKRFX (WESTON and BARRELL 1986) (not shown, positions 873–43)]; *2*, UL38 (UL38X, positions 51 098–52 141; third position G + C; see Sect. 5.3); *3*, UL106 (UL106X, positions 155 043–155 465; third position G + C); *4*, UL112 (UL112X, positions 161 638–160 466; third position G + C; mapping data; WRIGHT et al. 1988); *5*, UL123 (UL123X positions 172 331–172 816; overlaps major immediate-early gene exons 2 and 3); *6*, J1I and IRL1 (IRL1X, positions 189 176–188 106; see *1* above). US25X (former name HHRF1, positions 215 051–215 518; WESTON and BARRELL 1986) had an excessive overlap with US25 and was omitted without another frame being substituted in its place. The small frame Ul111A (marked as *A*) was included because it has a Kozak consensus ATG, a transcript has been identified in the region, and it is a conserved feature of a transforming region in HCMVs Towne and AD169 (RAZZAQUE et al. 1988; JAHAN et al. 1989). The frame is one amino acid shorter than the Towne sequence, having a relative 3-bp deletion, but the predicted amino acid sequence is otherwise identical

Table 2. Homologs of HCMV-reading frames in the sequenced herpesviruses. Internal HCMV-related sequences as well as EBV, VZV, and HSV-1 homologs are listed, together with FastA scores (PEARSON and LIPMAN 1988). HCMV homologous families containing three or more sequences are indicated only in Table 1. We have found from experience that FastA scores above 100 are often significant, except when sequences are highly biased in composition. Homologs which were not identified by library searches, but which were inferred from their collinearity with other conserved frames, are scored as *P* (positionally conserved). Listings scored as *P?* should be regarded as tentative at best. Listings with a *question mark* and a FastA score show borderline similarity in the absence of supporting evidence and should be regarded as speculative. In most cases the highest scores above 90 were listed. Compositionally biassed matches were excluded for the following frames: HCMV-TRL/IRL4, TRL/IRL13, UL32, UL44, and UL113. Nomenclature for EBV, VZV and HSV-1 frames is conventional (BAER et al. 1984; DAVISON and SCOTT 1986; MCGEOCH et al. 1988a); the EBV sequence designated as LP (leader protein) is translated from the spliced EBNA2 mRNA (WANG et al. 1987)

Frame	HCMV	Score	Homologs EBV	Score	VZV	Score	HSV	Score
HCMVUL15			BCRF2?	93				
HCMVUL25	HCMVUL35	235					UL9?	87
HCMVUL35	HCMVUL25	235						
HCMVUL45			BORF2	151	VZV19	178	UL39	238
HCMVUL46			BORF1?	P	VZV20?	P	UL38?	P
HCMVUL47	HCMVUL86?	96	BOLF1?	P	VZV21?	P	UL37?	P
HCMVUL48			BPLF1	143	VZV22	P	UL36	144
HCMVUL49			BFRF2	249	VZV23	P	UL35	P
HCMVUL50			BFRF1?	P?	VZV24?	P	UL34?	P
HCMVUL51			BFRF1?	P?	VZV25	97	UL33	106
HCMVUL52			BFLF1	138	VZV26	179	UL32	207
HCMVUL53	HCMVUL69?	95	BFLF2	263	VZV27	99	UL31	141
HCMVUL54	HCMVUL130?	90	BALF5	343	VZV28	326	UL30	423
HCMVUL55			BALF4	720	VZV31	1061	UL27	1052
HCMVUL56	HCMVUL112?	95	BALF3	321	VZV30	290	UL28	323
HCMVUL57			BALF2	352	VZV29	220	UL29	298
HCMVUL61			LP?	181				
HCMVUL69	HCMVUL53?	95	BMLF1	P	VZV4	P	UL54	127
HCMVUL70			BSLF1	293	VZV6	302	UL52	405
HCMVUL71			BSRF1	92	VZV7?	P	UL51?	P
HCMVUL72			BLLF2	P	VZV8	P	UL50	88
HCMVUL73			BLRF1	134				
HCMVUL75	HCMVUL25?	90	BXLF2	217	VZV37	P	UL22	P
HCMVUL76			BXRF1	219	VZV35	151	UL24	132
HCMVUL77			BVRF1	316	VZV34	278	UL25	291
HCMVUL80			BVRF2	347	VZV33	177	UL26	243
HCMVUL82	HCMVUL83	325						
HCMVUL83	HCMVUL82	325						
HCMVUL85			BDLF1	P	VZV41	114	UL18	138
HCMVUL86	HCMVUL47?	96	BcLF1	1876	VZV40	767	UL19	1225
HCMVUL87			BcRF1	542	VZV38?	P	UL21?	P
HCMVUL89			BD/BGRF1	1181	VZV42/45	1104	UL15	1206
HCMVUL92			BDLF4	213				
HCMVUL93			BGLF1?	P	VZV43?	P	UL17?	P
HCMVUL94			BGLF2	241	VZV44	P	UL16	P
HCMVUL95			BGLF3	112	VZV46	P	UL14	P
HCMVUL97			BGLF4	157	VZV47	112	UL13	97
HCMVUL98			BGLF5	191	VZV48	78	UL12	140
HCMVUL99			BBLF1?	P	VZV49?	P	UL11?	P
HCMVUL100			BBRF3	417	VZV50	224	UL10	215
HCMVUL101			BBLF2?	P	VZV51?	P	UL9?	P
HCMVUL102			BBLF3?	P	VZV52?	P	UL8?	P
HCMVUL103			BBRF2	102	VZV53	91	UL7	121
HCMVUL104			BBRF1	357	VZV54	375	UL6	309
HCMVUL105			BBLF4	704	VZV55	642	UL5	598

Frame	HCMV	—Homologs Score	EBV	Score	VZV	Score	HSV	Score
HCMVUL112	HCMVUL56?	95						
HCMVUL114			BKRF3	545	VZV59	461	UL2	489
HCMVUL116			BDLF3?	128				
HCMVUL122							IE110?	90
HCMVUS2	HCMVUS3	169						
HCMVUS3	HCMVUS2	169						

survey of HCMV proteins including map assignments in the AD169, Towne, and Davis strain genomes has been conducted previously by LANDINI and MICHELSON (1988).

5 IE Genes

The activation of IE genes is the initial step in a viral program of gene expression. Northern hybridization studies have shown that transcription from the HCMV genome during the immediate early phase of productive infection is limited to several discrete loci, with the most active region located near one end of UL (DEMARCHI 1981; WATHEN and STINSKI 1982; McDONOUGH and SPECTOR 1983; JAHN et al. 1984; WILKINSON et al. 1984). This major immediate-early (MIE) region has been studied in several CMV strains, and unlike the bulk of the CMV genome is CpG suppressed (HONESS et al. 1989). The MIE genes encode regulatory proteins, the expression of which requires only cellular factors, although virion components may also play a transactivating role (SPAETE and MOCARSKI 1985a; STINSKI and ROEHR 1985). More recently two other immediate-early loci have been sequenced and characterized in AD169 (KOUZARIDES et al. 1988; WESTON 1988).

5.1 MIE Gene Region

The first sequence data for this region were reported for HCMV Towne (STENBERG et al. 1984) and showed the four-exon arrangement of the major immediate-early (IE1) gene. Sequence analysis of the corresponding AD169 region revealed a similar arrangement with minor differences. Only two changes were observed at the amino acid level (AKRIGG et al. 1985). The organization of the equivalent murine CMV gene is grossly similar, but differs considerably at the sequence level (KEIL et al. 1987). Analysis of the HCMV IE promoter region exposed a complex array of 21-, 19-, 18-, and 16-bp repeats upstream of the TATA and CAAT boxes (THOMSEN et al. 1984; AKRIGG et al. 1985). The upstream sequence demonstrates a potent enhancer activity, detected by its ability to rescue enhancerless SV40 genomes (BOSHART et al. 1985). Homology with the core enhancer sequence TGGAAAG/TGGTTTG was noted in the 18-bp repeats and potential Sp1-binding sites were also found. The enhancer binds cellular factors (GHAZAL et al. 1987, 1988) and dissection has shown that the 19-bp elements can mediate cAMP induction (FICKENSCHER et al. 1989; HUNNINGHAKE et al. 1989). Similar enhancers were also found in murine and simian CMVs (DORSCH-HASLER et al. 1985; JEANG et al. 1987). Nuclear factor 1 binding sites are associated with the enhancer region in both human and simian CMVs (HENNIGHAUSEN and FLECKENSTEIN 1986; JEANG et al. 1987).

STINSKI et al. (1983) recognized two further IE regions beginning immediately downstream of IE1. The IE2 region has more recently been called IE2a and a further region recognized as IE2b (HERMISTON et al. 1987; STENBERG et al. 1985). Under immediate-early conditions, transcription of the IE2a region starts mainly from the IE1 promoter and a set of alternatively spliced transcripts is produced. In the predominant species the IE2a exon (HCMV-UL122 in AD169) is fused to the first three exons of IE1. HCMV-UL122 encodes 494 amino acids following the splice acceptor. This is in agreement with the size predicted of the IE2a exon reported for the Towne strain by PIZZORNO et al. (1988). A 1.7-kb unspliced mRNA can also originate from a promoter proximal to the IE2a frame (which also contains a Kozak consensus ATG; KOZAK 1981). This transcript is more abundant at early and late times postinfection (STENBERG et al. 1985). The product of the IE2a frame may be involved in autoregulation (PIZZORNO et al. 1988). A minor transcript extending into the IE2b region has been diagrammed (HERMISTON et al. 1987). We are unable to correlate this with the AD169 sequence using the available information. However, a potential splice donor occurs before the UL122 termination codon, and a polyA signal at position 167 503 is consistent with the predicted end point of the Towne transcript. It is likely that the reading frames on either side of this signal, UL119 and UL118, are spliced together to encode a membrane glycoprotein.

5.2 HCMV US3 IE Gene

Sequencing of the US region of HCMV revealed an enhancer element containing five 18-bp repeats with homology to the MIE 18-bp repeats and the core enhancer element (WESTON 1988). These repeats were located in the region -80 to -270 of an RNA cap site in the HCMV-US3 (HQLF1) gene. In the region -340 to -600 a further set of six novel 11-bp repeats was found. A 275-bp fragment containing the 18-bp repeats enhanced expression in an orientation-independent manner in HeLa cells, with an efficacy equivalent to the SV40 enhancer (WESTON 1988), while the MIE enhancer 18-bp repeats have recently been shown to be involved in positive autoregulation by IE1 (CHERRINGTON and MOCARSKI 1989). The significance of the 11-bp repeats is unknown. However, a hexanucleotide consensus (TRTCGC) derived from these repeats was noted to occur in the MIE enhancer (WESTON 1988). Transcription from the HCMV-US3 reading frame associated with the enhancer is highly active at IE times and produces a set of differentially spliced transcripts. The protein-coding sequence of HCMV-US3 contains signal, anchor, and N-linked glycosylation sequences, is homologous to HCMV-US2 (HQLF2), and may also be related to the RLII and US6 gene families (Sect. 8).

5.3 UL37 IE Gene

A second UL IE transcription unit was identified in the region of the AD169 *Hin*dIII J and Z fragments (WILKINSON et al. 1984). The sequence of this region together with mapping data for three mRNAs has been published (KOUZARIDES et al. 1988). A 3.4-kb IE transcript was shown to be spliced from four exons and, like HCMV-US3, encodes a potential glycoprotein. This mRNA is 3' coterminal with a 1.65-kb transcript which can be detected in the IE phase but is more abundant at the late stage of infection. The predicted product of the 1.65-kb mRNA is a member of the US22 homologous protein family (Sect. 7.2). A 1.7-kb transcript utilizing the same promoter as the 3.4-kb mRNA is most abundant at IE times but can also be detected late in infection. Of the mapped transcripts only this RNA contains the HCMV-UL38 (HZLF3) reading frame. However, expression of UL38 from this transcript would require the upstream UL37 exon 1 to be bypassed; alternatively, the frame may be read from an uncharacterized low-abundance transcript (KOUZARIDES et al. 1988). A 40-kDa protein synthesized in vitro from *Hin*dIII Z or J hybrid-selected mRNA is consistent with translation from UL38 (WILKINSON et al. 1984). Although a slightly longer reading frame completely overlaps UL38 on the opposite strand (UL38X, not shown), analysis of third position G + C contents suggests that of the two opposing frames UL38 is more likely to be coding (84.3% vs 62.8% G + C).

6 Early and Late Genes

Immediate-early proteins are required to activate genes which establish the early or delayed early (E or DE) phase of infection, the outcome of which is the replication of the viral genome. Late genes are expressed at high levels after DNA replication and are likely to encode most of the structural and assembly proteins of the virus. The distinction between E and late phases is blurred for some genes, and is further complicated by posttranscriptional regulation of gene expression (DEMARCHI 1983; GEBALLE et al. 1986a; GOINS and STINSKI 1986). In the following sections we attempt to correlate the available information on E and late genes with our sequence data. The organization of the following sections superficially resembles the viral timetable as convenient, but may be similarly inscrutable in places.

6.1 Major Early Transcripts

The most abundantly transcribed region of HCMV at early times postinfection is situated in the long repeats of the virus and encodes a 2.7-kb transcript of unknown function (GREENAWAY and WILKINSON 1987; HUTCHINSON et al. 1986; McDONOUGH et al. 1985). An early transcript of similar size also originates in RL of HCMV Towne (WATHEN and STINSKI 1982), one copy of which can be deleted without compromising viability in cultured human fibroblasts (SPAETE and MOCARSKI 1987).

GREENAWAY and WILKINSON (1987) determined a 6220-bp sequence in HCMV AD169 which encompasses the gene for the 2.7-kb transcript. Their sequence is equivalent to positions 1635–7859 of Fig. 3 viewed in the opposite orientation. (We refer only to TRL sequence positions for clarity.) It contains two ambiguities and differs from our sequence at nine positions. However, only one of these is located within the major early transcription unit; the doublet CC beginning at position 3386 of GREENAWAY and WILKINSON (1987) is a triplet in our sequence. The open reading frame corresponding to the predicted translation product of the major 2.7-kb transcript as mapped by these authors is TRL/IRL4. The translational start is suggested to be the fourth ATG from the start of the transcript and occurs at position 4294 in our sequence. This is not a Kozak ATG in that it does not have a purine at -3 or a G at $+4$ (KOZAK 1981, 1982). However, two upstream ATG codons fit the Kozak consensus. The first has the sequence CGGATGG and is followed by a stop codon after seven amino acids. The second has the sequence GAGATGA and begins a 35-amino-acid reading frame. These codons have been shown to inhibit translation from a downstream AUG and may therefore be cis-regulatory signals (GEBALLE et al. 1986a; GEBALLE and MOCARSKI 1988). Upstream Kozak consensus ATGs precede a number of other HCMV genes, and suggest a general phenomenon in HCMV translational regulation. However, this role has yet to be demonstrated directly and so far no products have been found for the major early transcript. A less-abundant 2.0-kb transcript has been mapped immediately downstream of the 2.7-kb transcript in the Eisenhardt strain of HCMV (HUTCHINSON et al. 1986). The predicted polyadenylation site is conserved in AD169, beginning at position 6552 in our sequence. However, a similar-sized transcript was not detected (MCDONOUGH et al. 1985). It is also not possible to suggest a 5' end from the Eisenhardt strain restriction map data. There are, however, no reading frames that might obviously be utilized in this region with the exception of TRL/IRL6. A minor 1.3-kb immediate-early RNA and a 1.2-kb late RNA have also been mapped to this general region (MCDONOUGH et al. 1985; HUTCHINSON et al. 1986); the latter is detected at early times postinfection but is most abundant in the late phase. The polyA signal for this message was located precisely in the Eisenhardt strain and begins at position 6365 of our sequence (HUTCHINSON et al. 1986). These authors also mapped the start of the transcript by nuclease protection and found no evidence for splicing. Further mapping and sequencing studies, the latter performed on genomic as well as cDNA clones, were used to predict a coding frame of 254 amino acids within the transcript (HUTCHINSON and TOCCI 1986). The region sequenced corresponds to positions 6300–7468 of Fig. 3 (displayed in the IRL orientation). However, in AD169 the 254-amino-acid reading frame is disrupted by three stop codons and two frameshifts relative to the Eisenhardt sequence and is identical in both repeats. Our data and those of GREENAWAY and WILKINSON are in agreement for the region spanned by the putative reading frame. We are unable to predict a reading frame which may be translated from this message in AD169. The first Kozak ATG occurs 164 nucleotides downstream of the transcription start predicted by HUTCHINSON and TOCCI (1986), but is followed by a stop codon after 42 intervening amino acid codons. Furthermore, although TRL/IRL7 is located in this message, it is over 500 bp from the predicted start. If these differences between the Eisenhardt and AD169 strains are genuine, sequencing from other strains would be useful in assessing their biological relevance.

6.2 Enzymes of Nucleotide and DNA Metabolism

6.2.1 Nucleotide Metabolism

HONESS (1984) postulated that differences in overall base compositions between herpesvirus genomes reflect the ability of the viruses to modulate and utilize the nucleotide pool available for DNA synthesis. This hypothesis appears to be borne out in the case of the two closely related α-herpesviruses, HSV-1 and VZV. The latter is AT rich and encodes a thymidylate synthase, which does not have a homolog in the G + C rich HSV-1 genome (THOMPSON et al. 1987; MCGEOCH et al. 1988a). A parallel exists in the less closely related γ-herpesviruses Epstein-Barr virus (EBV) and herpesvirus saimiri (HVS); the latter A + T rich virus encodes thymidylate synthase and dihydrofolate reductase, which both seem to be absent from the G + C rich EBV (HONESS et al. 1986; TRIMBLE et al. 1988; BAER et al. 1984). All four viruses also encode deoxyribonucleoside kinases, and hence can utilize the salvage pathway of dNTP synthesis (MCKNIGHT 1980; DAVISON and SCOTT 1986; LITTLER et al. 1986; GOMPELS et al. 1988a). These enzymes differ in their substrate specificity and their main role might be to allow the exploitation of specific cell types, such as may occur in latency. Genes for ribonucleotide reductase, a key enzyme in deoxyribonucleotide synthesis, have been found in HSV, VZV, and EBV as well as other herpesviruses, but have not so far been identified in HVS (GIBSON et al. 1984; DAVISON and SCOTT 1986; NIKAS et al. 1986). The HCMV genome is relatively G + C rich (Fig. 2) and it will be of interest to determine if its complement of enzymes is consistent with the theory of HONESS (1984). HCMV does not appear to encode a thymidine (deoxyribonucleoside) kinase (TK); the position in the AD169 genome equivalent to the TK locus in other herpesviruses is deleted relative to the other herpesviruses (Fig. 3). However, HCMV is sensitive to the nucleoside analog DHPG, and a resistant mutant of AD169 has been isolated which accumulates less of the triphosphate form of the drug (BIRON et al. 1986). This may indicate that a deoxyribonucleoside kinase is encoded at some other locus.

The partial conservation of a ribonucleotide reductase (RR) homolog is more puzzling. Mammalian cells contain an iron-tyrosyl radical enzyme, which is the type found in herpesviruses (SJOBERG et al. 1985; REICHARD 1989). The enzyme has an $\alpha_2\beta_2$-structure; the HCMV-UL45 gene product is homologous to the α-(large) RR subunit, and HCMV-UL45 is positionally conserved with the gene for this subunit in other herpesviruses. However, the gene for the β-(small) subunit does not appear to be conserved; HCMV-UL44 is positionally analogous to the small RR gene in other herpesviruses but encodes a set of late DNA-binding proteins (see Sect. 6.5). The small subunit contains the active tyrosyl radical and would be essential for function. Thus it is not clear at present if HCMV is capable of expressing a fully active ribonucleotide reductase. Although we have used loosely defined motifs to search all the predicted reading frames for a potential active site, no obvious candidates were identified. Several explanations could account for this. For example, if HCMV-UL45 is functionally conserved with the large subunit, it might usurp the place of its cellular counterpart which mediates allosteric control as well as being involved in catalysis. Herpesviral reductases appear to be unregulated, indicating that the function is either unnecessary or perhaps detrimental in the viral context (LANIKEN et al. 1982; AVERTT et al. 1983). It is also possible that synthesis of one or both of the cellular subunits is upregulated during viral infection (STINSKI 1977). The genes for the human RR subunits are unlinked; the α-subunit gene is on chromosome 11 (ENGSTROM et al. 1985), and the β-gene on chromosome 2 (YANG-FENG et al. 1987). Finally, it is worth mentioning that another key allosteric enzyme of nucleotide metabolism is dCMP deaminase; this enzyme converts dCMP to dUMP, which is the substrate for thymidylate synthase. Hence it might be an appropriate enzyme for herpesviral repertoires, particularly those which have devolved to an A + T bias.

6.2.2 DNA Replication

A set of seven HSV-1 genes has been shown to be essential for the replication of an HSV-origin-containing plasmid (WU et al. 1988; McGEOCH et al. 1988b). The HCMV homologs of four of these have been identified by sequence analysis. HCMV-UL54 encodes the DNA polymerase (KOUZARIDES et al. 1987a; HEILBRONN et al. 1987) and HCMV-UL57 the major DNA-binding protein (MDBP). The latter sequence shows 72% identity over a length of 1160 aligned amino acids to the MDBP of simian CMV (Colburn) (ANDERS and GIBSON 1988; ANDERS and GIBSON, personal communication). HCMV-UL105 encodes a homolog to HSV-UL5, which is probably a helicase enzyme (CRUTE et al. 1988, 1989). Helicases belong to a superfamily of proteins with functions in replication and/or recombination (HODGMAN 1988). A nucleotide-binding site in UL105 (MARTIGNETTI 1987), of the type GxxGxGK (where x = any amino acid), is common to the other members of the superfamily. HCMV-UL70 is the fourth HCMV gene with an obvious replication gene counterpart, in HSV-UL52. The product of HSV-UL52 is part of a helicase-primase complex in HSV-1-infected cells which also contains the HSV-UL5 and UL8 proteins (CRUTE et al. 1989). HCMV genes UL102 and UL101 are positionally equivalent to HSV-UL8 and UL9 respectively, although they show no clear-cut homology. However, HCMV-UL102 is a similar length to HSV-UL8 (798 and 750 residues respectively). HSV-UL9 encodes an origin-binding protein (OLIVO et al. 1988), and the positive identification of its HCMV counterpart may require the identification of an HCMV origin of replication.

6.2.3 DNA Repair

The gene for uracil-DNA glycosylase, which is involved in base excision repair, was identified in HSV-2 and is conserved in the sequenced herpesviruses (WORRAD and CARADONNA 1988; BAER et al. 1984; DAVISON and SCOTT 1986; MULLANEY et al. 1989). The corresponding HCMV-reading frame is HCMV-UL114, which is the last frame at this end of UL with detectable homology to sequenced human herpesviruses. A dUTPase gene is also conserved in herpesviruses, albeit less well than uracil-DNA glycosylase (PRESTON and FISHER 1984; DAVISON and SCOTT 1986; BAER et al. 1984). The HCMV homolog is HCMV-UL72.

6.2.4 Deoxyribonuclease

A deoxyribonuclease gene found in HCMV appears to be ubiquitous in herpesviruses, as homologs are found in HHV-6 (LAWRENCE et al., unpublished results), EBV (ZHANG et al. 1987), HSV (MCGEOCH et al. 1986), and VZV (DAVISON and SCOTT 1986). The role of this enzyme is currently unknown, but it may be involved in cleavage of viral concatemers and/or the processing of genome termini (CHOU and ROIZMAN 1989).

6.3 Phosphotransferase

The putative phosphotransferase encoded by HCMV-UL97 is conserved in the human herpesviruses and distantly related to the protein kinase family (CHEE et al. 1989a; SMITH and SMITH 1989). Interestingly, some of the most conserved amino acids in protein kinases are variant in the herpesvirus sequences. One motif where these differences occur is shared with bacterial phosphotransferases, which vary at the same amino acid positions as do the herpesvirus proteins (BRENNER 1987). Hence it remains to be shown if HCMV-UL97 and its homologs are in fact conventional kinases. Whatever its specific role, the preservation of this gene in all of the recognized herpesvirus lineages and HHV-6 implies an important or indispensable contribution to the viral life cycle. None of the other HCMV-reading frames we have screened have detectable homology to known protein kinase motifs, which are seen in the α-herpesvirus US-encoded kinases (MCGEOCH and DAVISON 1986).

6.4 Early Phosphoprotein Genes

The gene for a set of phosphoproteins sharing a common N-terminus has been mapped by WRIGHT et al. (1988). These authors mapped the termini of two spliced 2.2-kb early transcripts, raised an antiserum against a synthetic peptide predicted from a 5'-terminal portion of the 5'-exon sequence (KOUZARIDES et al. 1983; RASMUSSEN et al. 1985a) and used this to detect four proteins of 34, 43, 50, and 84 kDa in infected cells (WRIGHT et al. 1988). Pulse-chase experiments did not suggest that any of the proteins were derivative in nature. Although the mapping data are as yet incomplete, it would thus appear that all four proteins are coded in alternatively spliced mRNAs sharing a 5' exon. This exon corresponds to UL112 in our sequence. A 279-bp portion of the UL113 frame (positions 161 503–161 781) is flanked by potential acceptor and donor sites, and may correspond to a 280-bp exon mapped by STAPRANS and SPECTOR (1986). The downstream exons may also be derived from UL113, which extends to position 162 797. A polyA signal begins at position 162 909, but there is an alternative polyA sequence coinciding with the end of UL113 (ATTAAA, beginning at position 162 796). It therefore seems likely that one or both of these signals indicates the end of the transcription unit. The four proteins were found to be predominantly contained in the nuclear fraction of infected cells, and were not shown to be virion structural proteins in preliminary studies (WRIGHT et al. 1988).

6.5 Late DNA-Binding Proteins

Mocarski and coworkers utilized immunological screening of a λgt11 expression library to map a group of proteins known as the ICP36 family to the HCMV-UL44-reading frame (MOCARSKI et al. 1985; LEACH and MOCARSKI 1989). The ICP36 proteins gravitate to the nucleus, include phosphorylated and glycosylated species, and are DNA-binding proteins (PEREIRA et al. 1982; GIBSON 1983; MOCARSKI et al. 1985). Regulation of HCMV-UL44 gene expression is manifested in both early and late transcription from different TATA boxes, and delayed translation of early message (LEACH and MOCARSKI 1989; GEBALLE et al. 1986b). The significance of this complex control is unclear, although it is interesting that the 3'-end of the reading frame is overlapped by a gene encoding a small RNA in the same orientation. This gene is probably transcribed by RNA polymerase III (MARSCHALEK et al. 1989).

6.6 Capsid Proteins

The gene for the major capsid protein (MCP) was identified by sequence homology to the MCP sequences of other human herpesviruses and the assignment confirmed immunologically (CHEE et al. 1989b). The MCP is encoded by the HCMV-UL86 reading frame. Homology searches show that the predicted protein sequence of another frame, HCMV-UL47, is similar to a region of the human herpesvirus major capsids corresponding approximately to positions 1080–1170 of Fig. 3 in (CHEE et al. 1989b). Although this match may be fortuitous, the alignment of HCMV-UL47 to conserved capsid sequences makes it of interest. However, the sequence is not obviously conserved in the EBV, VZV, and HSV-1 reading frames collinear with HCMV-UL47.

A second capsid protein, which is a constituent of incomplete capsids, has been mapped in the UL region of three CMV strains (ROBSON and GIBSON 1989). Several lines of evidence implicate this protein in DNA packaging and/or capsid assembly (PRESTON et al. 1983; IRMIERE and GIBSON 1985; LEE et al. 1988; RIXON et al. 1988). The gene for the putative assembly protein is conserved in the human herpesviruses, and is predicted to encode proteins of 635, 605, 605, and 708 amino acids in HSV, VZV, EBV, and HCMV respectively (MCGEOCH et al. 1988a; DAVISON and SCOTT 1986; BAER et al. 1984) (Table 1). The sequence of a 1-kb cDNA derived from the Colburn strain of CMV shows homology only to the 3' half of HCMV-UL80, consistent with the 37-kDa size of the Colburn strain assembly protein which is probably processed at the carboxy terminus (ROBSON and GIBSON 1989). A larger transcript of 1.8-kb is also encoded at this locus. The 5' portion of the HCMV-UL80 frame is conserved in the other sequenced human herpesviruses. It thus seems likely that at least two seperate proteins are encoded by HCMV-UL80, with a TATA box at position 115 992 being used to produce the assembly protein transcript (ROBSON and GIBSON 1989). This TATA box is located within 15 bp which are identical in Colburn and AD169 (NECKER et al. 1988 cited in ROBSON and GIBSON 1989). It is also noteworthy that the ATG downstream of this TATA box does not fit the Kozak consensus in either of the two CMV sequences. In contrast to the major DNA-binding protein (Sect. 6.2.2), the sequences for the putative assembly protein are quite divergent. The Colburn sequence from the first methionine of the predicted cDNA reading frame exhibits approximately 40% identity to the carboxy-terminal 371 amino acids of HCMV-UL80.

6.7 Structural Phosphoprotein Genes

HCMV virions contain three main phosphoproteins which appear to be located in the virion tegument (ROBY and GIBSON 1986). The largest of these is approximately 150 kDa in size, constitutes approximately 20% of virion protein content (IRMIERE and GIBSON 1983), and is also modified by O-linked glycosylation (BENKO et al. 1988). A 6360-bp region containing the pp150 gene sequence (which corresponds to the reading frame HCMV-UL32) has been published and spans positions 37 157– 43 516 of Fig. 3 viewed in the opposite orientation. A late 6.2-kb mRNA was mapped in this region, and its termini delineated. Some processing at an alternative polyA site (ATTAAA) downstream of the orthodox signal was demonstrated. The major RNA species is predicted to encode pp150 although a range of smaller RNA species was also detected (JAHN et al. 1987).

The two other major phosphoproteins located in virions are pp71 and pp65, also known as the upper and lower matrix phosphoproteins respectively. The 65-kDa phosphoprotein is also glycosylated (CLARK et al. 1984; PANDE et al. 1984), and pp71 may be similarly modified. The genes for pp65 and pp71 are located in the HindIII L, c, b region of the genome and correspond to reading frames HCMV-UL83 and UL82 respectively. The sequence of a HindIII/BglII fragment containing these genes has been reported, and corresponds to nucleotides 117 276–121 377 of Fig. 3 viewed in the opposite orientation (RUGER et al. 1987). The published sequence is in error; position 212 (121 166 in the genome) is shown as a G but should be read as a C. This change does not affect the predicted coding sequences. Two transcripts which appear to be 3′ coterminal were mapped in this region. They are an abundant 4-kb mRNA and a low-level 1.9-kb mRNA. The 5′ ends of both transcripts have been located, but surprisingly no TATA box is proximal to the 4-kb transcription unit (RUGER et al. 1987). The 4-kb message should encode pp65, while the shorter mRNA would allow pp71 to be translated. The mRNA encoding pp65 (ICP27) in HCMV Towne appears to be produced efficiently both early and late in infection, but is not translated at high levels until the late phase (GEBALLE et al. 1986b; but see DEPTO and STENBERG 1989). The gene sequences for two further structural phosphoproteins have been reported (MEYER et al. 1988; DAVIS and HUANG 1985). The data of MEYER et al. (1988) represent positions 143 791–145 191 of our sequence in the HindIII R

Table 3. HCMV glycoprotein genes. A compilation of signal and anchor sequences and numbers of possible N-linked glycosylation sites in 54 reading frames. The selection of frames was based on criteria defined by McGeoch (1985). A questionmark after the number of NXT/S sites indicates that at least one of these sites is located on the putative cytoplasmic face of the sequence. Twenty-two of the frames lack at least a signal or an anchor sequence. Many of these may represent glycoprotein exons (Table 1), while some may encode unusual or non-N-linked glycoproteins like the pseudorabies gp50 (Petrovskis et al. 1986). It is also possible that some of the potential glycoproteins may be fixed to membranes by glycosyl-phosphatidylinositol anchors (Ferguson and Williams 1988)

Frame	Strand	Signal	NXT/S	Anchor
HCMVTRL/IRL3		MYCFLFLQKDTFFHEQFLARRRHAE	4	IGVLVVVCGFYFFLYLSMTVFLFFVLIII
HCMVTRL/IRL10		MYPRVMHAVCFLALSLVSYVAVCAE	3	EPITMLGAYSAWGAGSFVATLIVLLVVFFVIYAR
HCMVTRL/IRL11		MQTYSTPLTLVIVTSLFLFTTQGSS	23	HCAWVSGMMIFVGALVICFLR
HCMVTRL/IRL12		MRVACRRPHHLTYRHTAYTIIIFYI	9	SRTVWTIVLVCMACIVLFFAR
HCMVTRL/IRL13		MDWRFTVMWTILISALSESCNQTCS	3	
HCMVTRL14			3	
HCMVUL1		MGMQCNTKLLLPVALIPVVIIGT	9	HAVWAGVVSVALIALYMGSH
HCMVUL2	C		-	HAGWAAAVTVIMIYVLIHFNVPATLR
HCMVUL4		MVMMLRTWRLLPMVLLAAYCYCVFG	9	RGIFLITLVIWTVVWLKLLR
HCMVUL5			-	HTTWVTGFVLLGLLTLFASLFR
HCMVUL6		MHAKMNGWAGVRLVTHCLNTRSRTY	10	LAFTYGSWGVAMLLFAAVMVLVD
HCMVUL7			11	HLALVGVIVFIALIVVCIMGWWK
HCMVUL8			3	HYSWMLIAIILIFIIICLR
HCMVUL9		MYRYTWLLWWITILLRIQQFFYQWWK	5	HTMWIIPLVIVTTIIVLICFK
HCMVUL10		MLLRYITFHREKVLYLAIACFFGIY	3	HSAWILIVIIIIVILFFFK
HCMVUL11		MLLVFLGPVNSFMKGIRDVGFGKPP	5	HALWLAVVIVIIIIIFYFR
HCMVUL12	C	MLWAHCGRFLRYHLLPLLLCRLPFL	1	
HCMVUL13		MWSRVVFLRSSETQTGMGGGRLPPL	2	KIGLLAAGSVALTSLCHLLCYWCSE
HCMVUL14		MERRRGTVPLGWVFFVLCLSASSSC	2	DIVLVSAITLFFFLLALR
HCMVUL16		MMTMWCLTLFVLWMLRVVGMHVLRY	8	RYNTMTISSVLLALLCALLFAFLH
HCMVUL18		MLGIRAMLVMLDYYWIQLITNNDTR	13	RYMYLFSVSCAGITGTVSIILVSLSLLICYYR
HCMVUL20			13	HWALLSICTVAAGSIALLSLFCILLIGLR
HCVMUL37EX3	C	MSPVYNLLGSVGLLAFWYFSYRWI	16	
HCMVUL37EX1	C	MNKFSNTRIGFTCAVMAPRTLILTV	-	
HCMVUL40	C		3	ETWAMYTVGILALGSFSSFYSQIAR
HCMVUL42	C		1?	KWTFALLVVAILGIIFLAVVFTVVINR
HCMVUL50	C		2	RFATLGPLVLALLVLALLWR
HCMVUL55	C	MESRIWCLVVCVNLCIVCLGAAVSS	21	KNPFGAFTIILVAIAVVIITYLIYTR
HCMVUL67		MVRSLEEIIYIIYSDDSVVNISLAS	3	
HCMVUL73		MEWNTLVLGLLVLSVVAESSGNNSS	3	
HCMVUL74	C	MGRKEMMVRDVPKMVFLISISFLLV	20	ELSLSSFAAWWTMLNALILMGAFCIVLR

Gene	C	N-terminal		C-terminal
HCMVUL75	C	MRPGLPPYLTVFTVYLLSHLPSQRY	5	RLLMMSVYALSAIIGIYLLYR
HCMVUL118	C		8	RLLAYGVLAFLVFMVIILLYVTYMLAR
HCMVUL119	C	MCSVLAIALVVALLGDMHGVKSST	4	RAFMIVILTQVVFVVFIINASFIWSWTFR
HCMVUL120	C	MYRAGVTLLVVAVVSLGRWDVVTMA	9?	DLGLLYAVCLILSFSIVAALWK
HCMVUL121	C	MWGCGWSRIIVLLPLMCMALMARGT	1	DTYPTATALCGTLVVGIVLCLSLASTVR
HCMVUL124		MERNSLLVCQLLCLVARAAATSTAQ	.3	RIFMIVCLWCVWICLSTFLIAMFH
HCMVUL129	C	MLRLLLRHHFHCLLLCAVWATPCLA	-	
HCMVUL130	C	MPAPRGLLRATFLVLVAFGLLLHID	3	EIMKVLAILFYIVTGTSIFSFIAVLIAVVYSSCCK
HCMVUL132	C	MNNLWKAWVGLWTSMGPLIRLPDGI	3?	HVAWTIVFYSINTLLVLFIVYVTVD
HCMVUS2	C	MKPVLVLAILAVLFLRLADSVPRPL	1	RTLLVYLFSLVVLVLLTVGVSAR
HCMVUS3	C	MDLLIRLGFLLMCALPTPGERSSRD	1	HGFFAVTLYLCCGITLLVVILALLCSITYE
HCMVUS6	C	MRIQLLVATLVASIVATRVEDMAT	1	RWLTIILYFMWTYLVTLLQYCIVR
HCMVUS7	C	MRRWLLVGLGCCWVTLAHAGNPY	2?	LELGVVIAICMAMVLLGYVLAR
HCMVUS8	C	MILWSPSTCSFFWHWCLIAVSVLSS	2	HVALFSFGVQVACCVYLR
HCMVUS9	C	MLRRGSLRNPLAICLLWWLGVVAAA	2	DYGAILKIYFGLFCGACVITR
HCMVUS10	C		2	
HCMVUS11	C	MNLVMLILALWAPVAGSMPELSLTL	1	
HCMVUS34	C	MNLEQLINVLGLLWIAARAVSRVG	4	KSAQYTLMMVAVIQVFWGLYVK

fragment and show the gene for a 28-kDa protein encoded by a late 1.3-kb RNA. MARTINEZ et al. (1989) and MARTINEZ and ST. JEOR (1986) mapped a 25-kDa protein to the same locus and assigned a 1.6-kDa late mRNA as the message. These RNAs are likely to be initiated from one or both of two TATA boxes proximal to HCMV-UL99. An HCMV Towne 1.4-kb late mRNA localized to this region may also denote HCMV-UL99 (PANDE et al. 1988). However, the Towne protein migrates as a 32-kDa protein. If the same frame is in fact being used, nontrivial explanations for the difference could be invoked at the genetic, transcriptional, and protein-processing levels. It is interesting to note that a minor 27-kDa species was detected by PANDE et al. (1988) in infected cells and virions.

An example of a phosphoprotein gene that appears not to be conserved between HCMVs Towne and AD169 was mapped and sequenced from passage 36 of HCMV Towne (DAVIS et al. 1984; DAVIS and HUANG 1985). This gene encodes an abundant late transcript, and immunological evidence suggests that its product is a 67-kDa nonglycosylated phosphoprotein found in virions. The sequenced fragment corresponds very approximately to a region of AD169 HindIII D beginning at about position 95 500. There appear to be significant differences between the two genomes in this region. These include numerous point and frameshift mutations and a deletion of 61 bp in Towne relative to AD169. A consequence of some of these differences is the disruption of the putative Towne reading frame in AD169, although a portion of the predicted phosphoprotein sequence is preserved in HCMV-UL65. The reported sequence was not determined fully on both strands, and not all sequenced fragments were shown to be contiguous. Hence further comparative sequence analysis and transcript mapping will be necessary before these findings can be interpreted unambiguously, particularly as the equivalent region in AD169 contains some potential splice sites. A gene which is posttranscriptionally regulated by an mRNA 3'-end processing event was partially sequenced and shown to contain a potential stem-loop structure (GOINS and STINSKI 1986). This sequence maps to positions 96 753–97 076, and may therefore correspond to the 3' end of a transcription unit spanning HCMV-UL65. The putative stem-loop structure in the Towne sequence is conserved in AD169, although there are three deletions relative to AD169 clustering in the 3'-terminal 25 nucleotides of the published sequence.

6.8 Surface Glycoproteins

The importance of glycoproteins as surface antigens has made the major HCMV glycoproteins a focus for characterization and functional studies. A total of 54 reading frames have now been found in the sequence that have charcteristics of glycoprotein genes or of exons of glycoprotein genes. These are presented in Table 3, which shows the predicted signal sequences, the number of N-linked glycosylation sites, and the anchor sequences. Twenty-two of these frames lack either a signal or an anchor. In the following sections we consider two immunologically important glycoproteins, and two which have homology to host immunoglobulin superfamily proteins. Known IE glycoprotein genes and glycoprotein gene families are considered separately in Sects. 5 and 7 respectively.

6.8.1 Glycoproteins B and H

There are seven virion glycoproteins encoded by HSV-1 and one putative glycoprotein (US5) predicted from the sequence (McGEOCH et al. 1988a). Of these five have counterparts in the sequence of VZV (DAVISON and SCOTT 1986) and only two in the genome of EBV (BAER et al. 1984). In addition, EBV has the gp350/220 (BLLF1a, b), BILF1, and BLRF1 glycoproteins. The latter has a homolog in HCMV-UL73. Of the other herpesvirus glycoproteins, only homologs to gB (HCMV-UL55) (CRANAGE et al. 1986; KOUZARIDES et al. 1987b; MACH et al. 1986) and gH (HCMV-UL75) (CRANAGE et al. 1988; PACHL et al. 1989) have been found in the HCMV sequence, and so gB and gH are common to all of the well-studied herpesviruses. The conservation of gH in distantly related herpesviruses (GOMPELS et al. 1988b) and the production by an HSV-1 ts mutant of noninfectious virus lacking gH (DESAI et al. 1988) underpin the substantial body of immunological evidence that gH is essential for virus infectivity. Monoclonal antibodies to HCMV gH can neutralize virus in vitro unassisted by complement (RASMUSSEN et al. 1984; CRANAGE et al. 1988). Antibodies to gB are also able to neutralize virus in vitro, but require complement (CRANAGE et al. 1986). A virion envelope glycoprotein complex has been shown to contain gB, but the structural nature of this entity awaits definition (see, for example, FARRAR and GREENAWAY 1986; GRETCH et al. 1988a). The unmodified gB precursor in AD169 is predicted to be 102 kDa in size. This is processed and glycosylated to give a 145-kDa species which is proteolytically cleaved to produce a 55-kDa species, both of which can be detected in infected cells. However, the residual 90-kDa amino-terminal cleavage product is not detected (CRANAGE et al. 1986). The site of cleavage has been mapped to Arg_{450} in the gB of HCMV Towne and by analogy processing of the AD169 gB is likely to occur after Arg_{459} (SPAETE et al. 1988). These authors also compare the gene and protein sequences of gB and find identities of 94% and 95% respectively between the two HCMV strains. (A similar level of conservation is found between the gH sequences of these strains; PACHL et al. 1989.) There appear to be noteworthy differences in the kinetics of gB transcription in these two strains. The AD169 gB transcripts are produced late in infection (KOUZARIDES et al. 1987b) while the Towne gB mRNA is of the early class. However, in HCMV Towne infected cells gB is not detected immunologically until late in infection (RASMUSSEN et al. 1985b), implying that the two strains might use different strategies to achieve a similar result in the regulation of gB expression.

6.8.2 HLA Homolog

The identification of an HCMV glycoprotein with homology to class I major histocompatibility (MHC) antigens has implications for host-virus interactions (HCMV-UL18, BECK and BARRELL 1988). The crystal structure of a human class I histocompatibility molecule (HLA-A2) has been solved (BJORKMAN et al. 1987a), making it possible to predict that the HLA homolog is likely to have three extracellular domains analogous to the class I α1-, α2-, and α3-domains. The latter contains a β_2-microglobulin (β_2m)-binding loop which is partially conserved in the

HCMV sequence (BECK and BARRELL 1988). In cellular HLA molecules, the α3-domain and associated β_2m are both β-sandwich structures surmounted by the α1- and α2-domains which each contain a long α-helical region. A groove between these helices forms an antigen-binding cleft while surface residues may be involved in binding to a T-cell receptor (TCR) (BJORKMAN et al. 1987b). In contrast to the cellular sequences, both the α1- and α2-domains in the HCMV homolog are potentially heavily glycosylated as they contain a total of ten NXS/T motifs. Three or four of these motifs are located in the predicted helical and interhelical domains and hence might have a direct bearing on any antigen or TCR binding ability of the molecule. The protein expressed in vaccinia recombinants is in fact heavily glycosylated (H. BROWNE and A. MINSON, personal communication). In light of recent evidence that murine CMV can prevent the association of specific viral antigens with MHC (DEL VAL et al. 1989), a role for the HCMV HLA homolog in infected cells can be proposed. That is, the viral protein may compete with cellular HLA for the binding of one or more specific viral antigens, and consequently interfere with their presentation on the cell surface (TOWNSEND et al. 1989). While it is also possible that β_2m binding in the HCMV tegument may be due to the HLA homolog, no evidence for a link between the two has yet been presented (STANNARD 1989; GRUNDY et al. 1987a, b). Whatever the function of the protein, when co-expressed with β_2m from vaccinia vectors it is capable of associating with β_2m, which can then be detected on the cell surface (H. BROWNE and T. MINSON, personal communication). Finally, it should be noted that this gene does not have a homolog in the other sequenced human herpesviruses, and is found in a region which appears to be unique to β-herpesviruses.

6.8.3 T-Cell Receptor Homology

Even more provocative than the identification of a HLA homolog is the finding that HCMV-UL20, which is in close proximity to the HLA-like gene, encodes a protein with similarity to T-cell receptor γ-chains (BECK and BARRELL, unpublished observations). However, the match is marginal in nature, and alignment of a single region with both the constant (Cγ) and variable (Vγ) TCRγ-regions is possible. The former alignment shows approximately 16% identity over 194 amino acids, while the latter has approximately 27% identity over 82 amino acids. Although the Cγ alignment matches four cysteines, two on each side of the transmembrane domain, the remainder of the alignment is less convincing. In contrast, the Vγ alignment contains at least three localized clusters of homology including a highly conserved cysteine residue. However, a disulfide bond formed within Vγ may not be conserved; in HCMV-UL20 the second cysteine residue is located in the putative transmembrane domain. It is clear that no conclusions can be drawn regarding the significance of this match on the basis of the alignment. As in the case of the HLA homolog, sequence data from wild-type isolates might clarify the situation. If HCMV-UL20 is in fact a TCR homolog, the virus could exploit the interaction between TCRγ and CD3 to infect T cells, which might parallel the interaction of CD4 with the HIV gp120 protein (BORST et al. 1987; BRENNER et al. 1987). Furthermore, it is interesting to note that a feline retrovirus has been shown to encode a TCRβ-gene (FULTON et al. 1987).

7 Gene Families

In addition to gB and gH, several small glycoprotein genes were identified in HCMV, in US (WESTON and BARRELL 1986). These are arranged tandemly and tend to cluster as homologous blocks of reading frames, constituting a large proportion of the gene families found in HCMV. Interestingly, the HSV US glycoprotein genes are also clustered (DAVISON and MCGEOCH 1986; MCGEOCH et al. 1988a). We currently recognize nine sets of homologous genes in the AD169 genome. There are three pairs (UL25 and UL35; UL82 and UL83; and US2 and 3) and six larger groups. Of the latter, three occur in US where they account for a total of at least 21 genes (WESTON and BARRELL 1986); one family occurs in UL and RL; and two families are partitioned between the long and the short regions of the genome (Table 1). The discovery of redundant protein coding sequences outside repeat regions was unexpected and presents a contrast to those single genes encoding multiple products (for example, see Sects. 6.4 and 6.5). Their presence also appears to contradict the virally frugal gene layout of HCMV. As individual family members are likely to have subtle differences in function, this paradox may be difficult to resolve. The characteristics of four gene families are discussed below. Proteins have been recognized for three of these, while the fourth is homologous to a class of cellular receptors. The evolutionary implications of these findings are discussed in Sect. 8.

7.1 The RL11 Family

This family comprises fourteen members distributed in the long repeats and a portion of UL adjacent to TRL (Table 1; Fig. 1). The sequences are characterized by a motif which resembles the cellular Thy-1 in a region which is conserved with some other members of the immunoglobulin superfamily (C.A. HUTCHISON III, unpublished observations). The members of the RL11 Family are predicted to be membrane glycoproteins (Table 3). This prediction has been substantiated by the immunological detection of the Towne UL4-equivalent protein in infected cells and virions (CHANG et al. 1989a). The detected 48 kd protein is expressed during the early phase of infection, and its presence in virions has led to its classification as an early structural glycoprotein (CHANG et al. 1989a). Its published amino acid sequence is 84% identical to UL4 over 150 amino acids. Multiple alignment of the RL11 family suggests that UL4 (which does not contain an anchor sequence) may be spliced to UL5 (which has an anchor but no signal or N-glycosylation sites), as their respective RL11 homologous regions appear to dovetail somewhat. However, splicing was not observed in transcript mapping experiments (CHANG et al. 1989b). Nevertheless, CHANG et al. (1989a) detect a protein reduced in size from 48 kd to 27 kd protein when infected cells are treated with an inhibitor of N-linked glycosylation, although the theoretical size of UL4 alone is approximately 17 kd. While this difference could be attributable to other post-translational modifications, it is noteworthy that the theoretical size of RL11, which is homologous to both UL4 and UL5, is approximately 27 kd. The mapped transcripts, which are initiated from three different promoters, also contain the UL5 reading frame. Hence it may be of interest to further characterize the 27 kDA protein. UL8 is truncated similarly to UL5, and therefore is also a candidate for splicing. As both these frames also contain KOZAK consensus ATG codons, a potential exists for the expression of this gene family to be regulated in a complex manner.

7.2 The US6 Family

This family corresponds to family 2 described by WESTON and BARRELL (1986) and is characterized by two areas of sequence homology, the second of which (region 2 (WESTON and BARRELL 1986)) is less well conserved. The region 1 core motif can be defined as C(VY)x(DQKR) (7–10) WxxxGxF where the bracketed residues are alternatives and x is any residue. The region 2 motif is characterized by cysteine and proline residues: PCxxC (4–6) CxPxxxxPWxP. The six members of this family are predicted to be membrane glycoproteins (Tables 1 and 3). GRETCH et al. (1988b) have recently used a MAb to demonstrate that this family correlates with the gp47–52 virion envelope glycoprotein complex they described previously (GRETCH et al. 1988a). Northern hybridization revealed three early transcripts from this region, two of which were minor species. The 1.6-kb size of the major transcript was consistent with initiation from the HCMV-US11 (HXLF1) TATA box, and in vitro translation experiments suggested it was bicistronic in nature. GRETCH et al. (1988a) suggest on the basis of these data and amino acid composition analysis that the main constituents of gp47–52 might be HCMV-US10 and US11 proteins. However, no direct correlation was established between the abundance of the putative transcript and the composition of gp47–52.

7.3 The US22 Family

This family is distributed in UL, US and RS and sequences for eight of the thirteen recognized members have been published, including the family 4 members described by WESTON and BARRELL (1986). Genes attributed to this family contain one or more of three sequence motifs (KOUZARIDES et al. 1988). The first motif (ooCCxxxLxxoG, where o is any hydrophobic residue and x any residue) is found in all of the members except IRS/TRS1 and UL28. Interestingly, in HCMV-UL36 the junction of exons 1 and 2 occurs immediately before the motif (KOUZARIDES et al. 1988). As HCMV-UL42 ends within the motif (FLCCDKFLPG- COO⁻), it seems possible that this gene, and perhaps other members of the family apart from HCMV-UL36, encode spliced transcripts. The remainder of the pattern comprises two motifs which are largely hydrophobic and may overlap in function. The IRS/TRS1 genes, identical over most of their length, diverge shortly after the third motif. Apart from the conserved motifs, several of these sequences contain short runs of charged residues in their carboxy-terminal domains, and 6 of the 12 members of the US22 gene family have at least 1 N-linked glycosylation site. However, there does not appear to be any obvious correlation between these latter features. The only present correlation between this gene family and viral proteins comes from the identification of the HCMV-US22 gene product ICP22. This is an early protein localizing in the nucleus which is also detectable in the cytoplasm and may be secreted from infected cells (MOCARSKI et al. 1988). Interestingly, the MAb used identifying US22 does not appear to recognize any of its homologs.

7.4 The G-Protein Coupled Receptor (GCR) Family

Several HCMV-reading frames, mostly located in US, are predicted to be integral membrane proteins capable of spanning the membrane several times (Table 1). All of these have seven potential membrane-spanning regions. Three of the reading frames, HCMV-US27 and HCMV-US28 (originally named HHRF2 and HHRF3; WESTON and BARRELL 1986), and HCMV-UL33, show homology to the opsin family of cell surface receptors (CHEE et al., submitted). Members of this diverse family of receptors

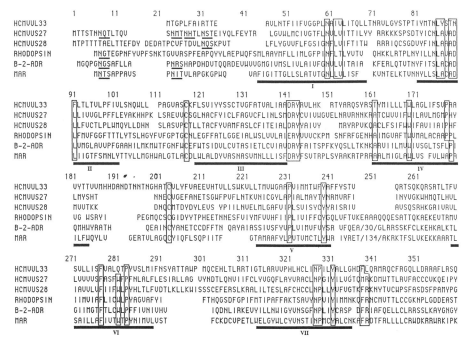

Fig. 4. An alignment of the three HCMV G-protein-coupled receptor homologs with bovine rhodopsin (NATHANS and HOGNESS 1983), human β-2-adrenergic receptor (B-2-ADR) (KOBILKA et al. 1987), and porcine muscarinic acetylcholine receptor (MAR) (KUBO et al. 1986). The NXT/S motifs are *underlined* in the N-terminal extracellular domain and identities which correspond in at least five of the six sequences are *boxed*. The seven membrane-spanning helical domains are indicated by *numbered bars* beneath the alignment. Each transmembrane domain and its disposition is defined by a motif unique within the sequence. The alignment has been truncated within the cytoplasmic C-terminal domains which possess receptor-specific functions, and sections of 30 and 134 amino acids have been excised from the B-2-ADR and MAR sequences respectively beginning at position 248. The two conserved cysteine residues at alignment positions 117 and 203 have been shown to be essential for function in bovine rhodopsin (KARNIK et al. 1988)

transduce different signals in a variety of systems, and have roles in vision, olfaction, memory and learning, and regulation of the circulatory system, among others (DOHLMANN et al. 1987; NATHANS 1987). The best-known subgroups of this family are the rhodopsins which absorb light via bound 11-*cis*-retinal, the β-adrenergic receptors which binds catecholamine hormones, and the muscarinic acetylcholine receptors. All of the above transduce signals through the membrane by activating G proteins. HCMV-US27, US28, and UL33 show the same membrane-spanning topography, are of similar size (362, 323, and 390 amino acids respectively), and are probably unspliced. US27 and US28 also have N-linked glycosylation sites at the N-terminus in common with the cellular members of the family. Apart from the overall similarity there is homology at the amino acid level mostly in and around the membrane-spanning sequences. An alignment of these sequences is shown in Fig. 4. The homology consists of short motifs that can uniquely define each membrane-spanning segment. At present the function of these genes is unknown. However, the downstream signal amplification by many of these receptors involves cAMP synthesis, which is suggestive in light of the presence of cAMP-responsive elements in the major immediate-early gene enhancer (Sect. 5.1).

8 Relationships to α and γ-Herpesvirus Genomes

The accumulated sequence data have begun to provide a broad evolutionary view of the herpesvirus family as a whole (HONESS 1984; HONESS et al. 1989). One feature in the evolution of herpesviruses is the movement of gene blocks within the genome, resulting in new arrangements of genes and presumably the disruption and formation of genes at recombinatorial junctions. Figure 5 shows the relationships of conserved sequences between the long unique regions of the sequenced human herpesviruses. The relationships between these regions of VZV, EBV, and HSV-1 have been analyzed previously (DAVISON and TAYLOR 1987; MCGEOCH et al. 1988a; MCGEOCH 1987). A comparison of the gene layout in HCMV *Hin*dIII F to equivalent regions in EBV and HSV-1 has also been published (KOUZARIDES et al. 1987b). As can be seen from Fig. 5, while the gene layouts of EBV and the α-herpesviruses are grossly more similar to each other than to HCMV, there do not appear to be any large blocks of genes that are not conserved between all three of the herpesvirus families. This is consistent with the notion that a core of herpesvirus genes is common to, and helps to define, the herpesvirus type. It also suggests that the three families of herpesviruses have diverged to such an extent that at the genetic level little else than this core set of genes remains in common between them. However, at the protein sequence level HCMV is more closely related to EBV than the α-herpesviruses, while the genes within each block show widely varying levels of conservation, ranging to undetectable or nonexistent (Table 2). While sequence comparisons with other herpesviruses help in establishing cladistic relationships, the following distinctive features of the HCMV genome give additional clues to its evolutionary past:

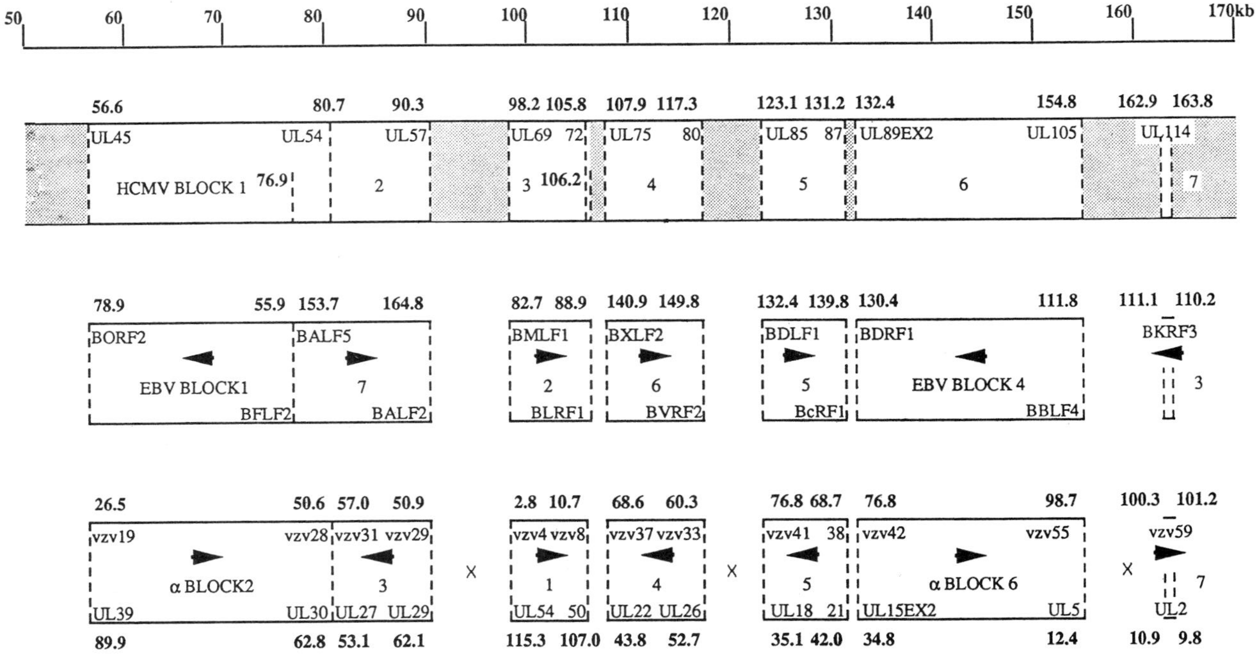

Fig. 5. Conserved blocks of sequence between HCMV and EBV, VZV, and HSV-1. The *uppermost map* represents a section of the HCMV UL indicated by the scale at the top of the diagram. The *middle map* depicts regions of EBV conserved with HCMV, and the *lower map* shows VZV and HSV-1 homologies, also to HCMV. Only the HCMV map is drawn to scale. All homologies found so far with the α- and γ-herpesviruses are located within the *unshaded* sections of the HCMV UL. The approximate boundary positions of the homology blocks within their respective genomes are marked in *boldtype* in kilobase pairs (positions are taken from Table 1 and BAER et al. 1984; DAVISON and SCOTT 1986; MCGEOCH et al. 1988a). Note that these numbers represent only the termini of the endmost detected homologous frames in each genome, and that some of these homologies are tentative (Table 2). The names of the frames are given. The orientation of each of the blocks in EBV and VZV (but not HSV-1) is shown relative to their published maps (BEAR et al. 1984; DAVISON and SCOTT 1986); *rightward arrowheads* denote collinearity. The order of the blocks within each genome is shown by a *block number*; these read from left to right across the genome in ascending order. Three of the five locations of nonhomologous reading frames found between the UL regions of HSV-1 and VZV are marked in the lower map (x) (MCGEOCH et al. 1988a)

The genes in HCMV that are conserved in the other herpesvirus families all appear to lie between approximately 50 to 170 kb in UL on the prototype genome. In contrast the extended HCMV gene families and the majority of the glycoprotein genes lie within US and in UL at left hand end of the prototype genome. Members of two families (the RL11 and US22 families) occur in RL and RS.

Two families (the US22 and GCR families) are partitioned between the short and the long regions of the genome. It also seems possible that the RL11, US2, and US6 families, together with HCMV-US34, are all members of a HCMV gene "super-family" which is also partitioned between the short and long regions. These sequences all encode glycoproteins (or putative glycoprotein exons) which are mostly in the range of 200 amino acids in length. Multiple sequence alignment reveals short regions of amino acid homology between US2 and US3 and some members of the RL11 family. For example, the RL11 family anchor sequences are characterized by the motif HxxW, which is also seen in US2 (Table 3). The distinguishing motifs of the RL11 and US6 families also show some similarity, and may also be echoed in HCMV-US34:

RL11 Family
  motif: Cxx (QEKR)   (7–10)   W   xxx   GxF
US6 Family
  motif: Cxx (NQEKTY) (4–6)   (YFLI) Nx (ST) xxxx   GxY
HCMV-US34: CLAE   VGVA   NAT   FLSRFNV GDF

Finally, the majority of the genes in families are present as tandemly repeated copies. These observations suggest that the HCMV gene repertoire has been expanding by gene duplication and divergence, a process which may be mediated by the HCMV DNA replication machinery (WEBER et al. 1988) and which may be related to expansion and contraction of repeat sequences (WHITTON and CLEMENTS 1984; DAVISON and McGEOCH 1986). Furthermore, there appears to have been at least one recombination event involving the long and short regions of HCMV which led to the distribution of gene families between both regions. A possible scenario for such an event might be an internal duplication of a terminal segment leading to the conversion of an ancestral non-inverting genome to a four-isomer genome. Genes partitioned between the repeats of the two new subsegments might then diverge, together with the expansion and contraction of the repeats. The characterization of other betaherpesvirus sequences may help to clarify the evolutionary history of HCMV, and it will be of interest to see if the propensity of HCMV for gene duplication is a general charcteristic of the β-herpesviruses.

9 Perspectives

This project is a contribution to a set of genomic sequences which now represents the three main branches of the herpesvirus family. The prior sequencing of EBV, VZV, and HSV-1 has greatly facilitated the analysis of the HCMV genome, and features which unify this highly divergent group of viruses are now coming into focus at the genetic level. The sequences have facilitated the correlation of biological and genetic experiments, and allowed much of this work to be generalized. The growing body of relational knowledge should make it increasingly informative to begin the characterization of herpesvirus genomes by sequencing. These data will continue to provide predictions which can be tested, and which promise to shed further light on the herpesviruses and their eukaryotic environment.

Acknowledgments. We thank Jon Oram and Peter Greenaway for providing the *Hind*III clones used in the sequence analysis and Bernard Fleckenstein for providing the cosmid clones used for determining the overlaps of the *Hind*III sites. We are grateful to Tony Minson and Helena Browne for advice and for making available results prior to publication, and to Mark Stinski for comments on parts of the manuscript. M.C. thanks the Commonwealth Scholarships Commission for support.

References

Addison C, Rixon FJ, Palfreyman JW, O'Hara M, Preston VG (1984) Characterisation of a herpes simplex virus type 1 mutant which has a temperature-sensitive defect in penetration of cells and assembly of capsids. Virology 138: 246–259

Akrigg A, Wilkinson GWG, Oram JD (1985) The structure of the major immediate early gene of human cytomegalovirus strain AD169. Virus Res 2: 107–121

Anders DG, Gibson W (1988) Location, transcript analysis, and partial nucleotide sequence of the cytomegalovirus gene encoding an early DNA-binding protein with similarities to ICP8 of herpes simplex virus type 1. J Virol 62: 1364–1372

Avertt DR, Lubbers C, Elion GB, Spector T (1983) Ribonucleotide reductase induced by herpes simplex virus type 1. Characterisation of a distinct enzyme. J Biol Chem 258: 9831–9838

Baer R, Bankier AT, Biggin MD, Deininger PL, Farrell PJ, Gibson TJ, Hatfull G, et al. (1984) DNA sequence and expression of the B95-8 Epstein-Barr virus genome. Nature 310: 207–211

Bairoch A (1988) Swiss-Prot protein sequence data bank release 8.0. Department de Biochimie Medicale, Centre Medical Universitaire, Geneva

Bankier AT, Barrell BG (1989) Sequencing single strand DNA using the chain termination method. In: Ward S, Howe C (eds) Nucleic acids sequencing: a practical approach. IRL, Oxford (in press)

Bankier AT, Weston KM, Barrell BG (1988) Random cloning and sequencing by the M13/dideoxynucleotide chain termination method. Methods Enzymol 155: 51–93

Batterson W, Furlong D, Roizman B (1983) Molecular genetics of herpes simplex virus VIII. Further characterization of a temperature-sensitive mutant defective in release of viral DNA and in other stages of the viral reproductive cycle. J Virol 45: 397–407

Beck S, Barrell BG (1988) Human cytomegalovirus encodes a glycoprotein homologous to MHC class-I antigens. Nature 331: 269–272

Benko DM, Haltiwanger RS, Hart GW, Gibson W (1988) Virion basic phosphoprotein from human cytomegalovirus contains O-linked N-acetyl glucosamine. Proc Natl Acad Sci USA 85: 2573–2577

Biron KK, Fyfe JA, Stanat SC, Leslie LK, Sorrell JB, Lambe CU, Coen DM (1986) A human cytomegalovirus mutant resistant to the nucleoside analog 9-{[2-hydroxy-1-(hydroxymethyl)ethoxy]methyl} guanine (BW B759U) induces reduced levels of BW B759U triphosphate. Proc Natl Acad Sci USA 83: 8769–8773

Bjorkman PJ, Saper MA, Samraoui B, Bennett WS, Strominger JL, Wiley DC (1987a) Structure of the human class I histocompatibility antigen, HLA-A2. Nature 329: 506–512

Bjorkman PJ, Saper MA, Samraoui B, Bennett WS, Strominger JL, Wiley DC (1987b) The foreign antigen binding site and T-cell recognition regions of class I histocompatibility antigens. Nature 329: 512–518

164   M. S. Chee et al.

Borst J, van de Griend RJ, van Oostveen JW, Ang S-L, Melief CJ, Seidman JG, Bolhuis RLH (1987) A T-cell receptor γ/CD3 complex found on cloned functional lymphocytes. Nature 325: 683–688

Boshart M, Weber F, Jahn G, Dorsch-Hasler K, Fleckenstein B, Schaffner W (1985) A very strong enhancer is located upstream of an immediate early gene of human cytomegalovirus. Cell 41: 521–530

Brenner S (1987) Phosphotransferase sequence homology. Nature 329: 21

Brenner MB, McLean J, Scheft H, Riberdy J, Ang S-L, Seidman JG, Devlin P, Krangel MS (1987) Two forms of the T-cell receptor γprotein found on peripheral blood cytotoxic T lymphocytes. Nature 325: 689–694

Chang C-P, Vesole DH, Nelson J, Oldstone MBA, Stinski MF (1989a) Identification and expression of a human cytomegalovirus early glycoprotein. J Virol 63: 3330–3337

Chang C-P, Malone CL, Stinski MF (1989b) A human cytomegalovirus early gene has three inducible promoters that are regulated differentially at various times after infection. J Virol 63: 281–290

Chee MS, Lawrence GL, Barrell BG (1989a) Alpha-, beta-, and gammaherpesviruses encode a putative phosphotransferase. J Gen Virol 70 (in press)

Chee MS, Rudolph S-A, Plachter B, Barrell BG, Jahn G (1989b) Identification of the major capsid protein gene of human cytomegalovirus. J Virol 63: 1345–1353

Chee MS, Satchwell SC, Preddie E, Weston KM, Barrell BG. Human cytomegalovirus encodes three G-protein coupled receptor homologues. Submitted for publication.

Cherrington JM, Mocarski ES (1989) Human cytomegalovirus ie1 transactivates the α promoter-enhancer via an 18-base-pair repeat element. J Virol 63: 1435–1440

Chou J, Roizman B (1989) Characterization of DNA sequence-common and sequence-specific proteins binding to cis-acting sites for cleavage of the terminal a sequence of the herpes simplex virus 1 genome. J Virol 63: 1059–1068

Clark BR, Zaia JA, Balce-Directo L, Ting Y-P (1984) Isolation and partial chemical characterization of a 64,000-dalton glycoprotein of human cytomegalovirus. J Virol 49: 279–282

Costa RH, Draper KG, Kelly TJ, Wagner EK (1985) An unusual spliced herpes simplex virus type 1 transcript with sequence homology to Epstein-Barr virus DNA. J Virol 54: 317–328

Cranage MP, Kouzarides T, Bankier AT, Satchwell SC, Weston KW, Tomlinson P, Barrell BG, et al. (1986) Identification of the human cytomegalovirus glycoprotein B gene and induction of neutralizing antibodies via its expression in recombinant vaccinia virus. EMBO J 5: 3057–3063

Cranage MP, Smith GL, Bell SE, Hart H, Brown C, Bankier AT, Tomlinson P, et al. (1988) Identification and expression of a human cytomegalovirus glycoprotein with homology to the Epstein-Barr virus BXLF2 product, varicella-zoster virus gpIII, and herpes simplex virus type 1 glycoprotein H. J Virol 62: 1416–1422

Crute JJ, Mocarski ES, Lehman IE (1988) A DNA helicase induced by herpes simplex virus type 1. Nucleic Acids Res 16: 6585–6596

Crute JJ, Tsurumi T, Zhu L, Weller SK, Olivo PD, Challberg MD, Mocarski ES, Lehman IR (1989) Herpes simplex virus 1 helicase-primase: a complex of three herpes-encoded gene products. Proc. Natl Acad Sci USA 86: 2186–2189

Davis MG, Huang E-S (1985) Nucleotide sequence of a human cytomegalovirus DNA fragment encoding a 67-kilodalton phosphorylated viral protein. J Virol 56: 7–11

Davis MG, Mar E-C, Wu Y-M, Huang E-S (1984) Mapping and expression of a human cytomegalovirus major viral protein. J Virol 52: 129–135

Davison AJ, McGeoch DJ (1986) Evolutionary comparisons of the S segments in the genomes of herpes simplex virus type 1 and varicella-zoster virus. J Gen Virol 67: 597–611

Davison AJ, Scott JE (1986) The complete DNA sequence of varicella-zoster virus. J Gen Virol 67: 1759–1816

Davison AJ, Taylor P (1987) Genetic relations between varicella-zoster virus and Epstein-Barr virus. J Gen Virol 68: 1067–1079

Del Val M, Munch K, Reddehase MJ, Koszinowski UH (1989) Presentation of CMV immediate-early antigen to cytolytic T lymphocytes is selectively prevented by viral genes expressed in the early phase. Cell 58: 305–315

DeMarchi JM (1981) Human cytomegalovirus DNA: restriction enzyme cleavage maps and map locations for immediate-early, early, and late RNAs. Virology 114: 23–38

DeMarchi JM (1983) Post-transcriptional control of human cytomegalovirus gene expression. Virology 124: 390–402

Depto AS, Stenberg RM (1989) Regulated expression of the human cytomegalovirus pp65 gene: octamer sequence in the promoter is required for activation by viral gene products. J Virol 63: 1232–1238

Desai PJ, Schaffer PA, Minson AC (1988) Excretion of non-infectious virus particles lacking glycoprotein H by a temperature-sensitive mutant of herpes simplex virus type 1: evidence that gH is essential for virion infectivity. J Gen Virol 69: 1147–1156

Dohlman HG, Caron MG, Lefkowitz RJ (1987) A family of receptors coupled to guanine nucleotide regulatory proteins. Biochemistry 26: 2657–2664

Dorsch-Hasler K, Keil GM, Weber F, Jasin M, Schaffner W, Koszinowski UH (1985) A long and complex enhancer activates transcription of the gene coding for the highly abundant immediate early mRNA in murine cytomegalovirus. Proc Natl Acad Sci USA 82: 8325–8329

Engstrom Y, Francke U (1985) Assignment of the structural gene for subunit M1 of human ribonucleotide reductase to the short arm of chromosome 11. Exp Cell Res 158: 477–483

Farrar GH, Greenaway PJ (1986) Characterization of glycoprotein complexes present in human cytomegalovirus envelopes. J Gen Virol 67: 1469–1473

Ferguson MAJ, Williams AF (1988) Cell-surface anchoring of proteins via glycosyl-phosphatidylinositol structures. Annu Rev Biochem 57: 285–320

Fickenscher H, Stamminger T, Ruger R, Fleckenstein B (1989) The role of a repetitive palindromic sequence element in the human cytomegalovirus immediate early enhancer. J Gen Virol 70: 107–123

Fleckenstein B, Muller I, Collins J (1982) Cloning of the complete human cytomegalovirus genome in cosmids. Gene 18: 39–46

Fulton R, Forrest D, McFarlane R, Onions D, Neil JC (1987) Retroviral transduction of T-cell antigen receptor β-chain and *myc* genes. Nature 326: 190–194

Geballe AP, Mocarski ES (1988) Translational control of cytomegalovirus gene expression is mediated by upstream AUG codons. J Virol 62: 3334–3340

Geballe AP, Spaete RR, Mocarski ES (1986a) A *cis*-acting element within the 5' leader of a cytomegalovirus β transcript determines kinetic class. Cell 46: 865–872

Geballe AP, Leach FS, Mocarski EM (1986b) Regulation of cytomegalovirus late gene expression: γ genes are controlled by posttranscriptional events. J Virol 57: 864–874

George DG, Barker WC, Hunt LT (1986) The protein identification resource (PIR). Nucleic Acids Res 14: 11–15

Ghazal P, Lubon H, Fleckenstein B, Hennighausen L (1987) Binding of transcription factors and creation of a large nucleoprotein complex on the human cytomegalovirus enhancer. Proc Natl Acad Sci USA 84: 3658–3662

Ghazal P, Lubon H, Hennighausen L (1988) Specific interactions between transcription factors and the promoter-regulatory region of the human cytomegalovirus major immediate-early gene. J Virol 62: 1076–1079

Gibson W (1983) Protein counterparts of human and simian cytomegalovirus. Virology 128: 391–406

Gibson T, Stockwell P, Ginsburg M, Barrell BG (1984) Homology between two EBV early genes and HSV ribonucleotide reductase and 38K genes. Nucleic Acids Res 12: 5087–5099

Goins WF, Stinski MF (1986) Expression of a human cytomegalovirus late gene is posttranscriptionally regulated by a 3'-end-processing event occurring exclusively late after infection. Mol Cell Biol 6: 4202–4213

Gompels UA, Craxton MA, Honess RW (1988a) Conservation of gene organization in the lymphotropic herpesviruses herpesvirus saimiri and Epstein-Barr virus. J Virol 62: 757–767

Gompels UA, Craxton MA, Honess RW (1988b) Conservation of glycoprotein H (gH) in herpesviruses: nucleotide sequence of the gH gene from herpesvirus saimiri. J Gen Virol 69: 2819–2829

Greenaway PJ, Wilkinson GWG (1987) Nucleotide sequence of the most abundantly transcribed early gene of human cytomegalovirus strain AD169. Virus Res 7: 17–31

Gretch DR, Kari B, Rasmussen L, Gehrz RC, Stinski MF (1988a) Identification and characterization of three distinct families of glycoprotein complexes in the envelopes of human cytomegalovirus. J Virol 62: 875–881

Gretch DR, Kari B, Gehrz RC, Stinski MF (1988b) A multigene family encodes the human cytomegalovirus glycoprotein complex gcII (gp47–52 complex). J Virol 62: 1956–1962

Grundy JE, McKeating JA, Griffiths PD (1987a) Cytomegalovirus strain AD169 binds β_2 microglobulin in vitro after release from cells. J Gen Virol 68: 777–784

Grundy JE, McKeating JA, Ward PJ, Sanderson AR, Griffiths PD (1987b) β_2 Microglobulin enhances the infectivity of cytomegalovirus and when bound to the virus enables class 1 HLA molecules to be used as a virus receptor. J Gen Virol 68: 793–803

Heilbronn R, Jahn G, Burkle A, Freese U-K, Fleckenstein B, zur Hausen H (1987) Genomic localization, sequence analysis, and transcription of the putative human cytomegalovirus DNA polymerase gene. J Virol 61: 119–124

Hennighausen L, Fleckenstein B (1986) Nuclear factor 1 interacts with five DNA elements in the promoter region of the human cytomegalovirus major immediate early gene. EMBO J 5: 1367–1371

Hermiston TW, Malone CL, Witte PR, Stinski MF (1987) Identification and characterization of the human cytomegalovirus immediate-early region 2 gene that stimulates gene expression from an inducible promoter. J Virol. 61: 3214–3221

Hodgman TC (1988) A new superfamily of replicative proteins. Nature 333: 22–23

Honess RW (1984) Herpes simplex and the 'herpes complex': diverse observations and a unifying hypothesis. J Gen Virol 65: 2077–2107

Honess RW, Bodemer W, Cameron KR, Niller H-H, Fleckenstein B, Randall RE (1986) The A + T-rich genome of herpesvirus saimiri contains a highly conserved gene for thymidylate synthase. Proc Natl Acad Sci USA 83: 3604–3608

Honess RW, Gompels UA, Barrell BG, Craxton M, Cameron KR, Staden R, Chang Y-N, Hayward GS (1989) Deviations from expected frequencies of CpG dinucleotides in herpesvirus DNAs may be diagnostic of differences in the states of their latent genomes. J Gen Virol 70: 837–855

Hunninghake GW, Monick MM, Liu B, Stinski MF (1989) The promoter-regulatory region of the major immediate-early gene of human cytomegalovirus responds to T-lymphocyte stimulation and contains functional cyclic AMP-response elements. J Virol 63: 3026–3033

Hutchinson NI, Tocci MJ (1986) Characterization of a major early gene from the human cytomegalovirus long inverted repeat; predicted amino acid sequence of a 30-kDa protein encoded by the 1.2 kb mRNA. Virology 155: 172–182

Hutchinson NI, Sondermeyer RT, Tocci MJ (1986) Organization and expression of the major genes from the long inverted repeat of the human cytomegalovirus genome. Virology 155: 160–171

Irmiere A, Gibson W (1983) Isolation and characterization of a noninfectious virion-like particle released from cells infected with human strains of cytomegalovirus. Virology 130: 118–133

Irmiere A, Gibson W (1985) Isolation of human cytomegalovirus intranuclear capsids, characterization of their protein constituents, and demonstration that the B-capsid assembly protein is also abundant in noninfectious enveloped particles. J Virol 56: 277–283

Jahan N, Razzaque A, Brady J, Rosenthal LJ (1989) The human cytomegalovirus mtrII colinear region in strain Tanaka is transformation defective. J Virol 63: 2866–2869

Jahn G, Knust E, Schmolla H, Sarre T, Nelson JA, McDougall JK, Fleckenstein B (1984) Predominant immediate-early transcripts of human cytomegalovirus AD169. J Virol 49: 363–370

Jahn G, Kouzarides T, Mach M, Scholl, B-C, Plachter B, Traupe B, Preddie E, et al. (1987) Map position and nucleotide sequence of the gene for the large structural phosphoprotein of human cytomegalovirus. J Virol 61: 1358–1367

Jeang K-T, Hayward GS (1983) A cytomegalovirus DNA sequence containing tracts of tandemly repeated CA dinucleotides hybridises to highly repetitive dispersed elements in mammalian cell genomes. Mol Cell Biol 3: 1389–1402

Jeang KT, Rawlins DR, Rosenfeld P, Shero JH, Kelly T, Hayward GS (1987) Multiple tandemly repeated binding sites for cellular nuclear factor 1 that surround the major immediate-early promoters of simian and human cytomegalovirus. J Virol 61: 1559–1570

Karnik SS, Sakmar TP, Chen H-B, Khorana HG (1988) Cysteine residues 110 and 187 are essential for the formation of correct structure in bovine rhodopsin. Proc Natl Acad Sci USA 85: 8459–8463

Keil GM, Ebeling-Keil A, Koszinowski UH (1987) Sequence and structural organization of murine cytomegalovirus immediate-early gene 1. J Virol 61: 1901–1908

Kobilka BK, Dixon RAF, Frielle T, Dohlman HG, Bolanowski MA, Sigal IS, Yang-Feng TL, et al. (1987) cDNA for the human β_2-adrenergic receptor: a protein with multiple membrane-spanning domains and encoded by a gene whose chromosomal location is shared with that of the receptor for platelet-derived growth factor. Proc Natl Acad Sci USA 84: 46–50

Kouzarides T, Bankier AT, Barrell BG (1983) Nucleotide sequence of the transforming region of human cytomegalovirus. Mol Biol Med 1: 47–58

Kouzarides T, Bankier AT, Satchwell SC, Weston K, Tomlinson P, Barrell BG (1987a) Sequence and transcription analysis of the human cytomegalovirus DNA polymerase gene. J Virol 61: 125–133

Kouzarides T, Bankier AT, Satchwell SC, Weston K, Tomlinson P, Barrell BG (1987b) Large-scale rearrangement of homologous regions in the genomes of HCMV and EBV. Virology 157: 397–413

Kouzarides T, Bankier AT, Satchwell SC, Preddie E, Barrell BG (1988) An immediate early gene of human cytomegalovirus encodes a potential membrane glycoprotein. Virology 165: 151–164

Kozak M (1981) Possible role of flanking nucleotides in recognition of the AUG initiator codon by eukaryotic ribosomes. Nucleic Acids Res 9: 5233–5252

Kozak M (1982) Analysis of ribosome binding sites from the s1 message of reovirus: initiation at the first and second AUG codons. J Mol Biol 156: 807–820

Kubo T, Fukuda K, Mikami A, Maeda A, Takahashi H, Mishina M, Haga T, et al. (1986) Cloning, sequencing and expression of complementary DNA encoding the muscarinic acetylcholine receptor. Nature 323: 411–416

Landini M-P, Michelson S (1988) Human cytomegalovirus proteins. Prog Med Virol 35: 152–185

Laniken H, Graslund A, Thelander L (1982) Induction of a new ribonucleotide reductase activity after infection of mouse L cells with pseudorabies virus. J Virol 41: 893–900

Leach FS, Mocarski ES (1989) Regulation of cytomegalovirus late-gene expression: differential use of three start sites in the transcriptional activation of ICP36 gene expression. J Virol 63: 1783–1791

Lee JY, Irmiere A, Gibson W (1988) Primate cytomegalovirus assembly: evidence that DNA packaging occurs subsequent to B capsid assembly. Virology 167: 87–96

Littler E, Zeuthen J, McBride AA, Trost-Sorensen E, Powell KL, Walsh-Arrand JE, Arrand JR (1986) Identification of an Epstein-Barr virus-coded thymidine kinase. EMBO J 5: 1959–1966

Mach M, Utz U, Fleckenstein B (1986) Mapping of the major glycoprotein gene of human cytomegalovirus. J Gen Virol 67: 1461–1467

Marschalek R, Amon-Bohm E, Stoerker J, Klages S, Fleckenstein B, Dingermann T (1989) CMER, an RNA encoded by human cytomegalovirus is most likely transcribed by RNA polymerase III. Nucleic Acids Res 17: 631–643

Martignetti JA (1987) Sequence analysis of HCMV. Dissertation, Cambridge University

Martinez J, St Jeor SC (1986) Molecular cloning and analysis of three cDNA clones homologous to human cytomegalovirus RNAs present during late infection. J Virol 60: 531–538

Martinez J, Lahijani RS, St Jeor SC (1989) Analysis of a region of the human cytomegalovirus (AD169) genome coding for a 25-kilodalton virion protein. J Virol 63: 233–241

McDonough SH, Spector DH (1983) Transcription in human fibroblasts permissively infected by human cytomegalovirus strain AD169. Virology 125: 31–46

McDonough SH, Staprans SI, Spector DH (1985) Analysis of the major transcripts encdoded by the long repeat of human cytomegalovirus strain AD169. J Virol 53: 711–718

McGeoch DJ (1985) On the predictive recognition of signal peptide sequences. Virus Res 3: 271–286

McGeoch DJ (1987) The genome of herpes simplex virus: structure, replication and evolution. J Cell Sci [Suppl] 7: 67–94

McGeoch DJ, Davison AJ (1986) Alphaherpesviruses possess a gene homologous to the protein kinase gene family of eukaryotes and retroviruses. Nucleic Acids Res 14: 1765–1777

McGeoch DJ, Dalrymple MA, Davison AJ, Dolan A, Frame MC, McNab D, Perry LJ, et al. (1988a) The complete sequence of the long unique region in the genome of herpes simplex virus type 1. J Gen Virol 69: 1531–1574

McGeoch DJ, Dolan A, Frame MC (1986) DNA sequence of the region in the genome of herpes simplex virus type 1 containing the exonuclease gene and neighbouring genes. Nucleic Acids Res 14: 3435–3448

McGeoch DJ, Dalrymple MA, Dolan A, McNab D, Perry L, Taylor P, Challberg MD (1988b) Structures of herpes simplex virus type 1 genes required for replication of virus DNA. J Virol 62: 444–453

McKnight SL (1980) The nucleotide sequence and transcript map of the herpes simplex virus thymidine kinase gene. Nucleic Acids Res 8: 5949–5963

Meyer H, Bankier AT, Landini MP, Brown CM, Barrell BG, Ruger B, Mach M (1988) Identification and procaryotic expression of the gene coding for the highly immunogenic 28-kilodalton structural phosphoprotein (pp28) of human cytomegalovirus. J Virol 62: 2243–2250

Mocarski ES, Roizman B (1982) Structure and role of the herpes simplex virus DNA termini in inversion, circularization and generation of virion DNA. Cell 31: 89–97

Mocarski ES, Pereira L, Michael N (1985) Precise localization of genes on large animal virus genomes: use of λgt11 and monoclonal antibodies to map the gene for a cytomegalovirus protein family. Proc Natl Acad Sci USA 82: 1266–1270

Mocarski ES, Pereira L, McCormick AL (1988) Human cytomegalovirus ICP22, the product of the HWLF1 reading frame, is an early nuclear protein that is released from cells. J Gen Virol 69: 2613–2621

Mullaney J, Moss HWMcL, McGeoch DJ (1989) Gene UL2 of herpes simplex virus type 1 encodes a uracil-DNA glycosylase. J Gen Virol 70: 449–454

Nathans J (1987) Molecular biology of visual pigments. Annu Rev Neurosci 10: 163–194

Nathans J, Hogness DS (1983) Isolation, sequence analysis, and intron-exon arrangement of the gene coding bovine rhodopsin. Cell 34: 807–814

Nikas I, McLauchlan J, Davison AJ, Taylor WR, Clements JB (1986) Structural features of ribonucleotide reductase. Proteins 1: 376–384

Olivo PD, Nelson NJ, Challberg MD (1988) Herpes simplex virus DNA replication: the UL9 gene encodes an origin-binding protein. Proc Natl Acad Sci USA 85: 5414–5418

Oram JD, Downing RG, Akrigg A, Doggleby CJ, Wilkinson GWG, Greenaway PJ (1982) Use of recombinant plasmids to investigate the structure of the human cytomegalovirus genome. J Gen Virol 59: 111–129

Pachl C, Probert WS, Hermsen KM, Masiarz FR, Rasmussen L, Merigan, TC, Spaete RR (1989) The human cytomegalovirus strain Towne glycoprotein H gene encodes glycoprotein p86. Virology 169: 418–426

Pande H, Baak SW, Riggs AD, Clark BR, Shively JE, Zaia JA (1984) Cloning and physical mapping of a gene fragment coding for a 64-kilodalton major late antigen of human cytomegalovirus. Proc Natl Acad Sci USA 81: 4965–4969

Pande H, Campo K, Churchill MA, Clark BR, Zaia JA (1988) Genomic localization of the gene encoding a 32-kDa capsid protein of human cytomegalovirus. Virology 167: 306–310

Pearson WR, Lipman DJ (1988) Improved tools for biological sequence comparison. Proc Natl Acad Sci USA 85: 2444–2448

Pereira L, Hoffman M, Gallo D, Cremer N (1982) Monoclonal antibodies to human cytomegalovirus: three surface membrane proteins with unique immunological and electrophoretic properties specify cross-reactive determinants. Infect Immun 36: 924–932

Pertuiset B, Boccara M, Cerbrian J, Berthelot N, Chousterman S, Puvion-Dutilleul F, Sisman J, Sheldrick P (1989) Physical mapping and nucleotide sequence of a herpes simplex virus type 1 gene required for capsid assembly. J Virol 63: 2169–2179

Petrovskis EA, Timmins JG, Armentrout MA, Marchioli CC, Yancey RJ Jr, Post LE (1986) DNA sequence of the gene for pseudorabies virus gp50, a glycoprotein without N-linked glycosylation. J Virol 59: 216–223

Pizzorno MC, O'Hare P, Sha L, LaFemina RL, Hayward GS (1988) trans-Activation and autoregulation of gene expression by the immediate-early region 2 gene products of human cytomegalovirus. J Virol 62: 1167–1179

Preston VG, Fisher FB (1984) Identification of the herpes simplex virus type 1 gene encoding the dUTPase. Virology 138: 58–68

Preston VG, Coates JAV, Rixon FJ (1983) Identification and characterization of a herpes simplex virus gene product required for encapsidation of virus DNA. J Virol 45: 1056–1064

Rasmussen LE, Nelson RM, Kelsall DC, Merigan TC (1984) Murine monoclonal antibody to a single protein neutralizes the infectivity of human cytomegalovirus. Proc Natl Acad Sci USA 81: 876–880

Rasmussen RD, Staprans SI, Shaw SB, Spector DH (1985a) Sequences in human cytomegalovirus which hybridize with the avian retrovirus oncogene v-myc are G + C rich and do not hybridize with the human c-myc gene. Mol Cell Biol 5: 1525–1530

Rasmussen L, Mullenax J, Nelson R, Merigan TC (1985b) Viral polypeptides detected by a complement-dependent neutralizing murine monclonal antibody to human cytomegalovirus. J Virol 55: 274–280

Razzaque et al. (1988) Localization and DNA sequence analysis of the transforming domain (mtrII) of human cytomegalovirus. Proc Natl Acad Sci USA 85: 5709–5713

Reichard P (1989) Interactions between deoxyribonucleotide and DNA synthesis. Annu Rev Biochem 57: 349–374

Rixon FJ, Cross AM, Addison C, Preston VG (1988) The products of herpes simplex virus type 1 gene UL26 which are involved in DNA packaging are strongly associated with empty but not with full capsids. J Gen Virol 69: 2879–2891

Robson L, Gibson W (1989) Primate cytomegalovirus assembly protein: genome location and nucleotide sequence. J. Virol. 63: 669–676

Roby C, Gibson W (1986) Characterization of phosphoproteins and protein kinase activity of virions, noninfectious enveloped particles, and dense bodies of human cytomegalovirus. J Virol 59: 714–727

Ruger B, Klages S, Walla B, Albrecht J, Fleckenstein B, Tomlinson P, Barrell BG (1987) Primary structure and transcription of the genes coding for the two virion phosphoproteins pp65 and pp71 of human cytomegalovirus. J Virol 61: 446–453

Saiki RK, Gelfand DH, Stoffel S, Scharf SJ, Higuchi R, Horn GT, Mullis KB, Erlich HA (1988) Primer-directed enzymatic amplification of DNA with a thermostable DNA polymerase. Science 239: 487–491

Sjoberg B-M, Eklund H, Fuchs JA, Carlson J, Standart NM, Ruderman JV, Bray SJ, Hunt T (1985) Identification of the stable free radical tyrosine residue in ribonucleotide reductase. FEBS Lett 183: 99–102

Smith RF, Smith TF (1989) Identification of new protein kinase-related genes in three herpes viruses, herpes simplex virus, varicella-zoster virus and Epstein-Barr Virus. J Virol 63: 450–455

Spaete RR, Mocarski ES (1985a) Regulation of cytomegalovirus gene expression: α and β promoters are trans activated by viral functions in permissive human fibroblasts. J Virol 56: 135–143

Spaete RR, Mocarski ES (1985b) The sequence of the cytomegalovirus genome functions as a cleavage/packaging signal for herpes simplex virus defective genomes. J. Virol. 54: 817–824

Spaete RR, Mocarski ES (1987) Insertion and deletion mutagenesis of the human cytomegalovirus genome. Proc Natl Acad Sci USA 84: 7213–7217

Spaete RR, Thayer RM, Probert WS, Masiarz FR, Chamberlain SH, Rasmussen L, Merigan TC, Pachl C (1988) Human cytomegalovirus strain Towne glycoprotein B is processed by proteolytic cleavage. Virology 167: 207–225

Staden R (1986) The current status and portability of our sequencing handling software. Nucleic Acids Res 14: 217–231

Staden R (1988) Methods to define and locate patterns of motifs in sequences. CABIOS 4: 53–60

Stannard LM (1989) β_2 microglobulin binds to the tegument of cytomegalovirus: an immunogold study. J Gen Virol 70: 2179–2184

Staprans SI, Spector DH (1986) 2.2-kilobase class of early transcripts encoded by cell-related sequences in human cytomegalovirus strain AD169. J Virol 57: 591–602

Stenberg RM, Thomsen DR, Stinski MF (1984) Structural analysis of the major immediate early gene of human cytomegalovirus. J Virol 49: 190–191

Stenberg RM, Witte PR, Stinski MF (1985) Multiple spliced and unspliced transcripts from human cytomegalovirus immediate-early region 2 and evidence for a common initiation site within immediate-early region 1. J Virol 56: 665–675

Stinski MF (1977) Synthesis of proteins and glycoproteins in cells infected with human cytomegalovirus. J Virol 23: 751–767

Stinski MF, Roehr TJ (1985) Activation of the major immediate early gene of human cytomegalovirus by cis-acting elements in the promoter-regulatory sequence and by virus-specific trans-acting components. J Virol 55: 431–441

Stinski MF, Thomsen DR, Stenberg RM, Goldstein LC (1983) Organization and expression of the immediate early genes of human cytomegalovirus. J Virol 46: 1–14

Tamashiro JC, Filpula D, Friedmann T, Spector DH (1984) Structure of the heterogeneous L-S junction region of human cytomegalovirus strain AD169 DNA. J Virol 52: 541–584

Thompson R, Honess RW, Taylor L, Morran J, Davison AJ (1987) Varicella-zoster virus specifies a thymidylate synthetase. J Gen Virol 68: 1449–1455

Thomsen DR, Stenberg RM, Goins WF, Stinski MF (1984) Promoter-regulatory region of the major immediate early gene of human cytomegalovirus. Proc Natl Acad Sci USA 81: 659–663

Townsend A, Ohlen C, Bastin J, Ljunggren H-G, Foster L, Karre K (1989) Association of class I major histocompatibility heavy and light chains induced by viral peptides. Nature 340: 443–448

Trimble JJ, Murthy CS, Bakker A, Grassmann R, Desrosiers RC (1988) A gene for dihydrofolate reductase in a herpesvirus. Science 239: 1145–1147

Wang F, Petti L, Braun D, Seung S, Kieff E (1987) A bicistronic Epstein-Barr virus mRNA encodes two nuclear proteins in latently infected, growth-transformed lymphocytes. J Virol 61: 945–954

Wathen MW, Stinski MF (1982) Temporal patterns of human cytomegalovirus transcription: mapping the viral RNAs synthesized at immediate early, early, and late times after infection. J Virol 41: 462–477

Weber PC, Challberg MD, Nelson NJ, Levine M, Glorioso JC (1988) Inversion events in the HSV-1 genome are directly mediated by the viral DNA replication machinery and lack sequence specificity. Cell 54: 369–381

Weller SK, Aschman DP, Sacks WR, Coen DM, Schaffer PA (1983) Genetic analysis of temperature-sensitive mutants of HSV-1: the combined use of complementation and physical mapping for cistron assignment. Virology 130: 290–305

Weston K (1988) An enhancer element in the short unique region of human cytomegalovirus regulates the production of a group of abundant immediate early transcripts. Virology 162: 406–416

Weston K, Barrell BG (1986) Sequence of the short unique region, short repeats and part of the long repeat of human cytomegalovirus. J Mol Biol 192: 177–208

Whitton JL, Clements JB (1984) The junctions between the repetitive and the short unique sequences of the herpes simplex virus genome are determined by the polypeptide-coding regions of two spliced immediate-early mRNAs. J Gen Virol 65: 451–466

Wilkinson GWG, Akrigg A, Greenaway PJ (1984) Transcription of the immediate early genes of human cytomegalovirus strain AD169. Virus Res 1: 101–116

Worrad DM, Caradonna S (1988) Identification of the coding sequence for herpes simplex virus uracil-DNA glycosylase. J. Virol. 62: 4774–4777

Wright DA, Staprans SI, Spector DH (1988) Four phosphoproteins with common amino termini are encoded by human cytomegalovirus AD169. J Virol 62: 331–340

Wu CA, Nelson NJ, McGeoch DJ, Challberg MD (1988) Identification of herpes simplex virus type 1 genes required for origin-dependent DNA synthesis. J Virol 62: 435–443

Yang-Feng TL, Barton DE, Thelander L, Lewis WH, Srinivasan PR, Francke U (1987) Ribonucleotide reductase M2 subunit sequences mapped to four different chromosomal sites in humans and mice: functional locus identified by its amplification in hydroxyurea-resistant cell-lines. Genomics 1: 77–86

Zhang CX, Decaussin G, de Turenne Tessier M, Daillie J, Ooka T (1987) Identification of an Epstein-Barr virus-specific deoxyribonuclease gene using complementary DNA. Nucleic Acids Res 15: 2707–2717

Human Cytomegalovirus Phosphoproteins and Glycoproteins and Their Coding Regions

G. Jahn and M. Mach

1 Introduction   171
2 The Two 150-kDa Structural Proteins of HCMV (pp150 and MCP)   172
3 The Phosphorylated Matrix Protein pp65   177
4 The Major Glycoprotein gp58   178
5 Conclusion   182
References   183

1 Introduction

Human cytomegalovirus (HCMV) phospho- and glycoproteins represent dominant antigens for the humoral immune response. This was suspected when the first immunoprecipitations and Western blot analyses were carried out using infected cells, purified virus, and human sera (Schmitz et al. 1980; Pereira et al. 1982, 1983; Nowak et al. 1984b; Landini et al. 1985) and when methods became available to investigate protein modification of viral-encoded polypeptides. A more detailed characterization of these proteins seems to be important for several reasons, such as the development of improved diagnostic reagents or the understanding of the immune response against the virus.

Various diagnostic tests are available for demonstration of HCMV antibodies. These serodiagnostics, however, need improvement since they are based on poorly defined viral antigens. Discrimination of primary and recurrent infection is often difficult and the detection of antibodies is usually of limited value in determining the time point of infection. In addition, more specific probes such as antibodies directed against defined early or late viral proteins are a prerequisite to study latency or the chronic state of HCMV infection. The proteins taken for antibody tests are usually prepared from cell-culture-adapted strains. These cell lysates do not necessarily represent the optimal antigens for antibody detection and may contain proteins bearing cross-reactivity with other herpesviruses. Future HCMV antibody test systems should be based on specific viral epitopes without cross-reactivity to other herpesviruses. In order to obtain such antigens in sufficient quality, it is necessary to characterize the viral proteins and their coding sequences. So far, the

Institut für Klinische und Molekulare Virologie der Universität Erlangen-Nürnberg, D-8520 Erlangen, FRG

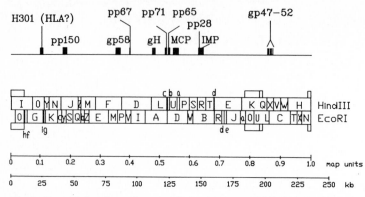

Fig. 1. Genomic locations of structural protein genes of HCMV. The restriction map for the enzymes *Hind*III and *Eco*RI is given for strain AD169. *pp*, phosphoproteins; *gp*, glycoproteins; *MCP*, major capsid protein; *IMP*, integrated membrane protein (LEHNER et al. 1989); H301 corresponds to a so far not identified potential glycoprotein (BECK and BARRELL 1988)

genes for five viral phosphoproteins have been identified (pp150: JAHN et al. 1987b; pp67: DAVIS et al. 1984; DAVIS and HUANG 1985; pp65: NOWAK et al. 1984a; RÜGER et al. 1987; pp28: MEYER et al. 1988) (Fig. 1).

Little is known about the immunological responses which limit the consequences of an HCMV infection in vivo. Most likely both the cellular and humoral arm of the immune system play an important role in curbing the severity of HCMV-induced disease. As has been shown for the other human herpesviruses the envelope glycoproteins are most likely important targets for the induction of neutralizing antibodies. However, the HCMV glycoproteins have until now been incompletely characterized. So far, between three and eight individual glycosylated envelope proteins have been identified by various investigators (BENKO and GIBSON 1986; FARRAR and GREENAWAY 1986; GIBSON 1983; STINSKI 1977). In addition, three families of glycoprotein complexes termed gC I–III have been described (GRETCH et al. 1988a; KARI et al. 1986). Of these polypeptides, proteins of 86 kDa (RASMUSSEN et al. 1984), 65 kDa (BRITT and AUGER 1985), 58 kDa (BRITT 1984), and 47–52 kDa (GRETCH et al. 1988a) are able to induce neutralizing antibodies in laboratory animals and may therefore represent targets of a protective humoral immune response. The coding regions for three glycoproteins (gp58: MACH et al. 1986; gp86(gH): CRANAGE et al. 1988; gp47–52: GRETCH et al. 1988b) have been identified on the viral genome (Fig. 1).

In this chapter we would like to describe results which were obtained in this laboratory with phosphoproteins of 150 kDa and 65 kDa, as well as with the glycoprotein of 58 kDa.

2 The Two 150-kDa Structural Proteins of HCMV (pp150 and MCP)

At least two prominent large proteins with an apparent molecular weight of about 150 kDa can be detected in virion preparations by sodium dodeyl sulfate polyacrylamide gel electrophoresis (SDS-PAGE). One of these polypeptides was identified as a phosphorylated structural component of the matrix (GIBSON 1983; ROBY and GIBSON 1986) and was named pp150 (NOWAK et al. 1984a, b). The other protein is the major capsid protein (MCP). This was mainly deduced from the similar electrophoretic mobility of the HCMV-MCP to that of the well-characterized MCP of a simian cytomegalovirus strain in one-dimensional and two-dimensional gel electrophoresis (GIBSON 1983). The pp150 and the MCP either comigrate in the SDS-PAGE as one band or they separate in different ways. NOWAK et al. (1984b) reported the upper band as the phosphorylated structural protein pp150. In contrast, GIBSON and IRMIERE (1984) described the phosphorylated matrix protein migrating faster than the nonphosphorylated major capsid protein. For their analyses, they used polyacrylamide gels containing increased concentrations of methylene bisacrylamid ("high-bis"). The inconsistent migration of the two 150-kDa proteins made it difficult to compare Western blot results from different laboratories. In immunoblots with human sera a 150-kDa protein showed stronger reactivity than any other structural protein of HCMV (LANDINI et al. 1985). To discriminate between immunoreactivities toward the MCP and the pp150, we used "high-bis" gels; in this system the phosphoprotein appeared always to be in the lower band (Fig. 2). Under these conditions, the strongest immune responses were consistently found with the phosphorylated matrix protein pp150, irrespective of the stage of infection (JAHN et al. 1987a). In general, the results of the Western blot analyses with purified viral proteins separated in the "high-bis" SDS-PAGE demonstrated that the pp150 is the most immunogenic structural protein in humans with respect to the humoral immune response. In order to obtain monospecific antisera we raised antibodies

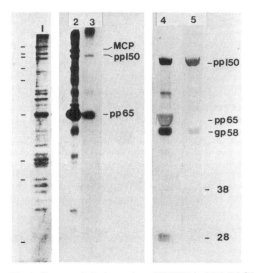

Fig. 2. Structural viral proteins of HCMV in SDS-PAGE and immunoblot. *Lane 1*, silver staining. *Left*, mol. wt. markers of 205, 160, 150, 116, 97, 66, 45, 38, and 29 kDa; *lane 2*, [^{35}S]methionine labeling; *lane 3*, ^{32}P$_i$-labeled virions; *lane 4*, immunoblot with high-titered human antiserum; *lane 5*, immunoblot with a serum of an infected newborn

against gel-purified viral proteins in rabbits. Again, the stronger immune reaction was seen against the pp150, even when the two 150-kDa proteins (pp150 and MCP) were injected simultaneously (JAHN et al. 1987a). The immunization results in rabbits were in line with the strong humoral immune response against pp150 in the natural infection of humans.

The large phosphorylated structural protein is reproducibly found in the purified virus particles in about equivalent amounts in wild-type and laboratory strains of HCMV. The gene for pp150 was mapped in the AD169 strain by screening a bacteriophage lambda gt11 cDNA expression library with a monospecific rabbit antiserum (JAHN et al. 1987b). Hybridization of the cDNA from the identified phage with cloned viral DNA mapped the gene to HindIII fragments J and N in the long unique segment. The DNA sequence of this region revealed two large open reading frames of 3144 and 2014 nucleotides respectively. The longer frame contained the DNA sequence homologous to the pp150-specific cDNA. This frame has the same orientation as the major late RNA detected in this region by Northern blot analyses. The open reading frame codes for a polypeptide of 1048 amino acids which corresponds to a 113-kDa protein. The size discrepancy between the numerical value and the molecular weight according to the SDS-PAGE raises the question of whether this single long frame codes for the entire mature pp150 in virions. The size discrepancy may be due to the high content of proline residues in the putative polypeptide, the basic nature of pp150, and the high degree of phosphorylation. Primer extension and nuclease protection experiments identified the transcription initiation site; it is preceded by a TATA consensus sequence. A poly (A) signal was localized 2.6 kb downstream of the open reading frame by S1 analyses. It is still possible that the mature mRNA of pp150 combines the identified long open reading frame with smaller frames near the 3' end of the transcript. However, a computer search for splice donor consensus sequences did not recognize such a signal within the entire long open reading frame.

Recently, PANDE et al. (1989) identified the genomic locus for pp150 in the Towne strain by a similar method. Their data demonstrated that the gene encoding the pp150 maps to an identical position at approximately 0.16–0.18 map units in the long unique region of both HCMV strains Towne and AD169.

Since the large phosphorylated matrix protein is the polypeptide most frequently reactive in immunoblotting analyses with human antisera, we were interested to obtain recombinant peptides of pp150 for diagnostic purposes. Computer analyses of the putative secondary structure of the polypeptide indicated a remarkable accumulation of hydrophilic residues in certain regions. This often coincided with β-pleated sheets and offered an explanation for the high antigenicity of the protein. Defined regions of pp150 were expressed as bacterial β-galactosidase fusion proteins and these recombinant proteins were tested for their immunoreactivity with human sera. The prokaryotic-expressed pp150 fragments were different in their computer-predicted antigenicity. However, it was not possible to predict the antigenic properties of the expressed peptides on the basis of hydrophilicity and β-turn indices only. The HCMV antibody-positive human sera so far tested recognized different pp150 hybrid polypeptides, irrespective of their computer-predicted antigenicity values. Particularly an expressed 450-bp fragment from the internal portion of the

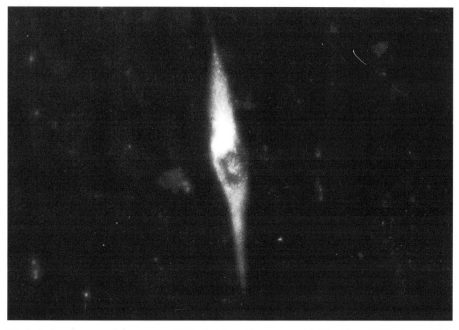

Fig. 3. Indirect immunofluorescence of HCMV-infected human foreskin fibroblasts HFF using a rabbit antiserum raised against the recombinant XP1/pp150 protein

pp150 open reading frame, called XP1, proved to be highly immunogenic (SCHOLL et al. 1988). This polypeptide was recognized by the HCMV antibody-positive sera tested in Western blot experiments and ELISAs, independently of the states of the infection.

The XP1 hybrid protein was taken to immunize rabbits. The high-titer monospecific antiserum obtained allowed the detection of HCMV-infected cells by immunofluorescence (Fig. 3) and immunoperoxidase techniques (SCHOLL et al. 1988). The antiserum was particularly useful to detect the viral antigen in sections of paraffin-embedded tissues by immunohistochemistry (BORISCH et al. 1988). In addition, a mouse monoclonal antibody directed against the XP1/pp150 recombinant protein is available which recognizes the viral protein under the same conditions like the rabbit antiserum (Fig. 4).

Taken together the matrix protein pp150 of HCMV or peptides thereof are good reagents for new diagnostic tests. The antibodies against genetically engineered pp150 worked nicely for in situ detection of viral antigens in tissues; the recombinant pp150 polypeptides were successfully used in antibody tests. Other herpesviruses do not possess such an antigenic phosphorylated structural protein in this size range. In *herpes simplex* for instance, the strongest reactivities with human positive sera are seen with the membrane glycoproteins such as gB or with the MCP VP5 of 150 kDa (KAHLON et al. 1986; EBERLE and MOU 1983). In contrast to other human herpesviruses, the MCP of HCMV appears to be of limited antigenicity according to Western blot analyses with sera from infected individuals. On the other hand the

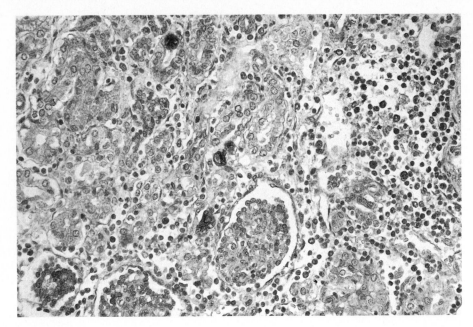

Fig. 4. Immunohistochemistry using a XP1/pp150 mouse monoclonal antibody for the detection of HCMV-infected cells in the kidney

MCPs of the herpesviruses are highly conserved. The homology of the amino acid sequences was found to be between 24% and 50% among HSV-1, VZV, and EBV. Recently the MCP gene of HCMV could be identified by comparing sequences of HCMV with the known genes for the MCPs of HSV, VZV, and EBV (CHEE et al. 1989). The open reading frame identified on the HCMV genome potentially codes for a polypeptide of 1370 amino acids with an estimated molecular weight of 154 kDa. The frame is localized in the long unique segment in *Hind*III fragments a and U (Fig. 1). The amino acid sequence shows a homology of 25% and 23%, respectively, to the HSV-1 and VZV MCPs and a homology of 29% was seen to the MCP of EBV.

To prove that the putative open reading frame does code for the MCP of HCMV, fragments were expressed in *Escherichia coli*. The resulting recombinant fragments of the MCP were tested for their immune reactivity with specific antibodies against the HCMV MCP (CHEE et al. 1989). In addition, the fusion proteins were used to raise antisera in rabbits. The sera detected the MCP of purified HCMV virions. The recombinant peptides of the MCP will also be helpful in searching for group-specific epitopes. This may be of importance for the development of new specific reagents for HCMV diagnostics in order to exclude cross-reactivity. On the other hand, defined MCP polypeptides may serve as reliable antigens to study the variation in the immune responses of the host to different herpesviruses.

3 The Phosphorylated Matrix Protein pp65

The most abundant structural constituent of laboratory strains of HCMV is the so-called lower matrix protein (GIBSON and IRMIERE 1984). The polypeptide was also named the major structural phosphoprotein (pp65) of HCMV (NOWAK et al. 1984a, b) or glycoprotein gp64 (CLARK et al. 1984; PANDE et al. 1984). Since the coding sequences of the proteins were identified independently on the AD169 and on the Towne genome, it is now obvious that the proteins are the same. The gene of pp65 could be mapped to the corresponding *Hind*III fragments L, b, and c of strain AD169 and to the *Hind*III fragments H and N of strain Towne (NOWAK et al. 1984a; CLARK et al. 1984). The partial amino acid sequence reported for the Towne strain (PANDE et al. 1984) matches perfectly to the sequence derived from the AD169 DNA sequence of the pp65 gene (RÜGER et al. 1987). DAVIS et al. (1984) mapped another phosphorylated viral protein of about 67 kDa to the *Eco*RI G fragment of the Towne strain. The coding region of this protein appeared close to the map position of pp65, but the sequence comparisons showed that the two phosphorylated structural polypeptides are not related (DAVIS and HUANG 1985; RÜGER et al. 1987). The gene of pp65 appeared to have unusual features. A characteristic TATA sequence was not identified in the promoter region and the mRNA of 4 kb appeared to be coterminal with a 1.9-kb transcript. Another structural phosphorylated protein of about 71 kDa in size corresponds to the single translational reading frame of this 1.9-kb RNA. The structure of the 4-kb mRNA implied that it is a potential bicistronic eukaryotic messenger.

It was not clear whether the second reading frame of the abundant 4 kb is used to synthesize the pp71 or whether pp71 is encoded by the 1.9 kb RNA (RÜGER et al. 1987). Recently DEPTO and STENBERG (1989) reported on the RNA expression and the promoter regulation of the pp65 gene. They detected the pp65 transcript at low levels prior to viral DNA replication. Maximal transcription, however, was found only after the initiation of viral DNA replication. From this the authors concluded that the pp65 gene is an early-late gene. The transactivation of the pp65 promoter was investigated in a transient expression assay. Transfection of the construct and subsequent superinfection with HCMV resulted in activation of the promoter at early times after infection. Cotransfection experiments with HCMV immediate-early (IE) constructs demonstrated that the pp65 promoter was activated only if both IE1 and IE2 regions were cotransfected. The authors were able to characterize the 5′ minimal sequence required for activation. Their studies suggested an important interaction between IE proteins and an 8-nucleotide sequence for the expression and regulation of the pp65 gene.

There is a marked difference in the relative abundance of the pp65 if recent clinical isolates and laboratory strains were compared (JAHN et al. 1987a; KLAGES et al. 1989). The major matrix phosphoprotein is by far the most abundant structural protein in laboratory strain AD169, which is found particularly enriched in the dense body fraction (GIBSON and IRMIERE 1984). Using a pp65 monoclonal antibody for immunoelectron microscopy the protein was detected exclusively in dense bodies of infected cells (LANDINI et al. 1987).

In low passage wild-type viruses the pp65 appeared to be a minor structural constituent and these viruses did not have significant amounts of dense bodies (JAHN et al. 1987a). All these data indicate that the pp65 is not abundant in virions and the concentration of this particular protein in HCMV particles corresponds to the accumulation of dense bodies. How an overproduction of a single matrix protein leads to the increased formation of defective particles almost exclusively containing this particular protein is not clear. The expression of pp65 can either be due to transcriptional or posttranscriptional regulation. The relative amounts of the pp65 encoding transcript in late RNA preparations of cells infected with laboratory strains and wildtype isolates were compared to the quantities of the expressed protein. Roughly estimated, the amount of the 4 kb RNA correlated with the amount of pp65. This was taken as evidence that the expression of pp65 was transcriptionally regulated (KLAGES et al. 1989). According to restriction enzyme analyses, the genomic region of the pp65 gene in various HCMV isolates showed only minor differences in the restriction pattern (CHANDLER and McDOUGALL 1986; KLAGES et al. 1989). This is in agreement with results of immunoblot analyses with a monoclonal pp65 antibody and various HCMV isolates, which all could be detected by the specific antibody. This protein seems to be highly conserved among the HCMV isolates and according the sequence data there is no counterpart in other herpesviruses. The humoral immune response of infected persons against the phosphoprotein pp65 is highly variable. Even though antibodies against pp65 are not always detectable by Western blot analyses, the polypeptide belongs to the few structural proteins most frequently recognized by sera of HCMV-positive individuals (LANDINI et al. 1985; JAHN et al. 1987a). The pp65 or parts of it may be added as reagents for future diagnostics or may be helpful to study functional aspects of the pp65.

4 The Major Glycoprotein gp58

The first glycoprotein of which more detailed information became available was the gp58. This protein has also been termed gA, gB, gp55/116 by various authors (PEREIRA et al. 1984; CRANAGE et al. 1986; BRITT 1984).

Monoclonal antibodies recognizing gp58 have been isolated from murine (NOWAK et al. 1984b; PEREIRA et al. 1984; BRITT 1984; RASMUSSEN et al. 1985) and more recently from human sources (MASUHO et al. 1987). Using these antibodies it was shown that the protein is present in the viral envelope in a disulfide-linked complex with at least one other protein. Polyacrylamide-gel-electrophoresis (PAGE) under reducing conditions following immunoprecipitations with monoclonal antibodies as well as monospecific antisera consistently resulted in the detection of at least two proteins. Whereas the gp58 migrates as a discrete band during PAGE the coprecipitated component(s) show(s) a highly diffuse signal in the molecular weight range of 116–150 kDa, depending on the gel system (Fig. 5). Using PAGE under nonreducing conditions, the complex has an apparent molecular weight of

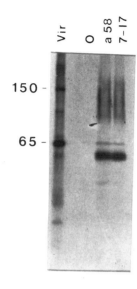

Fig. 5. Immunoprecipitation of HCMV antigens by a monospecific rabbit serum (a58) or a monoclonal antibody (7–17) against gp58. Human foreskin fibroblasts were infected with HCMV strain AD169, and 48 h after infection the cells were labeled with [^{35}S]methiomine for 24 h and extracellular virus was purified on glycerol tartrate gradients. The precipitated antigens were analyzed on a SDS-polyacrylamide gel and autoradiographed

approximately 250–300 kDa. In Western blots, however, both monoclonal antibodies (LAW et al. 1985) as well as monospecific rabbit antisera (MACH et al. 1987) detect exclusively the gp58. Under nonreducing conditions only the high molecular weight complex can be detected (MACH et al. 1987). This as well as results derived from peptide mapping (BRITT and AUGER 1986) indicated that the heterogeneous high molecular weight component of the gp58 complex is not antigenically related to gp58 and does not contain cross-reactive epitopes. The formation of disulfide-linked high molecular weight complexes seems to be a phenomenon common to HCMV glycoproteins. So far three families of glycoproteins containing at least five individual members have been identified (GRETCH et al. 1988a).

The gene encoding the gp58 was mapped to the right end of the *Hind*III F fragment of strain AD169 (MACH et al. 1986) (Fig. 1). The nucleotide sequence revealed an open reading frame in this area that has the characteristics typical of a membrane glycoprotein (CRANAGE et al. 1986). The primary translation product is a protein of 906 amino acids and has a numerical molecular weight of 102 kDa. Tunicamycin-treated infected fibroblasts synthesize a protein of similar size which can be immunoprecipitated by gp58-specific monoclonal antibodies (PEREIRA et al. 1984; RASMUSSEN et al. 1988). The mature glycosylated gp58 is derived from a glycosylated precursor of approximately 160 kDa via proteolytic cleavage (BRITT and AUGER 1986; BRITT and VUGLER 1989). It represents the carboxy-terminal part of the molecule. This was concluded from the fact that a monospecific rabbit antiserum recognized a gp58-β-galactosidase fusion protein containing the last nine amino acids of the open reading frame (MACH et al. 1986). In a more recent study these data were confirmed by the investigation of the gp58 equivalent of the Towne strain (SPAETE et al. 1988). HCMV strain Towne contains a protein that is 94% homologous on the DNA level and 95% homologous on the amino acid level to gp58 of strain AD169 (SPAETE et al. 1988). By amino acid sequencing the Towne gp58 was shown to contain the amino-terminal sequence STDGNN which corresponds to amino acids 461–466 of the primary translation product. The putative cleavage signal RTKR/S$_{461}$ is located directly upstream. Dibasic peptides serve as processing sites for a number of viral membrane glycoproteins such as the gp160 of HIV (VERONESE et al. 1985) or the hemagglutinin of influenza A viruses (WEBSTER and ROTT 1987). In the case of tick-brone encephalitis virus the membrane protein is processed at a site (RTRR/S, MANDL et al 1988) which is identical to the putative gp58 cleavage sequence of strain AD169.

Interestingly similar signals can be found in a number of homologous glycoproteins of mammalian herpesviruses. The primary translation products of gpII of varicella zoster virus (VZV) and gII of pseudorabies virus contain the motifs RSRR/S (KELLER et al. 1986) and RARR/S (ROBBINS et al. 1987), respectively. The corresponding proteins are derived from precursors by proteolytic cleavage and the amino acid sequence of the amino-terminal part of gpII confirmed the motif as the cleavage signal. Glycoprotein B, the homologous protein of herpes simplex virus (HSV), does not contain a similar sequence, which is in agreement with its size of approximately 120 kDa. A special situation seems to exist for the BALF-4 reading frame product of Epstein-Barr virus (EBV). The primary translation product contains the motif RRRRD (BAER et al. 1984). However, so far it has not been shown that the gene product is cleaved; instead a glycoprotein of 125 kDa has been identified as the gene product (EMINI et al. 1987). This would implicate that in addition to a dibasic motif other factors are necessary for the proteolytic processing of the herpesvirus envelope glycoproteins. The conservation of a basic amino acid at -4 as well as the small uncharged residue at + 1 is striking. Future experiments will have to establish which sequences meet the requirements for efficient proteolytic processing.·

During natural infection gp58 is the immunodominant antigen among the glycoproteins. Antibodies against this polypeptide can be detected at high frequencies in patients having medium or high titers of HCMV antibodies (LANDINI et al. 1985). However, when compared with other structural proteins such as the phosphoproteins of 150 kDa, 65 kDa, or 28 kDa the gp58 is a far less well recognized antigen. Detectable antibody levels against the other glycoproteins occur at significantly lower frequencies. This is in marked contrast to the situation in other human herpesviruses where antibodies against the glycoproteins can be readily detected in human sera and constitute a considerable fraction of the total amount of antibodies against the respective virus. Whether the rather weak immune response against gp58 has consequences for the outcome of an infection is not clear at present.

The fact that a number of murine and human monoclonal antibodies, which recognize gp58, have neutralizing activity turns this protein into a candidate for a subunit vaccine. At present only live, attenuated virus strains are available as immunogens (PLOTKIN et al. 1985). The efficacy of these vaccines is controversial and their use is precluded with certain populations. On the other hand it has been demonstrated that in the case of herpes simplex virus recombinant derived antigen preparations (BERMAN et al. 1984) or even synthetic peptides (EISENBERG et al. 1985) could evoke an immune response capable of neutralizing infectious virus in vitro and in vivo. It is therefore of great interest to learn more about the gp58 and the immune response against it in order to evaluate its importance for infection and/or reactivation. An important antigenic region of the molecule was identified recently

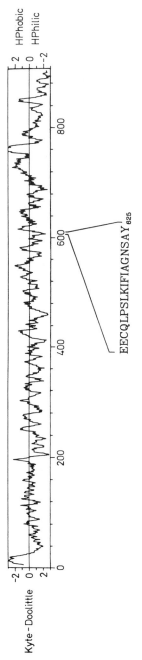

Fig. 6. The neutralizing epitope on gp58. A hydrophilicity profile according to KYTE and DOOLITTLE (1982) of the primary translation product is shown in the *upper part*. The maximal epitope recognized by the neutralizing antibody 7–17 is given

(UTZ et al. 1989) (Fig. 6). A series of overlapping expression plasmids was constructed which synthesize parts of the gp58 reading frame as fusion proteins with β-galactosidase. A number of monoclonal antibodies reactive with denatured gp58 were tested in Western blots for the recognition of the hybrid proteins. The panel included the neutralizing antibody 7–17 (BRITT 1984). The binding site of this antibody was determined to be located between amino acids 608 and 625 (UTZ et al. 1989) (Fig. 6). The sequences surrounding a BglII site at nucleotide 1847 (corresponding to amino acid 614) seemed to be critical for the recognition. Insertion of four amino acids at this point led to the destruction of the antibody-reactive site. Interestingly a second, nonneutralizing antibody (27–287) was able to compete for the binding site of 7–17. This antibody also partially inhibited the neutralizing activity of antibody 7–17 (UTZ et al. 1989). In another study the competitive inhibition of several monoclonal antibodies directed against related domains of gp58 was also observed (LUSSENHOP et al. 1988). In this case, however, only complement-dependent neutralizing antibodies which recognized conformational epitopes were studied.

The biological relevance of antibody inhibition of neutralizing antibodies remains unknown. Other studies have observed that nonneutralizing antibodies may inhibit the complete neutralization of a number of viruses and may account for the pathogenesis of several persistent viral infections (MASSEY and SCHOCHETMAN 1981). However, if neutralizing antibodies are an important component of the host response to HCMV, then even partial inhibition of this response will be detrimental to the host. Future strategies to develop subunit vaccines will also have to consider the fact that entire virion proteins might induce antagonistic antibodies.

5 Conclusion

Taken together it seems that the coding regions for the major immunogenic phosphoproteins of HCMV have been identified. The information can now be used to develop more specific and sensitive reagents for diagnostic purposes or the investigation of gene regulation of structural proteins. As far as the glycoproteins are concerned less information is available with regard to the actual number of proteins and/or their genomic location. The analyses of envelope glycoproteins, however, is a prerequisite for a better understanding of the immunological response following an HCMV infection or the development of a potential vaccine.

Acknowledgments. This work was supported by the Deutsche Forschungsgemeinschaft and the Bundesministerium für Forschung und Technologie. We thank W. BRITT, Birmingham Alabama, for providing monoclonal antibodies.

References

Baer R, Bankier AT, Biggin MD, Deininger PL, Farrell PJ, Gibson TJ, Hatfull G, et al. (1984) DNA sequence and expression of the B95-8 Epstein-Barr virus genome. Nature 310: 207–211

Beck S, Barrell BG (1988) Human cytomegalovirus encodes a glycoprotein homologous to MHC class-I antigens. Nature 331: 269–272

Benko DM, Gibson W (1986) Primate cytomegalovirus glycoproteins: lectin binding properties and sensitivities to glycosidases. J Virol 59: 703–713

Berman PW, Gregory T, Crase D, Kasky K (1984) Protection from genital herpes simplex virus type 2 infection by vaccination with cloned type 1 glycoprotein D. Science 227: 1490–1492

Borisch B, Jahn G, Scholl B-C, Filger-Brillinger J, Heymer B, Fleckenstein B, Müller-Hermelink HK (1988) Detection of human cytomegalovirus DNA and viral antigens in tissues of different manifestations of CMV infection. Virchows Arch [B] 55: 93–99

Britt WJ (1984) Neutralizing antibodies detect a disulfide-linked glycoprotein complex within the envelope of human cytomegalovirus. Virology 135: 369–378

Britt WJ, Auger D (1985) Identification of a 65000 dalton virion envelope protein of human cytomegalovirus. Virus Res 4: 31–36

Britt WJ, Auger D (1986) Synthesis and processing of the envelope gp155–116 complex of human cytomegalovirus. J Virol 58: 185–191

Britt WJ, Vugler LG (1989) Processing of the gp55–116 envelope glycoprotein complex (gB) of human cytomegalovirus. J Virol 63: 403–410

Chandler SH, McDougall JK (1986) Comparison of restriction site polymorphisms among clinical isolates and laboratory strains of human cytomegalovirus. J Gen Virol 67: 2179–2192

Chee M, Rudolph S-A, Plachter B, Barrell B, Jahn G (1989) Identification of the major capsid protein gene of human cytomegalovirus. J Virol 63: 1345–1353

Clark BR, Zaia JA, Balce-Directo L, Ting Y-P (1984) Isolation and partial chemical characterization of a 64.000 dalton glycoprotein of human cytomegalovirus. J Virol 49: 279–282

Cranage MP, Kouzarides T, Bankier AT, Satchwell S, Weston K, Tomlinson P, Barrell B, et al. (1986) Identification of the human cytomegalovirus glycoprotein B gene and induction of neutralizing antibodies via its expression in recombinant vaccinia virus. EMBO J 5: 3057–3063

Cranage MP, Smith GL, Bell SE, Hart H, Brown C, Bankier AT, Tomlinson P, et al. (1988) Identification and expression of a human cytomegalovirus glycoprotein with homology to the Epstein-Barr virus BXLF2 product, varicella-zoster virus gpIII, and herpes simplex virus type 1 glycoprotein. H J Virol 62: 1416–1422

Davis MG, Huang E-S (1985) Nucleotide sequence of a human cytomegalovirus DNA fragment encoding a 67-kilodalton phosphorylated viral protein. J Virol 56: 7–11

Davis MG, Mar E, Wu Y, Huang E-S (1984) Mapping and expression of a human cytomegalovirus major viral protein. J Virol 52: 129–135

Depto AS, Stenberg RM (1989) Regulated expression of the human cytomegalovirus pp65 gene: octamer sequence in the promoter is required for activation by viral gene products. J Virol 63: 1332–1338

Eberle R, Mou S-W (1983) Relative titers of antibodies to individual polypeptide antigens of herpes simplex virus type 1 in human sera. J Infect Dis 148: 436–443

Eisenberg R, Cerini C, Heilman C, Joseph A, Dietzschold B, Golub E, Lang D, et al. (1985) Synthetic glycoprotein D-related peptides protect mice against herpes simplex virus challenge. J Virol 56: 1014–1017

Emini E, Luka J, Armstrong M, Keller P, Ellis R, Pearson G (1987) Identification of an Epstein-Barr virus glycoprotein which is antigenically homologous to the varicella zoster glycoprotein II and the herpes simplex virus glycoprotein B. Virology 157: 552–555

Farrar HG, Greenaway PJ (1986) Characterization of glycoprotein complexes present in human cytomegalovirus envelopes. J Gen Virol 67: 1469–1473

Gibson W (1983) Protein counterparts of human and simian cytomegaloviruses. Virology 128: 391–406

Gibson W, Irmiere A. (1984) Selection of particles and proteins for use as human cytomegalovirus subunit vaccines. In: Plotkin S et al. (eds) CMV: pathogenesis and prevention of human infection. Liss, New York, pp 305–324

Gretch DR, Kari B, Rasmussen L, Gehrz RC, Stinski MF (1988a) Identification and characterization of three distinct families of glycoprotein complexes in the envelope of human cytomegalovirus. J Virol 62: 875–881

Gretch DR, Kari B, Gehrz R, Stinski M (1988b). A multigene family encodes the human cytomegalovirus glycoprotein complex gcII (gp47–52 complex). J Virol 62: 1956–1962

Jahn G, Scholl B-C, Traupe B, Fleckenstein B (1987a) The two major structural phosphoproteins (pp65 and pp150) of human cytomegalovirus and their antigenic properties. J Gen Virol 68: 1327–1337

Jahn G, Kouzarides T, Mach M, Scholl B-C, Plachter B, Traupe B, Preddie E, et al. (1987b) Map position and nucleotide sequence of the gene for the large structural phosphoprotein of human cytomegalovirus. J Virol 61: 1358–1367

Kahlon J, Lakeman FD, Ackermann M, Whitley RJ (1986) Human antibody response to herpes simplex virus-specific polypeptides after primary and recurrent infection. J Clin Microbiol 23: 725–730

Kari B, Lussenhop N, Goertz R, Wabuke-Bunoti M, Radeke R, Gehrz R (1986) Characterization of monoclonal antibodies reactive to several biochemical distinct human cytomegalovirus glycoprotein complexes. J Virol 60: 345–352

Keller PM, Davison AJ, Lowe R, Bennett C, Ellis R (1986) Identification and structure of the gene encoding gpII, a major glycoprotein of varicella zoster virus. Virology 152: 181–191

Klages S, Rüger B, Jahn G (1989) Multiplicity dependent expression of the predominant phosphoprotein pp65 of human cytomegalovirus. Virus Res 12: 159–168

Kyte J, Doolittle RF (1982) A single method for displaying the hydropathic character of a protein. J Mol Biol 157: 105–132

Landini MP, Re MC, Mirolo G, Baldassari B, LaPlaca M (1985) Human immune response to cytomegalovirus structural polypeptides studied by immunoblotting. J Med Virol 17: 303–311

Landini MP, Severi B, Furlini G, Badiali de Giorgi L (1987) Human cytomegalovirus structural components: intracellular and intraviral localization of p28 and p65–69 by immunoelectron microscopy. Virus Res 8: 15–23

Law K, Wilton-Smith P, Farrar GH (1985) A murine monoclonal antibody recognizing a single glycoprotein within a human cytomegalovirus virion envelope glycoprotein complex. J Med Virol 17: 255–266

Lehner R, Meyer H, Mach M (1989) Identification and characterization of a human cytomegalovirus gene coding for a membrane protein that is conserved among human herpesviruses. J Virol 63: 3792–3800

Lussenhop L, Goertz R, Wabuke-Bunoti M, Hehrz R, Kari B (1988) Epitope analysis of human cytomegalovirus glycoprotein complexes using murine monoclonal antibodies. Virology 164: 362–372

Mach M, Utz U, Fleckenstein B (1986) Mapping of the major glycoprotein gene of human cytomegalovirus. J Gen Virol 67: 1461–1467

Mach M, Utz U, Fleckenstein B (1987) The major glycoprotein of human cytomegalovirus. In: Chanock R, Lerner R, Brown F, Ginsberg H (eds) Vaccines 87. CSH, pp 306–310

Mandl CW, Heinz FX, Kunz C (1988) Sequence of the structural proteins of tick borne encephalitis virus (Western subtype) and comparative analysis with other flaviviruses. Virology 166: 197–205

Massey RJ, Schochetman G (1981) Viral epitopes and monoclonal antibodies. Isolation of blocking antibodies that inhibit virus neutralization. Science 213: 447–449

Masuho Y, Matsumoto Y-I, Sugano T, Fujinaga S, Minamishia Y (1987) Human monoclonal antibodies neutralizing human cytomegalovirus. J Gen Virol 68: 1457–1461

Meyer H, Bankier AT, Landini MP, Brown CM, Barrell BG, Rüger B, Mach M (1988) Identification and procaryotic expression of the gene coding for the highly immunogenic 28 kD structural phosphoprotein (pp28) of human cytomegalovirus. J Virol 62: 2243–2250

Nowak B, Gmeiner A, Sarnow P, Levine AJ, Fleckenstein B (1984a) Physical mapping of human cytomegalovirus genes: identification of DNA sequences coding for a virion phosphoprotein of 71 kD and a viral 65 kD polypeptide. Virology 134: 91–102

Nowak B, Sullivan C, Sarnow P, Thomas R, Bricaut F, Nicolas IC, Fleckenstein B, Levine AJ (1984b) Characterization of monoclonal antibodies and polyclonal immune sera directed against human cytomegalovirus virion proteins. Virology 132: 325–338

Pande H, Baak SW, Riggs AD, Clark BR, Shively JE, Zaia JA (1984) Cloning and physical mapping of a gene fragment coding for a 64-kilodalton major late antigen of human cytomegalovirus. Proc Natl Acad Sci USA 81: 4965–4969

Pande H, Campo K, Churchill MA, Zaia JA (1989) Genomic locus for a 140 kDa structural protein (pp150) of human cytomegalovirus in strains Towne and AD169. Virus Res. 12: 11–18

Pereira L, Hoffman M, Cremer N (1982) Electrophoretic analysis of polypeptides immune precipitated from cytomegalovirus-infected cell extracts by human sera. Infect Immun 36: 933–942

Pereira L, Stagno S, Hoffman M, Volanakis JE (1983) Cytomegalovirus-infected cell polypeptides immune-precipitated by sera from children with congenital and perinatal infections. Infect Immun 39: 100–108

Pereira L, Hoffman M, Tatsuno M, Dondero D (1984) Polymorphism of human cytomegalovirus glycoproteins characterized by monoclonal antibodies. Virology 139: 73–86

Plotkin SA, Weibel RE, Alpert G, Starr SE, Friedman HM, Preblud SR, Hoxie J (1985) Resistance of seropositive volunteers to subcutaneous challenge with low-passage human cytomegalovirus. J Infect Dis 151: 737–739

Rasmussen L, Nelson R, Kelsa U, Merigan TC (1984) Murine monoclonal antibody to a single protein neutralizes the infectivity of human cytomegalovirus. Proc Natl Acad Sci USA 81: 876–880

Rasmussen L, Mullenax J, Nelson R, Merigan TC (1985) Viral polypeptides detected by complement-dependent neutralizing murine monoclonal antibody to human cytomegalovirus. J Virol 55: 274–280

Rasmussen L, Nelson M, Neff M, Merigan TC (1988) Characterization of two different human cytomegalovirus glycoproteins which are targets for virus neutralizing antibody. Virology 163: 308–318

Robbins AK, Dorney DJ, Wathen MW, Whealy ME, Gold C, Watson RJ, Holland LE, et al. (1987) The pseudorabies virus gII gene is closely related to the gB glycoprotein gene of herpes simplex virus. J Virol 61: 2691–2701

Roby C, Gibson W (1986) Characterization of phosphoproteins and protein kinase activity of virions, noninfectious enveloped particles, and dense bodies of human cytomegalovirus. J Virol 59: 714–727

Rüger B, Klages S, Walla B, Albrecht J, Fleckenstein B, Tomlinson P, Barrell B (1987) Primary structure and transcription of the genes coding for the two virion phosphoproteins pp65 and pp71 of human cytomegalovirus. J Virol 61: 446–453

Schmitz H, Müller-Lantzsch N, Peteler G (1980) Human immune response to proteins of cytomegalovirus. Intervirology 13: 154–161

Scholl B-C, von Hintzenstern J, Borisch B, Traupe B, Bröker M, Jahn G (1988) Prokaryotic expression of immunogenic polypeptides of the large phosphoprotein (pp150) of human cytomegalovirus. J Gen Virol 69: 1195–1204

Spaete R, Thayer R, Probert W, Masiarz F, Chamberlain S, Rasmussen L, Merigan TC, Packl C (1988) Human cytomegalovirus strain Townie glycoprotein B is processed by proteolytic cleavage. Virology 167: 207–225

Stinski M (1977) Synthesis of proteins and glycoproteins in cells infected with human cytomegalovirus. J Virol 23: 751–767

Utz U, Britt W, Vugler L, Mach M (1989) Identification of a neutralizing epitope on the glycoprotein gp58 of human cytomegalovirus. J Virol 63, 1995–2001

Veronese FP, DeVico AL, Copeland TD, Oroszlan S, Gallo RC, Sarngadharan MG (1985) Characterization of gp41 as the transmembrane protein coded by the HTLV-III/LAV envelope gene. Science 229: 1402–1405

Webster RG, Rott R (1987) Influenza virus A pathogenicity: the pivotal role of hemagglutinin. Cell 50: 665–666

Immune Response

Cellular and Molecular Basis of the Protective Immune Response to Cytomegalovirus Infection*

U. H. KOSZINOWSKI, M. DEL VAL, and M. J. REDDEHASE

1 Introduction 189
2 Murine Model for the Study of Protective Immunity to CMV Disease 190
2.1 Cell-Type-Specific MCMV Morphogenesis and Its Relation to Pathogenicity 190
2.2 Manifestations of CMV Disease in the Immunocompetent and the Immuno-
     compromised Host 191
2.3 Protective Immunity Mediated by T-Lymphocytes of the CD8 Subset 193
2.4 Antihemopoietic Effect of CMV Infection and Its Prevention 197
2.5 Persistent Infection in the CD4-Subset-Depleted Host 201
3 Molecular Identification of MCMV Antigens That Elicit Protective Immunity 202
3.1 Immediate-Early Antigens Dominate the CTL Response to MCMV Infection 202
3.2 MCMV IE Genes and Gene Products 204
3.3 Regulatory Function of pp89 205
3.4 Identification of pp89 as an Antigen for CTL 206
3.5 Protective Immunity Mediated by CD8$^+$ Effector T-Lymphocytes Specific for pp89 207
3.6 Molecular Basis of the Recognition of pp89 by CTL 208
3.6.1 Antigenic Site in pp89 208
3.6.2 A Pentapeptide as Minimal Antigenic Determinant of pp89 211
4 Temporal Regulation of the Presentation of the pp89-Derived Antigenic Determinant 212
5 Conclusions 214
References 215

1 Introduction

Cytomegalovirus (CMV) infection can occur throughout life. Similar to other herpesviruses, after primary infection CMV remains in the host in a latent state. Infection of the immunocompetent host does not cause clinical symptoms, whereas infection of the immunocompromised host can cause severe and even fatal disease. Morbidity and mortality associated with primary CMV infection or with reactivation from latency is common in immunosuppressed transplant recipients and in patients with immunodeficiency caused by HIV infection. CMV pneumonia is considered the immediate cause of death in these patients.

Department of Virology, Institute for Microbiology, University of Ulm, D-7900 Ulm, FRG
*This work was supported by The Deutsche Forschungsgemeinschaft grant Ko 571/8 and SFB 322. M.
Del Val received a fellowship by the Alexander-von-Humboldt Foundation

Chemotherapy with the guanosine analog 9-(1,3-dihydroxy-2-propoxymethyl) guanine (ganciclovir, DHPG) can limit viral spread, but is associated with serious side effects. In absence of an improvement of the immunological status, maintenance therapy with ganciclovir does not eliminate the virus, and even progression of infection is possible (DREW 1988). Passive immunization with anti-CMV immunoglobulin does not show consistent benefits in the prevention of infection (SULLIVAN 1987). Combined regimens of chemotherapy and immunotherapy appear to be more successful than either therapy alone (REED et al. 1988; EMANUEL et al. 1988).

Clinical evidence suggests that CMV infection is controlled by the cellular immune response (QUINNAN et al. 1982). Therefore, treatments aimed to reconstitute specific cellular immune functions may be more effective in controlling CMV disease.

Crucial for an approach to prevent CMV disease by cellular immunotherapy is a better understanding of the pathogenesis of the infection, of the possible contribution of different T-lymphocyte subsets to its control, and of the viral antigens recognized by specific T-lymphocytes with protective effects in vivo. Owing to the principle difficulties in studying the in vivo function of T-lymphocytes in humans, an animal model of CMV infection is needed. The strict species specificity of cytomegaloviruses prevents infection experiments with human CMV (HCMV) and, therefore, the infection of the mouse with murine CMV (MCMV) was chosen for a model.

The objective of this study was to analyze the induction and the antigen specificity of T-lymphocytes in mice infected with MCMV. The antiviral in vivo effector function of T-lymphocytes was tested in an experimental regimen designed to reflect the clinical conditions found in the immunocompromised patient. The gene encoding an antigen recognized by protective T-lymphocytes was identified and was then used to construct a recombinant experimental vaccine. It is demonstrated that vaccination with a nonstructural viral protein can induce a protective T-lymphocyte response.

2 Murine Model for the Study of Protective Immunity to CMV Disease

MCMV infection offers the advantage of studying lethal CMV disease, protection against it, and the conditions for establishing persistent and latent infection in the natural host.

2.1 Cell-Type-Specific MCMV Morphogenesis and Its Relation to Pathogenicity

If we wish to understand the pathobiology of CMV, it is worth recalling that early investigators described for several species the presence in salivary glands of enlarged cells containing pronounced intranuclear inclusions (COLE and KUTTNER 1926;

KUTTNER 1927; KUTTNER and WANG 1934; McCORDOCK and SMITH 1936). The viruses causing this cytopathic effect were from then on known as salivary gland viruses until they were renamed cytomegaloviruses (WELLER et al. 1960). The cell type involved could not be isolated and cultivated, and it was not until 1954 that SMITH succeeded in propagating the mouse salivary gland virus in cell culture in murine embryonic fibroblasts. Ultrastructural examination revealed marked differences between in vivo and in vitro virion morphogenesis (LUSSIER et al. 1974). Virus production in salivary glands of the chronically infected host proved restricted to a particular cell type, the acinar glandular epithelial cells that undergo necrosis during termination of chronic infection (HENSON and STRANO 1972). In this cell type high numbers of exclusively monocapsid virions can be seen in cytoplasmic vacuoles, each of which is filled with ca. 1000 virions, which is in the range of 10^4–10^5 virions/cell. As opposed to this, two modes of virion assembly occur simultaneously in embryonic fibroblasts in cell culture; some nucleocapsids bud at the inner nuclear membrane and are released as monocapsid virions, whereas most nucleocapsids gather in the cytoplasm to extensive aggregates which bud into cytoplasmic vacuoles and leave the cell by exocytosis as multicapsid virions (HUDSON et al. 1976; WEILAND et al. 1986). This in vitro type of morphogenesis has been related to reduced pathogenicity. It has been reported that "attenuation" is readily established in fibroblast cell culture and can be reversed by only one in vivo passage (OSBORN and WALKER 1971; CHONG and MIMS 1981).

2.2 Manifestations of CMV Disease in the Immunocompetent and the Immunocompromised Host

QUINNAN and MANISCHEWITZ (1987) have concluded that genetically determined resistance to lethal MCMV infection is not immunologically mediated, but is dependent on the permissivity of host cells to support virus replication, and major histocompatibility complex (MHC)-related differences in the permissivity of macrophages have been reported by PRICE et al. (1987). Yet, it is clinical experience with human CMV infection that lethal manifestations of CMV disease develop only during immunodeficiency. Specifically, interstitial CMV pneumonia is a risk after immunodepletion by whole-body irradiation in leukemia patients receiving bone marrow transplantation (MEYERS 1984). It was therefore our aim to establish a model that conforms to the clinical reality. Three basic conditions have to be fulfilled: first, the selected mouse strain should be susceptible to infection. Second, the infection should be controlled in the case of immunocompetence. Third, lethal CMV disease should develop during an immunodeficient state.

When fully immunocompetent, adult mice of the susceptible strain BALB/c (MHC-d) are experimentally infected by a subcutaneous route with purified, fibroblast-culture-derived MCMV, Smith strain, no morbidity or mortality is seen (lethal dose > 10^7 plaque-forming units, PFUs). Virus replication persists for ca. 6–8 weeks selectively in salivary gland tissue, is confined to acinar glandular epithelial cells, and is followed by the establishment of latency. On the contrary,

BALB/c mice inoculated by the intraperitoneal route with a virulent salivary gland virus preparation die of MCMV disease (50% lethal dose ca. 10^5 PFUs). This discrepancy raises the question of which mode of infection more closely reflects the natural conditions and should thus be preferred for use in models for the study of CMV pathogenesis. Even though at first glance one might argue that fibroblast-culture-derived MCMV is not the naturally occurring virus, the restricted tissue distribution of virus replication resulting from this mode of infection closely resembles the situation in chronically infected feral mice in which a disseminated virulent MCMV infection was seen only after immunosuppression (GARDNER et al. 1974), as it was the case also in experimental models of CMV recurrence (MAYO et al. 1977; JORDAN et al. 1977; SHANLEY et al. 1979).

As a model, it was therefore decided to use the intraplantar infection with fibroblast-culture-derived MCMV for the study of CMV disease and its prevention in BALB/c mice immunodepleted by 6 Gy irradiation using a ^{137}Cs source.

By day 10 after infection of immunodepleted mice, a swelling of the footpad became visible that developed into necrosis of the tissue. Histological examination revealed a highly exudative process with extensive hemorrhages, but no cellular infiltration except of a few neutrophilic granulocytes. Ultrastructural analysis demonstrated productive infection followed by disintegration mainly of connective tissue fibroblasts and adventitial cells. From the local site of infection, the virus disseminated to vital tissues. By in situ DNA-DNA hybridization using cloned genomic fragments of MCMV DNA, single foci of colonization were demonstrated in the lungs at day 6 p.i., corresponding to a virus content of 100–1000 PFUs, and the titers for other organs were similar. Focal spread of the infection in tissues then led to a log-linear increase in the virus titers approaching 10^6–10^7 PFUs at the peak of mortality, as exemplified for salivary glands, lungs, liver, spleen, and adrenal glands. All irradiated infected mice inevitably died in the period between day 10 and day 18 after infection. The terminal stage of disease was signified by a severe wasting syndrome, aplasia, hepatitis with focal liver necroses caused by productive infection of hepatocytes, adrenalitis with necroses mainly in the reticular zone of the cortex, and interstitial pneumonia with infected interstitial fibroblasts, pneumocytes, and endothelial cells (REDDEHASE et al. 1985, 1988). Productive infection of pulmonary macrophages, described by BRODY and CRAIGHEAD (1974) for mice that developed pulmonary cytomegalic inclusion disease after immunosuppression with antilymph-ocyte antiserum, was not seen in the irradiated host, in which cellular infiltration of lung tissue was absent. In salivary gland tissue, infection was not confined to acinar glandular epithelial cells but had spread to fibroblasts also. In fibroblasts infected in vivo (REDDEHASE et al. 1985), including those in salivary gland tissue (WEILAND, personal communication), and also in other cell types as documented for paren-chymal cells of the adrenal cortex (REDDEHASE et al. 1988), virion morphogenesis was as described for embryonic fibroblasts in cell culture.

In our interpretation, the virion morphogenesis observed in embryonic fi-broblasts in cell culture is not a sign of in vitro attenuation, but reflects a "fibroblast type" of virion morphogenesis that is the rule also in vivo in the immunodeficient host for fibroblasts and most other cell types including epithelial cells, for instance pneumocytes, whereas the type of morphogenesis seen in acinar glandular epithelial cells appears to be the exception. It is a not yet fully explained, but interesting, observation (SELGRADE et al. 1981) that salivary gland virus isolated early after infection or from immunosuppressed mice is more virulent than embryo fibroblast culture-derived MCMV, whereas virus recovered from salivary gland tissue during the persistent phase in immunocompetent mice is less virulent, suggesting that the virulence of the virus produced in salivary gland tissue is influenced by the immune response. Along the same line of reasoning, salivary glands of immunologically immature, weanling mice are a source of virulent isolates (OSBORN and WALKER 1971). Virus recovered during the acute phase of infection from liver or spleen is also of low virulence (EIZURA and MINAMISHIMA 1979). It is worthy of consideration that, regardless of the virulence of the seeding virus, the virus produced in the respective tissue is responsible for the focal spread of infection. In light of these arguments, the simplistic view that virus produced in vivo is virulent and that virus produced in culture is attenuated has to be revised.

In conclusion, the infection model fulfills the three basic conditions formulated above, and should allow identification of the immune mechanisms that restrict virus replication to salivary gland tissue and prevent virus dissemination and disease.

2.3 Protective Immunity Mediated by T-Lymphocytes of the CD8 Subset

Enhanced susceptibility of the athymic mutant *nu/nu* (nude) as compared with the heterozygous euthymic *nu/+* mice has indicated a role for T-lymphocytes in the resistance to MCMV infection (SELGRADE et al. 1976; STARR and ALLISON 1977). In *nu/nu* mice, the T-lymphocyte subsets $CD4^+CD8^-$ and $CD4^-CD8^+$ are deficient, while a $CD4^-CD8^-$ population is amplified (MACDONALD et al. 1986). It is now established that T-lymphocytes of this new subset express γ/δ T-cell receptors and are capable of performing a cytolytic function (MOINGEON et al. 1987; MATIS et al. 1987). The resistance of *nu/nu* mice was further reduced by in vivo depletion of asialo-GM_1-expressing lymphocytes (BUKOWSKI et al. 1983, 1984). This finding, in concert with the observation of an elevated susceptibility of "natural killer" (NK)-deficient *bg/bg* (beige) mutant mice (SHELLAM et al. 1981), provided arguments for an involvement also of NK cells in the control of MCMV infection.

A population present in the spleen of adult, normal mice and effective upon adoptive transfer in protecting 3- to 5-day-old, that is immunologically immature, mice from lethal MCMV disease was identified as lymphocytes with the phenotype $Thy-1^-$, asialo-GM_1^+, $NK1^+$, $Ly-5^+$, characteristic of NK cells (BUKOWSKI et al. 1985). Yet, in these experiments, more than 10^7 splenocytes were required to see protection, and an earlier report (STARR and ALLISON 1977) adds the information that transfer even of 10^8 unprimed splenocytes failed to protect lethally infected adult mice. The studies of STARR and ALLISON (1977) and of HO (1980) provided evidence for an amplification of antiviral effector cells during infection. These cells were classified as T-lymphocytes by the expression of the Thy-1 surface antigen and by restriction of their function through MHC genes. Upon adoptive transfer they prevented liver pathology and mortality in immunocompetent recipients that were lethally infected by the intraperitoneal route. In accord with the clinical experience that disseminated CMV infection occurs in patients regardless of the presence of antiviral antibody in sera (CRAIGHEAD 1969), STARR and ALLISON (1977) reported the failure of infused immune serum to protect. In view of these results it could already be proposed that control of virus dissemination in tissue is a function mainly of specific cellular immunity mediated by T-lymphocytes.

Interpretation problems are inherent with the use of transfer recipients that are immunocompetent or only partly immunodeficient. First, a direct antiviral effect of lymphocyte subpopulations cannot be assessed with certainty, as donor cells may operate indirectly by stimulating cells of the recipient to perform an antiviral function, and, second, an occupation of lymphoid tissues by resident cells impedes the homing of transfused effector cells and can thereby limit their efficacy. Inconsistencies in the literature concerning the involvement of lymphocyte subpopulations in the control of infection may relate to this.

Immunodepletion of transfer recipients by whole-body irradiation permits homing of transfused donor lymphocytes to lymphoid sites and infiltration into infected host tissues. This provides the basis for testing a modulation of disseminated, lethal infection by transfer of defined lymphocyte subpopulations, with the aim of working out a regimen for cytoimmunotherapy of CMV disease in the irradiated host. The same approach can be taken also as an in vivo assay for estimating the strength of the antiviral immunity established in infected donor mice. Two protocols were employed in our studies, the "prophylactic" and the "therapeutic" adoptive transfer. The protocols differ in that for the prophylactic transfer donor lymphocytes were infused before the infection with the idea that the colonization of host tissues by virus can then be prevented, whereas, for the therapeutic transfer, infusion was done at day 6 p.i., that is, at a time when the infection was already established in tissues and when antiviral effector cells were thus needed for limiting its focal spread (REDDEHASE et al. 1985, 1987a, b, 1988).

The confinement of viral replication to salivary gland tissue after intraplantar infection of immunocompetent BALB/c mice is accompanied by a strong response in the draining popliteal lymph node, during which T-lymphocytes with the phenotype Thy-1$^+$, CD5$^+$, CD8$^+$ are generated that can proliferate in vitro without further antigen contact in the presence of interleukin-2 to Thy-1$^+$, CD5$^-$, CD8$^+$ cytolytic clones with MHC-restricted antiviral specificity (REDDEHASE et al. 1984a). In view of the coincidence of these events it was reasoned that T-lymphocytes of the CD8 subset, specifically sensitized by viral antigens and found in the regional lymph node that drains the local site of infection, are responsible for the observed pattern of virus replication in host tissues. Upon prophylactic adoptive transfer, as few as 10^4 sensitized lymph node lymphocytes, taken from donors at the peak of the immune response during acute infection, diminished virus replication in recipient tissues, and 10^7 lymphocytes proved efficient in preventing infection of tissues except of salivary gland tissue. Yet, even though dissemination of MCMV to the salivary glands was not prevented, local virus production was reduced by a factor of 10^2 (REDDEHASE et al. 1985) and, as it was the case in the immunocompetent host, infection was then confined to acinar glandular epithelial cells while sparing the fibroblasts. This cell-type selectivity of the antiviral control implied that salivary gland tissue is accessible to effector lymphocytes, and that persistent infection is based on an as yet undefined immune escape mechanism of the glandular epithelial cells. Because of the high productivity of the virion morphogenesis in this cell type, few infected cells can account for the virus titer determined for the whole gland. Evidence for a function of the effector cells in controlling the focal spread of virus in tissue was provided by the antiviral effect assessed with the therapeutic transfer protocol, albeit ca. 100-fold more cells were needed to cope with established infection (REDDEHASE et al. 1985, 1987a). In accord with the in vitro requirement of interleukin-2 for the proliferation of antiviral cytolytic T-lymphocytes, the in vivo antiviral efficacy in both the prophylactic and the therapeutic transfer protocol could be improved by in vivo application of interleukin-2 (REDDEHASE et al. 1987a).

While a preceding priming with antigen, as accomplished by infection, was required for an in vivo amplification of T-lymphocytes with anti-MCMV specificity, the state of activity of T-lymphocytes at the time of the transfer appeared to be less decisive for the in vivo function: acutely sensitized lymph node lymphocytes without detectable ex vivo cytolytic activity (REDDEHASE et al. 1985, 1987a), cytolytic lines of

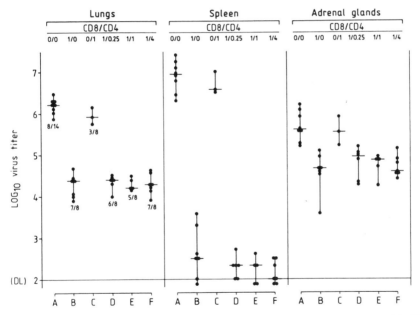

Fig. 1. Identification of the memory T-lymphocyte subset operating in a short-term antiviral immunotherapy model. Memory cells of either T-lymphocyte subset or defined mixtures of both were transferred i.v. into irradiated (6 Gy) and infected (10^5 PFUs of fibroblast culture-derived MCMV) recipients at day 6 p.i., i.e., according to the therapeutic schedule. Spleens of 10-month-old latently infected BALB/c mice, infected the day after birth i.p. with 100 PFUs of fibroblast culture-derived MCMV, were taken as the source of memory T-lymphocytes. *Closed circles* signify individual titers in tissues determined at day 14 p.i., and median values are marked by *horizontal bars*. The detection level (DL) was 100 PFUs/organ. The proportion of recipients that had survived until the day of assay is given in the *left panel. Columns: A*, no transfer of lymphocytes (code 0/0); *B*, transfer of 10^6 T-lymphocytes depleted of the CD4 subset (code 1/0); *C*, transfer of 10^6 T-lymphocytes depleted of the CD8 subset (code 0/1); *D–F*, transfer of mixtures of both subsets composed as indicated. (From REDDEHASE et al. 1988)

T-lymphocytes derived thereof by propagation in vitro with interleukin-2 (REDDEHASE et al. 1987b), as well as memory T-lymphocytes recovered from the spleen of latently infected mice months after primary infection (REDDEHASE et al. 1988) proved equally effective upon adoptive transfer. Concordantly, in all three cases, the antiviral effector cells belonged to the CD4$^-$CD8$^+$ subset of T-lymphocytes, while T-lymphocytes of the CD4$^+$CD8$^-$ subset had no antiviral effect on their own and were also not required as helper cells, as was concluded from therapeutic cotransfer of the two subsets into irradiated recipients (Fig. 1). These data are contrary to findings by SHANLEY (1987), who reported for *nu/nu* recipients an antiviral function of the CD4 subset in the adrenal glands and a failure of either

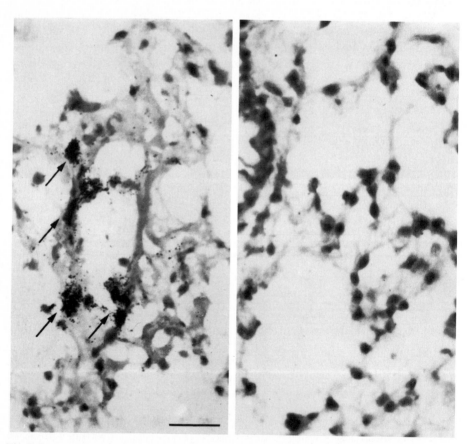

Fig. 2a, b. In situ demonstration of the antiviral effect of CD8-positive T-lymphocytes. Infected cells in frozen thin sections (5–10 μm) of lung tissue were visualized at day 14 postinfection by in situ hybridization of viral nucleic acid with a mixture of plasmid-cloned MCMV DNA fragments as specific probe. A polyclonal short-term T-lymphocyte line was obtained from the draining popliteal lymph node during the acute response to intraplantar infection by in vitro propagation of sensitized T-lymphocytes in interleukin-2 for 8 days. The population was found to be composed ca. half and half of CD8$^+$CD4$^-$ and CD8$^-$CD4$^+$ T-lymphocytes, and was depleted of either subset before prophylactic adoptive transfer. **a** Transfer of 2 × 10^5 CD4-positive T-lymphocytes. **b** Transfer of 2 × 10^5 CD8-positive T-lymphocytes. *Arrows* in **a** point to clusters of infected cells. Both sections are shown at the same magnification. *Bar,* 30 μm. (From REDDEHASE et al. 1987b)

subset in controlling the infection of the lungs. The independence of the CD8$^+$ effector T-lymphocytes was affirmed by transfer into irradiated recipients that were in addition depleted of the CD4 subset by infusion of anti-CD4 antibody to make sure that no help was delivered by residual or reconstituted CD4$^+$ T-lymphocytes of the recipient (REDDEHASE et al. 1988). For a cytolytic antiviral activity in vitro, CD8$^+$ memory T-lymphocytes need to be restimulated by antigen (Ho and ASHMAN 1979; REDDEHASE et al. 1984b), and from this requirement it is expected that transferred memory cells must encounter antigen in the recipient to function. Infiltration by CD8$^+$ memory T-lymphocytes of infected adrenal cortical tissue, a site to which intravenously infused lymphocytes have to migrate specifically, could be demonstrated by immunohistological staining (REDDEHASE et al. 1988).

It is worth emphasizing that the antiviral activity of the CD8$^+$ effector T-lymphocytes was not accompanied by cell-mediated histopathology, but was protective in that it prevented virus-mediated histopathology (Fig. 2) and mortality (REDDEHASE et al. 1987b).

2.4 Antihemopoietic Effect of CMV Infection and Its Prevention

From previous studies one could conclude that the extent of the involvement of the liver (HENSON et al. 1966; STARR and ALLISON 1977; BUKOWSKI et al. 1984; SELGRADE et al. 1984), the spleen (BUKOWSKI et al. 1984; MERCER and SPECTOR 1986), the adrenal glands (SHANLEY and PESANTI 1986), or the lungs (JORDAN 1978; SHANLEY and PESANTI 1985) is indicative of a lethal outcome of MCMV disease, and, for clinical CMV, pneumonia has long been considered the cause of death from opportunistic or recurrent CMV infection in the immunocompromised patient (NEIMAN et al. 1973; MEYERS 1984). In view of the disseminated fatal MCMV infection affecting several vital organs, and the finding that survival after cytoimmunotherapy correlated with diminished virus replication in any tissue looked at (REDDEHASE et al. 1985, 1987a, b, 1988), it was difficult to ascribe mortality to the histopathology in a particular organ. In a 2 months follow-up of the course of disease in mice that had survived an otherwise lethal MCMV infection as the result of immunotherapy with CD8$^+$ T-lymphocytes, a persistent infection was seen in the salivary glands of most recipients, some of which showed considerable virus replication also in the lungs, without signs of morbidity (REDDEHASE et al. 1987b). This observation raised doubt of whether interstitial pneumonia alone is responsible for mortality.

Studies on clinical CMV and in mouse models indicated that CMV infection interferes with hemopoiesis (OSBORN and SHAHIDI 1973; PETURSSON et al. 1984; BALE et al. 1987), and infection of cells of different hemopoietic lineages, either productive (TEGTMEYER and CRAIGHEAD 1968; OLDING et al. 1975; MIMS and GOULD 1978; BRAUTIGAM et al. 1979; REISER et al. 1986; BRAUN and REISER 1986) or restricted to the expression of immediate-early or early gene products (RICE et al. 1984; EINHORN and ÖST 1984; SCHRIER et al. 1985), has been reported, which may explain depressed immune responsiveness (CARNEY and HIRSCH 1981; LOH and HUDSON 1982; RODGERS et al. 1985; SCHRIER et al. 1986; KAPASI and RICE 1988).

Irradiation   Irradiation & Infection

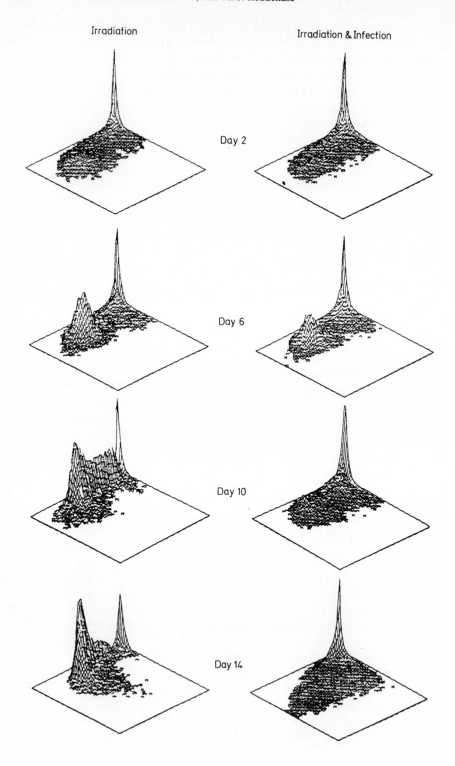

Day 2

Day 6

Day 10

Day 14

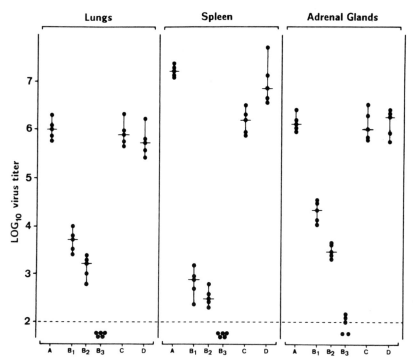

Fig. 4. Antiviral efficacy of T-lymphocyte subsets and bone marrow cells. Lymphocyte subsets were obtained as described for Fig. 2 and transferred according to the prophylactic schedule. Virus titers in tissues were measured at day 14 after infection in five surviving recipients/group. Individual titers are signified by *closed circles*, and median values are marked by *horizontal bars*. The *dashed line* represents the detection level. *A*, no transfer of lymphocytes; B_1, B_2, B_3, transfer of 10^4, 10^5, and 10^6 CD8$^+$ T-lymphocytes, respectively; *C*, transfer of 10^6 CD4$^+$ T-lymphocytes; *D*, transfer of 10^6 bone marrow cells depleted of T-lymphocytes. (From MUTTER et al. 1988)

Irradiation of mice with the sublethal dose of 6 Gy causes a profound immunodepletion, but does not wipe out all bone marrow stem cells, and, therefore, bone marrow and immune system can be replenished by autoreconstitution. This hemopoietic activity should be most sensitive to an intervention, if that exists, by CMV infection. The cellularity of the bone marrow after irradiation alone versus after irradiation and infection was monitored by a dual-parameter light scatter analysis, and in both cases the bone marrow was found to be almost depleted of

Fig. 3. CMV infection prevents autoreconstitution of bone marrow in the irradiated host. *Left column*, kinetics of bone marrow autoreconstitution after total-body irradiation with a dose of 6 Gy, visualized by dual-parameter light scatter analysis of bone marrow cellularity. The main peak that develops with time at a position of intermediate size (*left-pointing axis*) and low granularity (*right-pointing axis*) represents mononuclear cells. *Right column*, kinetics of bone marrow autoreconstitution after irradiation and intraplantar infection with MCMV. Five individuals per group and per time point were analyzed and ranked according to increasing progress in bone marrow autoreconstitution. For the sake of brevity, the bone marrow profiles are depicted only for the animals with the median (No. 3) rank. (From MUTTER et al. 1988)

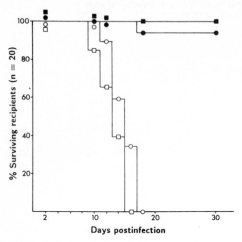

Fig. 5. Antiviral CD8[+] T-lymphocytes and bone marrow cells both protect against lethal CMV disease. Mortality in 20 irradiated (6 Gy) infected recipients/group ($n = 20$) was monitored for 30 days after no transfer of cells (*open squares*), transfer of 10^6 bone marrow cells depleted of T-lymphocytes (*closed squares*), transfer of 10^6 CD4[+] T-lymphocytes (*open circles*), and transfer of 10^6 CD8[+] T-lymphocytes (*closed circles*). (From MUTTER et al. 1988)

nucleated cells at day 2 after irradiation. By day 6 after irradiation, autoreconstitution became visible under both conditions as an emerging peak of bone marrow cells. While, however, after irradiation alone, the generation of bone marrow cells proceeded to normal, hemopoiesis discontinued in irradiated and infected mice, resulting in an aplasia (Fig. 3). From this general failure in hemopoiesis concerning all lineages, it was reasoned that the proliferation of an early progenitor or of the stem cell itself must be affected. A stagnation was seen in the generation of spleen colony-forming units, the CFU-S[14] (MUTTER et al. 1988), which represent the earliest type of multipotential, self-generating hemopoietic stem cell for which an assay is available to date, namely the formation of clonally derived multilineage colonies in the spleen of lethally irradiated recipients by day 14 after intravenous infusion (MAGLI et al. 1982). Interestingly, this intervention of infection with early hemopoiesis and the aplasia resulting from it could be prevented by antiviral T-lymphocytes, and, again, the CD8 subset proved to be the effector subset. This finding raised the question of which function of antiviral CD8[+] T-lymphocytes was decisive for survival: the prevention of tissue lesions in vital organs or the prevention of bone marrow aplasia.

The decision came from the transplantation of syngeneic bone marrow cells. Even though bone marrow cells did not limit virus multiplication in tissues, all recipients survived the infection, because the hemopoietic system was restored (Figs. 4, 5). It was therefore concluded that aplasia resulting from the virus-induced failure in hemopoiesis is the primary cause of death from CMV disease in the immunocompromised murine host, and that its prevention is the critical protective function of antiviral CD8[+] T-lymphocytes.

2.5 Persistent Infection in the CD4-Subset-Depleted Host

Manifestations of CMV disease have been reported as episymptoms of AIDS (DREW and MINTZ 1984). The conditions for superimposed CMV disease during HIV infection differ from those in bone marrow transplant recipients in that the immunosuppression caused by HIV selectively affects the CD4$^+$ T-lymphocytes, while sparing the CD8$^+$ T-lymphocytes (KLATZMANN et al. 1984; SATTENTAU and WEISS 1988). It was therefore of interest to explore to what extent the residual CD8 subset can cope with a CMV infection on its own. As a model for CMV disease in the CD4-subset-deficient host, it was studied how the course of MCMV infection, that is, the succession of acute phase, persistent phase, and latent phase, is altered in mice that are depleted of the CD4 subset (JONJIĆ et al. 1989). The problem falls into two main questions: first, can antiviral CD8$^+$ effector cells be generated from their precursors without help delivered by the CD4 subset, and, second, if so, is the CD4 subset also dispensable for an enduring CD8-subset-mediated control of a persistent or latent infection in absence of antiviral antibody?

To address these questions, BALB/c mice were depleted of the CD4 subset by intravenous infusion of anti-CD4 monoclonal antibody already at the day before the infection, and the depleting antibody was from then on administered weekly to maintain a state of selective CD4-subset deficiency throughout an observation period of 10 weeks. In accord with previous experience (COBBOLD et al. 1984), the depletion was rapid and complete, so that at the time of infection the T-lymphocyte population consisted entirely of CD8$^+$ T-lymphocytes. During long-term depletion, continued absence of CD4$^+$ T-lymphocytes could be confirmed, but a new T-lymphocyte subset with the phenotype CD4$^-$CD8$^-$ was then seen amplified, a phenomenon described recently also for noninfected mice (ERMAK and STEGER 1988).

Confirming the conclusions made in other models of experimental CD4-subset deficiency (COBBOLD et al. 1984; WOFSY et al. 1985; GORONZY et al. 1986; BULLER et al. 1987; AHMED et al. 1988), the production of anti-MCMV antibody proved strictly helper dependent, as mice depleted of the CD4 subset remained seronegative throughout. This finding implies that the newly arising CD4$^-$CD8$^-$ lymphocytes do not substitute for CD4$^+$ T-lymphocytes in providing help to B-lymphocytes.

The strength of the CD8-subset-mediated immunity established at 6 weeks after the infection in presence or absence of the CD4 subset was compared by using the adoptive transfer as an assay for in vivo antiviral function, with the result that CD4$^-$ T-lymphocytes recovered from the spleen were equally effective. Since, however, after long-term depletion of the CD4 subset, the lymphocyte population comprised a CD4$^-$CD8$^+$ and a CD4$^-$CD8$^-$ subset, it became necessary to consider the possibility that the antiviral function was performed also by the CD4$^-$CD8$^-$ subset and not only, as one would anticipate (BULLER et al. 1987; AHMED et al. 1988), by CD8$^+$ effector cells generated independently of the CD4 subset. Depletion in vitro of the CD8$^+$ T-lymphocytes and transfer of the remaining CD4$^-$CD8$^-$ lymphocytes did not reveal any direct antiviral activity of this subset, and affirmed again that antiviral effector cells belong to the CD8 subset. The failure of the CD4$^-$CD8$^-$

lymphocytes in controlling infection is in line with the results obtained in *nu/nu* mice, in which this subset is amplified (MACDONALD et al. 1986), and yet the resistance to MCMV infection reduced (SELGRADE et al. 1976; STARR and ALLISON 1977).

Even though the clearance of productive infection in tissues was delayed in CD4-subset-depleted mice, virus production had ceased by 10 weeks after infection at all sites tested, except in salivary gland tissue, where virus replication was confined to the acinar glandular epithelial cells as described above for chronic infection. The interesting new aspect is that the host was now seronegative, which was taken to mean that antibody is not required for terminating productive infection in most tissues and also not for preventing a redissemination of salivary gland-derived virus to already cleared sites. Again, this control proved a function of CD8$^+$ effector cells, as additional depletion of the CD8 subset in long-term CD4-subset-depleted mice led to continued virus production in the lungs.

In conclusion, while in immunocompetent mice viral latency is established, CD4-subset-deficient mice cannot eliminate virus production in the salivary glands and thus remain persistently infected. As opposed to the prolonged, but finally declining, acute infection of the lungs, the infection of acinar glandular epithelial cells in salivary gland tissue was truly persistent in that virus production continued undiminished for a long period. If we understand latency in a clinical sense as a state during which virus is not replicating at any site, but can be induced to recurrence, then CD4-subset-deficient mice fail to establish latency. Yet, it is incorrect to interpret this as an incompetence of the CD8 subset to aid the establishment of a latent infection of host cells. There is evidence for the spleen being a site of MCMV latency (OLDING et al. 1975; MAYO et al. 1977; WISE et al. 1979; JORDAN et al. 1982; JORDAN and MAR 1982; MERCER et al. 1988), and the spleen was, in fact, one of the first sites at which productive infection discontinued under the influence of antiviral CD8$^+$ effector cells (REDDEHASE et al. 1985, 1987a, b, 1988; JONJIĆ et al. 1989). The basis of the persistent infection in salivary gland tissue rather appears to be an as yet undefined immune escape mechanism of acinar glandular epithelial cells. In light of the special virion morphogenesis seen in this cell type, it can be speculated that viral protein processing and surface presentation required for the reçognition by MHC class I-restricted CD8$^+$ effector cells may differ also.

3 Molecular Identification of MCMV Antigens That Elicit Protective Immunity

3.1 Immediate-Early Antigens Dominate the CTL Response to MCMV Infection

Cytolytic activity against infected cells that present viral antigens is an in vitro testable function of CD8$^+$ T-lymphocytes, defining the cytolytic T-lymphocytes (CTLs), and the induction of virus-specific CTLs has been described also for the infection with MCMV (QUINNAN et al. 1978; HO and ASHMAN 1979; SETHI and BRANDIS 1979). Although it is not proven yet that limitation of viral spread in tissue results from in situ cytolysis of infected cells by CTLs, it is a tacit understanding that viral proteins serving as target antigens for CD8$^+$ CTLs in vitro are relevant also for the protective function of antiviral CD8$^+$ effector cells in vivo. If cytolysis should be the mechanism of viral clearance in tissue, CTLs must lyse infected cells before the release of the majority of progeny virions and the disintegration of cells caused by the lytic infection itself. MCMV gene expression is regulated in a cascade fashion with three distinct phases: immediate-early (IE) genes encode proteins required for the expression of early genes, which, after DNA replication, is followed by the expression of late genes and the production of infectious virus. It was therefore of interest to identify in which phase of viral transcription antigens are expressed that induce antiviral CTLs and elicit protective immunity.

For comparing the relative importance of different MCMV-encoded antigens in the in vivo induction of CTLs, a limiting dilution assay was established to estimate the frequencies of in vivo sensitized interleukin-2 receptive CTL precursors (IL-CTL-P) by in vitro expansion to detectable CTL clones. Restimulation by antigen in vitro is a selective process depending on the antigen preparation used, and leads to a preferential proliferation of those CTLs that are specific for the antigens which are efficiently presented in vitro. To define the immunodominant viral antigens recognized by CTLs in vivo, culture conditions had to be developed that provided the clonal expansion of all sensitized precursors to CTL clones of detectable size, independently of their antigen specificity. In vitro expansion with interleukin-2 in absence of restimulating antigen selects cells only on the basis of in vivo activation, reflected by acquired responsiveness to interleukin-2, and excludes in vitro selection of certain clonotypes based on antigen specificity (REDDEHASE et al. 1984a). With this approach, it was determined that about half of the CTLs induced in a draining popliteal lymph node by day 8 after intraplantar infection are specific for antigens synthesized when viral replication in infected cells is arrested in the IE phase by metabolic inhibitors (REDDEHASE et al. 1984b; REDDEHASE and KOSZINOWSKI 1984). Statistical clonal analysis of polyclonal CTL populations indicated that early- and late-phase proteins can also serve as antigens (REDDEHASE et al. 1984b), and cloned CTL lines with selective specificity for an IE antigen (REDDEHASE et al. 1986a, 1987c), an early antigen (DEL VAL et al. 1989), and virion structural antigens (REDDEHASE et al. 1986a, 1987c) could be established. From the observation that the collective CTL frequency for all other antigens is about the same as the frequency of IE-antigen-specific CTLs, it was concluded that IE proteins are immunodominant (REDDEHASE and KOSZINOWSKI 1984), which, at that time, was surprising, as IE proteins are neither structural components of the virus particle nor integral cell membrane proteins, but are regulatory proteins located predominantly in the nucleus of the infected cell (KEIL et al. 1985; KOSZINOWSKI et al. 1987a).

The first evidence for an in vivo antiviral function of IE-antigen-specific effector cells came from panning studies demonstrating that depletion of IE-antigen-specific CTL activity in polyclonal T-lymphocytes abolishes their capacity to control infection (REDDEHASE et al. 1987b). This indicated that IE antigens not only dominate the CTL response in a quantitative sense, but are also decisive for antiviral function.

3.2 MCMV IE Genes and Gene Products

In order to understand the molecular basis of the recognition of IE antigens, the IE genes and the proteins they encode had to be defined. As the first step, the HindIII fragments of the DNA of the Smith strain of MCMV were cloned and the physical map of the genome was established. The MCMV DNA was found to consist of a long unique sequence spanning 235 kilobase pairs without detectable terminal or internal repeat units and to lack the inverted repeat sequences described for HCMV and other herpesviruses (EBELING et al. 1983). The cloned subgenomic fragments served to define the regions of IE transcription. At IE times, viral RNA species ranging in size from 1.05 to 5.1 kb are transcribed from the adjoining DNA fragments HindIII K and HindIII L, located at between 0.769 and 0.817 map units, and low levels of transcription result from the two terminal fragments (KEIL et al. 1984). IE polypeptides are defined as those synthesized in the presence of actinomycin D after release from a protein synthesis block mediated by cyclohex- imide. Murine immune serum predominantly immunoprecipitates two polypeptides of 89 and 76 kDa, with the 76-kDa polypeptide representing a posttranslational modification product of the 89-kDa protein. The major IE protein is not glycosylated but phosphorylated, and is therefore referred to as pp89 (KEIL et al. 1985). A more detailed analysis revealed that the region of IE transcription can be subdivided into three transcription units. Transcription unit IE1 gives rise to an abundant 2.75-kb mRNA which directs the synthesis of pp89. Smaller mRNA species derived from the same transcription unit are translated into smaller proteins antigenically related to pp89. Upstream of IE1 and separated by a long enhancer sequence (DORSCH-HÄSLER et al. 1985), a second transcription unit, named IE2, could be located. From IE2, a 1.75-kb mRNA of moderate abundance is transcribed in the opposite direction. Hybrid selection and in vitro translation identified a 43- kDa polypeptide as an IE2 product. A third transcription unit, IE3, which shares with IE1 the transcription start site and the first three exons, is located directly downstream of IE1 and gives rise to RNA species of low abundance (KEIL et al. 1987a). To locate precisely the gene encoding pp89, transcription unit IE1 was sequenced and the structural organization of the gene, named IEI, was determined. Nuclease digestion experiments revealed that gene IEI is composed of four exons of 300, 111, 191, and 1703 nucleotides separated by introns of 825, 95, and 122 nucleotides, respectively. The first AUG is located in the second exon and a single open reading frame of 1785 nucleotides predicts a protein of 595 amino acids with a calculated molecular mass of 66.713 kDa (KEIL et al. 1987b).

The comparison of the corresponding regions encoding IE proteins in HCMV and MCMV reveals a certain degree of homology. In both viruses the IE promoters are regulated by a very long and complex enhancer sequence (BOSHART et al. 1985; DORSCH-HÄSLER et al. 1985). A single promoter is used at IE times of infection for transcription of one very abundant mRNA and a number of minor RNA species.

The major mRNA originates from four exons. In both viruses the first exon is not translated, the second exon contains the first AUG, and the fourth exon represents the major component of the mRNA (STENBERG et al. 1984; KEIL et al. 1987b). Downstream of the abundantly expressed major IE gene, and sharing with it the first three exons, another transcription unit is located (IE2 of HCMV and IE3 of MCMV). In HCMV, IE2 transcripts include an additional coding sequence, which contains a splice site used to generate the majority of the transcripts (STENBERG et al. 1985). For MCMV the situation is less clear. There is evidence for at least one IE3 exon which can be used to select mRNA for in vitro translation of IE3 products. The fact that the first three exons of IE1 also hybridize with the same mRNA (KEIL et al. 1987b), along with the finding that antisera with specificity for the amino-terminal sequences of pp89 also precipitate the IE3 product (MESSERLE, unpublished results), further corroborate the structural homology of this gene complex between HCMV and MCMV. A difference concerns the location of the third IE transcription unit. Whereas in MCMV the IE2 unit is located close to the enhancer, no such transcription unit is found in HCMV, and the HCMV IE3 region located further downstream of the HCMV IE1/IE2 complex (STENBERG et al. 1984) has no counterpart in MCMV.

Despite the overall similarity in the organization of the corresponding IE genes of HCMV and MCMV, there is no significant homology with regard to the nucleotide and the amino acid sequences.

3.3 Regulatory Function of pp89

Similar to HCMV and other herpesviruses, MCMV gene expression is coordinately regulated. It is known that IE proteins are required for transcription of the early-phase genes, but the contribution of the individual IE gene products was open to question. To study transcriptional activation mediated by pp89, its coding region was stably introduced into L cells. pp89 constitutively expressed in L-cell transfectants stimulated the expression of cotransfected recombinant constructs containing the bacterial chloramphenicol acetyltransferase gene under the control of viral promoters (KOSZINOWSKI et al. 1986). In a different approach, the effect of the IE*I* gene product on cell cycle regulation was studied. For that purpose, plasmids containing the isolated gene were microinjected into growth-arrested NIH 3T3 fibroblasts. As a consequence of pp89 synthesis, the expression of the c-*fos* protooncogene was stimulated, and at later times cellular DNA synthesis was triggered. These results suggest that pp89 can stimulate cells to enter the cell cycle (SCHICKEDANZ et al. 1988).

In order to activate transcription, pp89 should directly or indirectly be able to interact with DNA. The conditions that permit the interaction of pp89 with DNA were studied. It was found that cellular DNA-binding factors markedly improve the association of pp89 with DNA. These factors could be identified as core histones, to which pp89 has a high-binding affinity (MÜNCH et al. 1988). In this context, it is of interest to note that the N-terminal region of pp89 contains an amino acid sequence homology with histone H2B (KEIL et al. 1987b). Gene IE*I* deletion mutants revealed that this region contributes to histone binding, although deletion of this sequence does not abolish it (MÜNCH ,unpublished). Taken together, these data indicate that pp89 is a regulatory protein. Since an induction of transcription of MCMV early genes by pp89 alone has not been shown yet, the role of pp89 in the coordinate regulation of MCMV transcription is still unknown.

3.4 Identification of pp89 as an Antigen for CTL

Antigenic peptides bound to MHC glycoproteins are recognized by T-lymphocytes via the idiotypic α/β-chain antigen receptor, the T-cell receptor (TCR) (MARRACK and KAPPLER 1987; DAVIS and BJORKMAN 1988). During viral infection, it is to be expected that the immune response comprises polyclonal T-lymphocytes that recognize peptides derived from more than one viral protein and presented by different MHC molecules. Given these variables of the trimolecular interaction between MHC molecule, antigenic peptide, and TCR, it appeared necessary to isolate a CTL clone with specificity for an IE antigen, to identify the presenting MHC molecule, and to characterize the antigenic protein that contains the antigenic determinant.

As a source to isolate CTL clones, BALB/c mice infected as newborns with MCMV were used, because they harbor memory CTL in lymphoid tissues when latency is established after a long period of persistent viral replication. Such memory CTL can be restimulated in vitro by adding infectious virus, and mesenteric lymph nodes turned out to be a superior source of memory CTL specific for IE antigens (REDDEHASE et al. 1984b). A cloned CTL line could be established that recognizes target cells which express IE antigens after enhanced, selective de novo synthesis of IE proteins, as it is achieved by infection with MCMV in the consecutive presence of cycloheximide and actinomycin D (REDDEHASE et al. 1986a). This CTL clone, referred to as clone IE1, displays the morphological phenotype of a large granular lymphocyte, and expresses an α/β TCR/CD3 complex and the surface phenotype CD4$^-$, CD5$^-$, CD8$^+$, Thy1$^+$. CTL clone IE1 can be grown in medium containing interleukin-2 in the absence of restimulating antigen, retaining antigen specificity as an intrinsic property (REDDEHASE et al. 1987c). Clone IE1 defines an IE antigenic determinant presented by the class I glycoprotein encoded by the L^d gene of the murine MHC (REDDEHASE et al. 1986a; KOSZINOWSKI et al. 1987b).

To test which of the IE genes encodes the antigen recognized by this CTL clone, fragments of MCMV DNA were transfected into L cells. Because L cells express the H-2^k haplotype of the murine MHC, it was necessary to cotransfect also the murine L^d gene. Transfection of a 10.8-kb fragment that includes the transcription units ie1 and IE3 and a part of IE2 resulted in cell lines that were lysed by clone IE1 (KOSZINOWSKI et al. 1987b). Using smaller fragments of MCMV DNA for transfection, the transcription unit ie1 was identified as the sequence encoding the IE antigen recognized by CTL clone IE1 (KOSZINOWSKI et al. 1987a). To test whether this finding obtained with a single CTL clone is representative of the polyclonal CTL response generated after MCMV infection in vivo, polyclonal CTL derived from draining lymph node T-lymphocytes by in vitro expansion with interleukin-2 were probed, and recognition of the IE1 transfectant was seen. Frequency analysis revealed that only ca. 25% of the IE-specific CTL clones also recognized the transfectant (KOSZINOWSKI et al. 1987a). This result may be explained a different ways. One possibility is that, in addition to presentation of IE1 products by the L^d molecule, the other two MHC molecules, namely K^d and D^d, also present antigenic determinants encoded by IE1. Another possibility is that clones in the polyclonal CTL population recognize other IE antigens not expressed by the transfectant.

The finding that cell lines transfected with the IE1 transcription unit are recognized by CTL still did not provide formal proof for the tacit assumption that the major IE protein pp89 represents the dominant antigen for the cellular immune response (REDDEHASE et al. 1984b). Several differently spliced mRNA are transcribed from transcription unit IE1, encoding, in addition to pp89, related minor proteins ranging in size from 31 to 67kDa. To prove that pp89 is recognized by CTL, it was necessary to express it selectively. To this end, gene IEI encoding pp89 was restructured by site-directed mutagenesis into an intron-free continuous coding sequence. This open reading frame was integrated into vaccinia virus DNA (VOLKMER et al. 1987). The resulting vaccinia-recombinant MCMV-IEI-VAC specified a protein indistinguishable from pp89 with regard to size, posttranslational processing, and intracellular transport. After infection with MCMV-IEI-VAC, L^d-transfectants were recognized by CTL clone IE1 and also by polyclonal MCMV-specific CTL. The recombinant virus could also be used to sensitize pp89-specific CTL in vivo. Altogether, these data provided evidence that a nonstructural herpesviral protein can stimulate a CTL response (VOLKMER et al. 1987).

3.5 Protective Immunity Mediated by CD8⁺ Effector T-Lymphocytes Specific for pp89

The fact that MCMV-*iel*-VAC was both antigenic and immunogenic provided the basis to test the potential protective effect of this recombinant as an experimental vaccine. This was of particular interest because vaccinia recombinants with protective potential had been generated so far only by insertion of genes coding for viral structural proteins. Protection by a nonstructural protein had not yet been tested. For initial information, the antiviral capacity of CD8⁺ T-lymphocytes derived from donors infected with MCMV-IEI-VAC or whole MCMV was compared. Effector cells from both sources limited viral spread in host tissues after adoptive transfer, but the cells from donors infected with MCMV were more effective. This different efficacy was not surprising, first, because MCMV stimulates a CTL response also to other MCMV antigens in addition to pp89, and, second, because infection with a vaccinia recombinant stimulates mainly CTLs specific for vaccinia antigens while only a minor fraction of cells are directed against the insert gene product. The important question was whether the immune response against the candidate protein was sufficient for protection against a lethal challenge with MCMV. Active immunization with a nonlethal dose of MCMV provided a protection that was not exclusively based on CD8⁺ effector T-lymphocytes, as it was not abolished when the CD8 subset was eliminated in vivo by infusion of anti-CD8

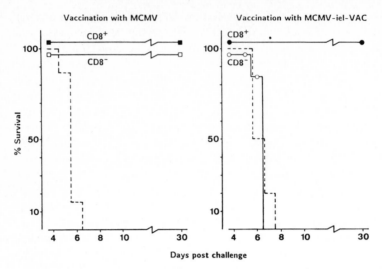

Fig. 6. Protection against challenge infection. Groups of six to ten mice were immunized either by intraplantar infection with a nonlethal dose (2×10^5 PFUs) of fibroblast culture-derived MCMV, by i.v. infection with 2×10^7 PFUs of MCMV-IE*I*-VAC or, for control, of wild-type vaccinia virus. Three weeks later the mice received an i.p. challenge infection with $5 LD_{50}$ of a highly virulent salivary gland isolate of MCMV. *Left panel*, no immunization (*broken line*), vaccination with MCMV (*closed squares*), or vaccination with MCMV and in vivo depletion of $CD8^+$ T-lymphocytes on the day of the challenge (*open squares*). *Right panel*, immunization with wild-type vaccinia virus (*broken line*), vaccination with MCMV-*ieI*-VAC (*closed circles*), or vaccination with MCMV-*ieI*-VAC and in vivo depletion of $CD8^+$ T-lymphocytes on the day of the challenge (*open circles*). (From JONJIĆ et al. 1988)

monoclonal antibody before the challenge (Fig. 6, left). On the other hand, vaccination with MCMV-IE*I*-VAC also provided protection, but this protection proved to be mediated entirely by effector T-lymphocytes of the CD8 subset (Fig. 6, right). Passive immunization demonstrated that serum recovered from mice infected with MCMV, but not from those infected with MCMV-IE-VAC, contained protective antibodies. In essence, different mechanisms of protection appear to be operative in mice infected with MCMV, but sensitization with a single nonstructural viral protein, the IE protein pp89, is sufficient for protective cellular immunity mediated by the CD8 subset of T-lymphocytes (JONJIĆ et al. 1988).

3.6 Molecular Basis for the Recognition of pp89 by CTL

3.6.1 Antigenic Site in pp89

According to current concepts of antigen processing and presentation for T-lymphocytes, most protein antigens undergo intracellular fragmentation, yielding short peptides (GERMAIN et al. 1986, 1988). After binding to MHC glycoproteins and expression at the cell surface, selected peptides of a protein are recognized by the TCR. On this basis, in order to define the antigenic regions of pp89 recognized by

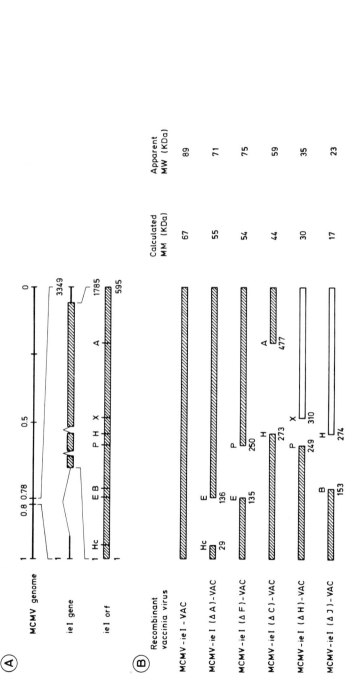

Fig. 7A, B. Structure of the deletion mutants of gene IE*I* encoding pp89. **A** The MCMV IE*I* gene, which is located between 0.78 and 0.80 map units of the MCMV genome, has a length of 3349 base pairs and comprises four exons, the first of which is noncoding. The continuous open reading frame IE*I* (IE*I* orf), 1785 base pairs in length, was derived from the IE*I* gene by site-directed mutagenesis. **B** Deletion mutants of the IE*I* orf, which are drawn to the same scale as the IE*I* orf, were constructed and cloned into vaccinia virus. Relevant restriction enzyme cleavage sites are indicated: *Hc, Hinc*II; *E, Eco*RV; *B, Bgl*II; *P, Pvu*II; *H, Hind*III; *X, Xba*I; *A, Asp*718. The *numbers below the constructs* refer to amino acid positions in pp89. For the mutated proteins, the residues of the authentic pp89 sequence flanking the deletions are indicated. *Hatched bars* represent the pp89 sequence expressed, whereas *open bars* in △**H** and △**J** indicate DNA sequences present in the recombinants but not expressed due to a frame shift that created new stop codons. For each recombinant virus, the molecular mass (*MM*) or the encoded protein was calculated from the amino acid sequence and is shown in comparison with the apparent molecular weight (*MW*) of the expression products that were detected after immunoprecipitation and SDS-polyacrylamide gel electrophoresis. (From DEL VAL et al. 1988)

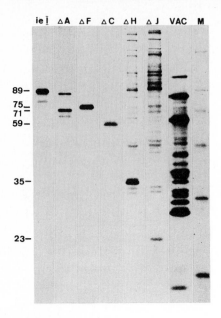

ie I ΔA ΔF ΔC ΔH ΔJ VAC M

89—
75—
71—
59—

35—

23—

Fig. 8. Expression of deletion mutants of pp89 in cells infected with recombinant vaccinia viruses. L cells were labeled for 2 h with [^{35}S]methionine starting at 12 h after infection with the indicated recombinants, and cell lysates, except that of recombinant ΔA, were immunoprecipitated with rabbit antiserum to peptide P(34–53). For the immunoprecipitation of the ΔA product, which lacks the 34–53 region, MCMV immune serum was used. SDS-polyacrylamide gel electrophoresis of the immunoprecipitates and of a representative lysate containing the proteins specified by the vaccinia virus vector (*VAC*) is shown. Apparent molecular masses of the pp89 fragments are indicated in kilodaltons. *M*, standards: 200, 92.5, 69, 46, 30, and 14.3 kDa (From DEL VAL et al. 1988)

CTLs, deletion mutants of the IE*I* open reading frame were constructed and integrated into the vaccinia virus genome for subsequent expression. It was decided to construct internal in-frame deletion mutants with the idea that, if several domains with antigenic and immunogenic properties did exist, all mutant proteins should be detected by some CTLs in a polyclonal population, whereas CTL clones should recognize only those mutants that still contain the relevant antigenic sequence. In Fig. 7, the structure of some of the mutants is depicted and Fig. 8 demonstrates that the expected mutant proteins are expressed in cells after infection with the recombinant viruses. It was found that the deletion mutants ΔF and ΔJ were not recognized by MCMV-specific CTLs, while all other mutants were recognized. This indicated that only the region from amino acids 154 to 249 was essential for antigenicity. The collection of deletion mutants was also used to sensitize mice in order to define the immunogenicity of the mutated proteins. Although the antigenic region must contain the immunodominant epitope of pp89, it was not yet excluded that the pp89 sequence contains additional epitopes which may become antigenic only in absence of the dominant epitope. Such conditions have been shown for a protein that is recognized in association with an MHC class II molecule (GAMMON et al. 1987; ADORINI et al. 1988). The results demonstrated that the only region of pp89 required for sensitization of BALB/c CTLs in the context of any of the H-2^d class I molecules was the same shown before to contain the antigenic sequences.

The data presented so far provided only negative evidence as to the location within the protein of epitopes recognized by CTLs. Because the antigenic sequences of a protein recognized by CTLs can be defined with externally added synthetic peptides (TOWNSEND et al. 1986), the region defined by the deletion mutants was screened for antigenic sequences using the algorithm for predicting antigenic sites by sequence motifs as proposed by ROTHBARD and TAYLOR (1988). When target cells were pulsed with different peptides, only the peptide P (161–179) was detected by both the polyclonal CTL population and the L^d-restricted CTL clone IE1 (DEL VAL et al. 1988). The recognition of the sequence at residues 161–179 presented by the L^d molecule does not exclude the possibility that CTLs from the BALB/c strain can also recognize other epitopes in pp89. However, if additional epitopes do exist, they should be located within or directly adjacent to residues 154–249. The location of the antigenic site excluded the possibility that products of transcription unit IE3 contribute to this response, because the antigenic region is encoded entirely by the fourth exon of gene IE1, which is not shared by IE3 transcripts.

3.6.2 A Pentapeptide as Minimal Antigenic Determinant of pp89

Peptides which are antigenic for T-lymphocytes are ligands of two receptors, the MHC glycoprotein and the TCR. In this trimolecular interaction, amino acids of the peptide must specify the contact with both receptors. The crystallographic structure determined for an MHC class I molecule has revealed a potential combining site that could accommodate an extended peptide of about 8 residues or a helical peptide of about 20 residues (BJORKMAN et al. 1987). The agretope site of an antigenic peptide provides the contact with the MHC molecule and the epitope contacts the TCR (ALLEN et al. 1987; ROTHBARD et al. 1988). With the sequence pattern *HFMPT*, the pp89 peptide H$_2$N-^{161}-GRLMYDMYP*HFMPT*NLGPS-^{179}-COOH contains a predicted linear motif. By screening a series of related peptides reduced in length from both termini (Table 1), the nonapeptide YP*HFMPT*NL was found to represent the optimal antigenic peptide for clone IE1. In addition, this analysis precisely identified the predicted motif *HFMPT* as the minimal antigenic peptide comprising both the complete epitope for recognition by the TCR of clone IE1 and an agretope sufficient for specifying the contact with the L^d molecule.

Titration of the nonapeptide YP*HFMPT*NL, the heptapeptide P*HFMPT*N, and the pentapeptide *HFMPT* revealed 10^3-fold differences in the antigenic potencies. These differences were also reflected by the time needed for optimal target formation; which was a few minutes for the nonapeptide and 2 h or more for the pentapeptide. Since, however, once the target was formed, cells that were prepared with any of the three peptides were lysed to the same extent by clone IE1, it was concluded that reducing the length of the peptide mainly affected the peptide-MHC glycoprotein association. The results obtained were not compatible with the assumption that residues flanking the antigenic pentameric core enhance the affinity to the L^d molecule by providing additional MHC-binding sites. The deletion of Tyr1 from peptide YP*HFMPT*NL diminished and the deletion of Leu9 destroyed the antigenicity, and the resulting octapeptides P*HFMPT*NL and YP*HFMPT*N both also failed to compete with the nonapeptide. These data and results obtained with longer as well as with shorter peptides (Table 1) follow the same consistent pattern, namely that starting with the pentameric motif and up to nonapeptide size symmetrical additions of residues improved the antigenicity, whereas addition of single residues at either end had a negative effect. The results suggest that individual

Table 1. Delimitation of the antigenic motif for CTL clone IE1

Peptide		Peptide concentration [log M]		
		Recognition (competition)	Detection limit	Detection saturation
11-mer:	MYP*HFMP*TNLG	+	-7 to -6	-4 to -3
10-mers:	MYP*HFMP*TNL	+	-9 to -8	-7 to -6
	YP*HFMP*TNLG	+	-8 to -7	-6 to -5
9-mers:	MYP*HFMP*TN	$-(-)$		
	YP*HFMP*TNL	+	-12 to -10	-9 to -7
	P*HFMP*TNLG	$+(-)$	-4 to -3	-2
8-mers:	YP*HFMP*TN	$-(-)$		
	P*HFMP*TNL	$+(-)$	-4 to -3	
7-mers:	YP*HFMP*T	$-$		
	P*HFMP*TN	+	-8 to -7	-4
	*HFMP*TNL	+	-5 to -4	
6-mers:	YP*HFMP*	$-$		
	P*HFMP*T	+	-2 to -3	
	*HFMP*TN	+	-2	
	*FMP*TNL	$-$		
5-mer:	*HFMP*T	+	-3	
4-mers:	*HFMP*	$-$		
	*FMP*T	$-$		

Dose response titrations of peptides giving the peptide molarities in solution required for detectable target formation (detection limit) and for optimal target formation (detection saturation). Peptide sequences are shown in *one-letter code* with the predicted motif set in italic. Clone IE1 CTL served as effector cells in a standard 3-h cytolytic (^{51}Cr release) assay. L/L^d fibroblast transfectants were incubated for 1 h with peptides at defined molarities to serve as target cells. The ability of peptides to compete with the optimal antigenic nonapeptide YP*HFMP*TNL was tested by adding the competitor peptide in 1000-fold excess 30 min before addition of the antigenic peptide. (From REDDEHASE et al. 1989)

residues flanking the antigenic core are not necessarily agretope residues in the sense of MHC receptor-binding sites, but affect, positively or negatively, the antigenic potency by determining the conformation of the peptide (REDDEHASE et al. 1989).

4 Temporal Regulation of the Presentation of the pp89-Derived Antigenic Determinant

Considering the high coding capacity of MCMV (EBELING et al. 1983), the finding that the majority of MCMV-specific CTLs raised in vivo recognize IE antigens was surprising at first glance (REDDEHASE and KOSZINOWSKI 1984). Yet, it may represent an efficient immune mechanism, provided that it leads to the lysis of infected cells by

CTL in the IE phase of the virus replication cycle, thus preventing production and release of infectious progeny virions. The validity of this assumption was tested by studying the kinetics of recognition of pp89 by CTLs throughout the virus replication cycle in permissively infected cells.

According to TOWNSEND et al. (1986), it is assumed that viral proteins are first processed in the cytoplasm of infected cells and then presented by MHC class I molecules at the cell membrane for their recognition by CTLs. Lysis of infected cells by pp89-specific CTLs took place when MCMV gene expression was selectively arrested in the IE phase, while, despite continued presence of pp89, cells were refractory to lysis during the early phase. In the late phase, reexpression of IE genes led to new synthesis of pp89 and to antigenicity for CTL clone IE1. These findings suggested that recognition of pp89 by CTLs might require ongoing synthesis of pp89 (REDDEHASE et al. 1986b). However, when this phenomenon was studied further, it was found that infected cells lost the ability to present pp89 to CTLs even after only 60 min of early gene transcription despite undiminished pp89 synthesis, thus indicating that early gene expression interferes with pp89 antigen presentation (DEL VAL et al. 1989).

For several viruses, including SV40 (GOODING 1982), adenoviruses (BERNARDS et al. 1983; BURGERT and KVIST 1985), and herpesviruses (JENNINGS et al. 1985; MASUCCI et al. 1987), an interference with the recognition of viral antigens by MHC class I-restricted CTL was detected that could be ascribed to decreased expression of MHC class I molecules at the cell membrane. However, throughout MCMV infection, surface expression of class I antigens was not modified (REDDEHASE et al. 1986b). Specifically, no difference in class I antigen presentation to CTLs was observed between the cells that presented pp89 and those that did not, suggesting that the mechanism operating in MCMV-infected cells was different.

Little is known about the steps involved in processing of viral antigens in infected cells. Because incubation of uninfected cells with adequate synthetic peptides derived from a viral protein can render them targets for virus-specific CTLs, it was proposed that antigen processing involves limited intracellular proteolytic cleavage of the viral proteins (TOWNSEND et al. 1986). This hypothesis has recently been strengthened by the finding that increased susceptibility of a protein to degradation correlates with improved presentation to CTLs (TOWNSEND et al. 1988). However, in the case of pp89, it was found that prevention of pp89 recognition by MCMV early gene products did not affect the stability of pp89 (DEL VAL et al. 1989). This indicates that early gene products interfere with pp89 processing by as yet undefined mechanisms.

If the same conditions apply to the infection in vivo, a limited expression of both IE and early genes in cells latently infected with MCMV would prevent recognition of these cells by pp89-specific CTLs and allow their escape and survival in the face of a specific and effective cellular immune response. In addition, during productive infection, this mechanism should delay efficient recognition of permissively infected cells by protective pp89-specific CTLs to the late phase of the virus replication cycle, during which infectious progeny is already released. As a consequence, the efficacy of virus clearance by CTLs would be diminished, thus providing a clear advantage to the virus.

5 Conclusions

By using the infection of immunodeficient mice as a model for CMV disease, experimental evidence for a protective role of CD8[+] T-lymphocytes in the control of acute and persistent CMV infection was provided. Prophylactic transfer of low numbers of sensitized T-lymphocytes did prevent fatal disease, and even a therapeutic lymphocyte transfer could be performed, resulting in a protective effect when the virus had already colonized vital organs.

A viral nonstructural protein, the regulatory IE protein pp89, was identified as an immunodominant antigen recognized by CTLs. The engineering of a recombinant vaccinia virus provided the opportunity to study an experimental vaccine, which selectively expressed this molecule. The results affirm that nonstructural viral proteins have to be considered as candidate antigens for recombinant vaccines against CMV. Protein antigens may contain a large number of antigenic epitopes. The generation of deletion mutants of the gene IE*I*, which encodes pp89, along with the screening of synthetic peptides, were successfully applied to define precisely an antigenic determinant of this protein recognized by CTLs.

Considering the central role of MHC glycoproteins in the presentation of antigens for recognition by T-lymphocytes, it may appear premature to extrapolate from experimental studies in a selected mouse inbred strain to the situation in humans. Since, however, the CTL response to the IE*I* gene product was surprisingly dominant and because the structure and regulation of MCMV IE*I* gene (KEIL et al. 1987b) closely resemble those of the IE1 gene of HCMV (STENBERG et al. 1984), it had been predicted that the HCMV IE1 gene product should represent a major CTL antigen in HCMV infection (KOSZINOWSKI et al. 1987a). The finding that the isolated HCMV IE1 product is detected by human CTLs and indeed represents a major CTL antigen (BORYSIEWICZ et al. 1988) confirmed the prediction, and thus justifies the use of MCMV infection as a model for human CMV disease.

Despite these major advances there are important areas of further study. More information is needed on the largely unknown intracellular events of protein processing and epitope selection, as well as on the presentation of antigens at the surface of infected cells. The interference of MCMV early gene products with the presentation of pp89 provides an example for the regulation of antigen presentation by viral gene expression, and calls for study of the underlying mechanisms.

In the specific case of CMV, when immunodepletion is part of the therapeutic regimen, vaccination and the isolation of CMV-specific lymphocytes for reinfusion after the immunosuppressive therapy could have a potential benefit. The availability of a protein vaccine, free of the risk inherent to infectious recombinant vaccines, would markedly improve the practicability of such an approach. The limiting factor, however, is that the conditions that provide efficient priming of CD8[+] T-lymphocytes by soluble proteins are not known yet. There has been some success in the induction of a primary response to protein fragments and synthetic peptides (WABUKE-BUNOTI et al. 1981; HEBER-KATZ and DIETZSCHOLD 1986; MOORE et al. 1988). However, because function and specificity of CD8[+] T-lymphocytes are restricted through the polymorphic MHC glycoproteins (ZINKERNAGEL and

DOHERTY 1979), the use of selected antigenic peptides may be beneficial to only a few individuals, unless peptides are found that are recognized after presentation by many MHC class I molecules, as has been described for a peptide recognized in the context of several MHC class II molecules (SINIGAGLIA et al. 1988). Therefore, a vaccine should still contain the complete protein to provide the chance that in every individual one of the different protein fragments could serve as an antigen. Altogether, the requirements that govern the response of CD8$^+$ T-lymphocytes to protein antigens of viruses and other pathogens represent important fields of future research.

References

Adorini L, Appella E, Doria G, Nagy ZA (1988) Mechanisms influencing the immunodominance of T cell determinants. J Exp Med 168: 2091–2104
Ahmed R, Butler LD, Bhatti L (1988) T4$^+$ T helper cell function in vivo: differential requirement for induction of antiviral cytotoxic T-cell and antibody responses. J Virol 62: 2102–2106
Allen PM, Matsueda GR, Evans RJ, Dunbar JB Jr, Marshall GR, Unanue ER (1987) Identification of the T cell and Ia contact residues of a T cell antigenic epitope. Nature 327: 713–715
Bale JF, O'Neil ME, Giller R, Perlman S, Koszinowski UH (1987) Murine cytomegalovirus genomic material in marrow cells: relation to altered leukocyte counts during sublethal infection of mice. J Infect Dis 155: 207–212
Bernards R, Schrier PI, Houweling A, Bos JL, van der Eb AJ, Zijlstra M, Melief CJM (1983) Tumorigenicity of cells transformed by adenovirus type 12 by evasion of T-cell immunity. Nature 305: 776–779
Bjorkman PJ, Saper MA, Samraoui B, Bennett WS, Strominger JL, Wiley DC (1987) Structure of the human class I histocompatibility antigen HLA-A2. Nature 329: 506–518
Borysiewicz LK, Hickling JK, Graham S, Sinclair J, Cranage MP, Smith GL, Sissons JGP (1988) Human cytomegalovirus-specific cytotoxic T cells. Relative frequency of stage specific CTL recognizing the 72 kD immediate early protein and glycoprotein B expressed by recombinant vaccinia virus. J Exp Med 168: 919–932
Boshart M, Weber F, Jahn G, Dorsch-Häsler K, Fleckenstein B, Schaffner W (1985) A very strong enhancer is located upstream of an immediate early gene of human cytomegalovirus. Cell 41: 521–530
Braun RW, Reiser HC (1986) Replication of human cytomegalovirus in human peripheral blood T cells. J Virol 60: 29–36
Brautigam AR, Dutko FJ, Olding LB, Oldstone MBA (1979) Pathogenesis of murine cytomegalovirus infection: the macrophage as a permissive cell for cytomegalovirus infection, replication and latency. J Gen Virol 44: 349–359
Brody AR, Craighead JE (1974) Pathogenesis of pulmonary cytomegalovirus infection in immunosuppressed mice. J Infect Dis 129: 677–689
Bukowski JF, Woda BA, Habu S, Okumura K, Welsh RM (1983) Natural killer cell depletion enhances virus synthesis and virus-induced hepatitis in vivo. J Immunol 131: 1531–1537
Bukowski JF, Woda BA, Welsh RM (1984) Pathogenesis of murine cytomegalovirus infection in natural killer cell-depleted mice. J Virol 52: 119–128
Bukowski JF, Warner JF, Dennert G, Welsh RM (1985) Adoptive transfer studies demonstrating the antiviral effect of natural killer cells in vivo. J Exp Med 161: 40–52
Buller RML, Holmes KL, Hügin A, Frederickson TN, Morse HC III (1987) Induction of cytotoxic T-cell responses in vivo in the absence of CD4 helper cells. Nature 328: 77–79
Burgert HG, Kvist S (1985) An adenovirus type 2 glycoprotein blocks cell surface expression of human histocompatibility class I antigens. Cell 41: 987–997
Carney WP, Hirsch MS (1981) Mechanism of immunosuppression in cytomegalovirus mononucleosis. II. Virus-monocyte interactions. J Infect Dis 144: 47–54
Chong KT, Mims CA (1981) Murine cytomegalovirus particle types in relation to sources of virus and pathogenicity. J Gen Virol 57: 415–419

Cobbold SP, Jayasuriya A, Nash A, Prospero TD, Waldmann H (1984) Therapy with monoclonal antibodies by elimination of T-cell subsets in vivo. Nature 312: 548–551

Cole R, Kuttner AG (1926) A filterable virus present in the submaxillary glands of guinea pigs. J Exp Med 44: 855–873

Craighead JE (1969) Immunologic response to cytomegalovirus infection in renal allograft recipients. Am J Epidemiol 90: 506–513

Davis MM, Bjorkman PJ (1988) T-cell antigen receptor genes and T-cell recognition. Nature 334: 395–402

Del Val M, Volkmer H, Rothbard JB, Jonjić S, Messerle M, Schickedanz J, Reddehase MJ, Koszinowski UH (1988) Molecular basis for cytolytic T lymphocyte recognition of the murine cytomegalovirus immediate-early protein pp89. J Virol 62: 3965–3972

Del Val M, Münch K, Reddehase MJ, Koszinowski UH (1989) Presentation of CMV immediate-early antigen to cytolytic T lymphocytes is selectively prevented by viral genes expressed in the early phase. Cell 58: 305–315

Dorsch-Häsler K, Keil GM, Weber F, Jasin M, Schaffner W, Koszinowski UH (1985) A long and complex enhancer activates transcription of the gene coding for the highly abundant immediate early mRNA in murine cytomegalovirus. Proc Natl Acad Sci USA 82: 8325–8329

Drew WL (1988) Cytomegalovirus infection in patients with AIDS. J Infect Dis 158: 449–456

Drew WL, Mintz L (1984) What is the role of cytomegalovirus in AIDS? Ann NY Acad Sci 439: 320–324

Ebeling A, Keil GM, Knust E, Koszinowski UH (1983) Molecular cloning and physical mapping of murine cytomegalovirus DNA. J Virol 47: 421–433

Einhorn L, Öst Å (1984) Cytomegalovirus infection of human blood cells. J Infect Dis 149: 207–214

Eizura Y, Minamishima Y (1979) Co-variation of pathogenicity and antigenicity in murine cytomegalovirus. Microbiol Immunol 23: 559–564

Emanuel D, Cunningham I, Jules-Elysee K, Brochstein JA, Kernan NA, Laver J, Stover D, et al. (1988) Cytomegalovirus pneumonia after bone marrow transplantation successfully treated with the combination of ganciclovir and high-dose intravenous immune globulin. Ann Intern Med 109: 777–782

Ermak TH, Steger HJ (1988) CD4⁻CD8⁻ T cells: amplification in spleens of mice following in vivo treatment with monoclonal antibody anti-L3T4. Eur J Immunol 18: 231–235

Gammon G, Shastri N, Cogswell J, Willbur S, Sadegh-Nasseri S, Krzych U, Miller A, Sercarz EE (1987) The choice of T cell epitopes utilized on a protein antigen depends on multiple factors distant from as well as at the determinant site. Immunol Rev 98: 53–74

Gardner MB, Officer JE, Parker J, Estes JD, Rongey RW (1974) Induction of disseminated virulent cytomegalovirus infection by immunosuppression of naturally chronically infected wild mice. Infect Immun 10: 966–969

Germain RN (1986) The ins and outs of antigen processing and presentation. Nature 332: 687–689

Germain RN (1988) Antigen processing and CD4⁺ T cell depletion in AIDS. Cell 54: 441–444

Gooding LR (1982) Characterization of a progressive tumor from C3H fibroblasts transformed in vitro with SV40 virus. Immunoresistance in vivo correlates with phenotypic loss of H-2Kᵏ. J Immunol 129: 1306–1312

Goronzy J, Weyand CM, Fathman CG (1986) Long-term humoral unresponsiveness in vivo, induced by treatment with monoclonal antibody against L3T4. J Exp Med 164: 911–925

Heber-Katz E, Dietzschold B (1986) Immune response to synthetic herpes simplex virus peptides: the feasibility of a vaccine. Curr Top Microbiol Immunol 130: 51–64

Henson D, Strano AJ (1972) Mouse cytomegalovirus: necrosis of infected and morphologically normal submaxillary gland acinar cells during termination of chronic infection. Am J Pathol 68: 183–202

Henson D, Smith RD, Gehrke J (1966) Nonfatal mouse cytomegalovirus hepatitis: combined morphological, virological, and immunological observations. Am J Pathol 49: 871–888

Ho M (1980) Role of specific cytotoxic lymphocytes in cellular immunity against murine cytomegalovirus. Infect Immun 27: 767–776

Ho M, Ashman RB (1979) Development in vitro of cytotoxic lymphocytes against murine cytomegalovirus. Aust J Exp Biol Med Sci 57: 425–428

Hudson JB, Misra V, Mosmann TR (1976) Properties of the multicapsid virions of murine cytomegalovirus. Virology 72: 224–234

Jennings SR, Rice PL, Kloszewski ED, Anderson RW, Thompson DL, Tevethia SS (1985) Effect of herpes simplex virus types 1 and 2 on surface expression of class I major histocompatibility complex antigens on infected cells. J Virol 56: 757–766

Jonjić S, del Val M, Keil GM, Reddehase MJ, Koszinowski UH (1988) A nonstructural viral protein expressed by a recombinant vaccinia virus protects against lethal cytomegalovirus infection. J Virol 62: 1653–1658

Jonjić S, Mutter W, Weiland F, Reddehase MJ, Koszinowski UH (1989) Site-restricted persistent cytomegalovirus infection after selective long-term depletion of CD4-positive T lymphocytes. J Exp Med 169: 1199–1212

Jordan MC (1978) Interstitial pneumonia and subclinical infection after intranasal inoculation of murine cytomegalovirus. Infect Immun 21: 275–280

Jordan MC, Mar VL (1982) Spontaneous activation of latent cytomegalovirus from murine spleen explants. Role of lymphocytes and macrophages in release and replication of virus. J Clin Invest 70: 762–768

Jordan MC, Shanley JD, Stevens JG (1977) Immunosuppression reactivates and disseminates latent murine cytomegalovirus. J Gen Virol 37: 419–423

Jordan MC, Takagi JL, Stevens JG (1982) Activation of latent murine cytomegalovirus in vivo and in vitro: a pathogenic role for acute infection. J Infect Dis 145: 699–705

Kapasi K, Rice GPA (1988) Cytomegalovirus infection of peripheral blood mononuclear cells: effects on interleukin-1 and -2 production and responsiveness. J Virol 62: 3603–3607

Keil GM, Ebeling-Keil A, Koszinowski UH (1984) Temporal regulation of murine cytomegalovirus transcription and mapping of viral RNA synthesized at immediate early times after infection. J Virol 50: 784–795

Keil GM, Ebeling-Keil A, Koszinowski UH (1987a) Immediate-early genes of murine cytomegalovirus: location, transcripts, and translation products. J Virol 61: 526–533

Keil GM, Ebeling-Keil A, Koszinowski UH (1987b) Sequence and structural organization of murine cytomegalovirus immediate-early gene 1. J Virol 61: 1901–1908

Keil GM, Fibi MR, Koszinowski UH (1985) Characterization of the major immediate-early polypeptides encoded by murine cytomegalovirus. J Virol 54: 422–428

Klatzmann D, Barre-Sinoussi F, Nugeyre MT, Dauguet C, Valmer E, Griscelli C, Brun-Vezinet F, et al. (1984) Selective tropism of lymphoadenopathy-associated virus (LAV) for helper-inducer T lymphocytes. Science 225: 59–63

Koszinowski UH, Keil GM, Volkmer H, Fibi MR, Ebeling–Keil A, Münch K (1986) The 89,000-M$_r$ murine cytomegalovirus immediate-early protein activates gene transcription. J Virol 58: 59–66

Koszinowski UH, Keil GM, Schwarz H, Schickedanz J, Reddehase MJ (1987a) A nonstructural polypeptide encoded by immediate-early transcription unit 1 of murine cytomegalovirus is recognized by cytolytic T lymphocytes. J Exp Med 166: 289–294

Koszinowski UH, Reddehase MJ, Keil GM, Schickedanz J (1987b) Host immune response to cytomegalovirus: products of transfected viral immediate-early genes are recognized by cloned cytolytic T lymphocytes. J Virol 61: 2054–2058

Kuttner AG (1927) Further studies concerning the filterable virus present in the submaxillary glands of guinea pigs. J Exp Med 46: 935–956

Kuttner AG, Wang S-H (1934) The problem of the significance of the inclusion bodies found in the salivary glands of infants, and the occurrence of inclusion bodies in the submaxillary glands of hamsters, white mice, and wild rats (Peiping). J Exp Med 60: 773–791

Loh L, Hudson JB (1982) Murine cytomegalovirus-induced immunosuppression. Infect Immun 36: 89–95

Lussier G, Berthiaume L, Payment P (1974) Electron microscopy of murine cytomegalovirus: development of the virus in vivo and in vitro. Arch Gesamte Virusforsch 46: 269–280

MacDonald HR, Blanc D, Less RK, Sordat B (1986) Abnormal distribution of T cell subsets in athymic mice. J Immunol 136: 4337–4339

Magli MC, Iscove NN, Odartchenko N (1982) Transient nature of early haematopoietic spleen colonies. Nature 295: 527–529

Marrack P, Kappler J (1987) The T-cell receptor. Science 238: 1073–1079

Masucci MG, Torsteinsdottir S, Colombani J, Brautbar C, Klein E, Klein G (1987) Down-regulation of class I HLA antigens and of the Epstein-Barr virus-encoded latent membrane protein in Burkitt lymphoma lines. Proc Natl Acad Sci USA 84: 4567–4571

Matis LA, Cron R, Bluestone JA (1987) Major histocompatibility complex-linked specificity of γ/δ receptor-bearing T lymphocytes. Nature 330: 262–264

Mayo DR, Armstrong JA, Ho M (1977) Reactivation of murine cytomegalovirus by cyclophosphamide. Nature 267: 721–723

McCordock HA, Smith MG (1936) The visceral lesions produced in mice by the salivary gland virus of mice. J Exp Med 63: 303–310

Mercer JA, Spector DH (1986) Pathogenesis of acute murine cytomegalovirus infection in resistant and susceptible strains of mice. J Virol 57: 497–504

Mercer JA, Wiley CA, Spector DH (1988) Pathogenesis of murine cytomegalovirus infection: identification of infected cells in the spleen during acute and latent infections. J Virol 62: 987–997

Meyers JD (1984) Cytomegalovirus infection following marrow transplantation: risk, treatment, and prevention. Birth Defects 20: 101–117

Mims CA, Gould J (1978) The role of macrophages in mice infected with murine cytomegalovirus. J Gen Virol 41: 143–153

Moingeon P, Jitsukawa S, Faure F, Troalen F, Triebel F, Graziani M, Forestier F, et al. (1987) A γ-chain complex forms a functional receptor on cloned human lymphocytes with natural killer-like activity. Nature 325: 723–726

Moore MW, Carbone FR, Bevan MJ (1988) Introduction of soluble protein into the class I pathway of antigen processing and presentation. Cell 54: 777–785

Münch K, Keil GM, Messerle M, Koszinowski UH (1988) Interaction of the 89K murine cytomegalovirus immediate-early protein with core histones. Virology 163: 405–412

Mutter W, Reddehase MJ, Busch FW, Bühring H-J, Koszinowski UH (1988) Failure in generating hemopoietic stem cells is the primary cause of death from cytomegalovirus disease in the immunocompromised host. J Exp Med 167: 1645–1658

Neiman P, Wasserman PB, Wentworth BB, Kao GF, Lerner KG, Storb R, Buckner CD, et al. (1973) Interstitial pneumonia and cytomegalovirus infection as complications of human marrow transplantation. Transplantation 15: 478–485

Olding LB, Jensen FC, Oldstone MBA (1975) Pathogenesis of cytomegalovirus infection. I. Activation of virus from bone marrow-derived lymphocytes by in vitro allogenic reaction. J Exp Med 141: 561–571

Osborn JE, Shahidi NT (1973) Thrombocytopenia in murine cytomegalovirus infection. J Lab Clin Med 81: 53–63

Osborn JE, Walker DL (1971) Virulence and attenuation of murine cytomegalovirus. Infect Immun 3: 228–236

Petursson SR, Chervenick PA, Wu B (1984) Megakaryocytopoiesis and granulopoiesis after murine cytomegalovirus infection. J Lab Clin Med 104: 381–390

Price P, Winter JG, Nikoletti S, Hudson JB, Shellam GR (1987) Functional changes in murine macrophages infected with cytomegalovirus relate to H-2 determined sensitivity to infection. J Virol 61: 3602–3606

Quinnan GV Jr, Manischewitz JF (1987) Genetically determined resistance to lethal murine cytomegalovirus infection is mediated by interferon-dependent and -independent restriction of virus replication. J Virol 61: 1875–1881

Quinnan GV, Manschiewitz JE, Ennis FA (1978) Cytotoxic T lymphocyte response to murine cytomegalovirus infection. Nature 273: 541–543

Quinnan GV, Kirmani N, Rook AH, Manischewitz J, Jackson L, Moreschi G, Santos GW, et al. (1982) HLA-restricted T-lymphocyte and non T-lymphocyte cytotoxic responses correlate with recovery from cytomegalovirus infection in bone-marrow-transplant recipients. N Engl J Med 307: 7–13

Reddehase MJ, Koszinowski UH (1984) Significance of herpesvirus immediate early gene expression in cellular immunity to cytomegalovirus infection. Nature 312: 369–371

Reddehase MJ, Keil GM, Koszinowski UH (1984a) The cytolytic T lymphocyte response to the murine cytomegalovirus. I. Distinct maturation stages of cytolytic T lymphocytes constitute the cellular immune response during acute infection of mice with the murine cytomegalovirus. J Immunol 132: 482–489

Reddehase MJ, Keil GM, Koszinowski UH (1984b) The cytolytic T lymphocyte response to the murine cytomegalovirus. II. Detection of virus replication stage-specific antigens by separate populations of in vivo active cytolytic T lymphocyte precursors. Eur J Immunol 14: 56–61

Reddehase MJ, Weiland F, Münch K, Jonjić S, Lüske A, Koszinowski UH (1985) Interstitial murine cytomegalovirus pneumonia after irradiation: characterization of cells that limit viral replication during established infection of the lungs. J Virol 55: 264–273

Reddehase MJ, Bühring H-J, Koszinowski UH (1986a) Cloned long-term cytolytic T-lymphocyte line with specificity for an immediate-early membrane antigen of murine cytomegalovirus. J Virol 57: 408–412

Reddehase MJ, Fibi MR, Keil GM, Koszinowski UH (1986b) Late-phase expression of a murine cytomegalovirus immediate-early antigen recognized by cytolytic T lymphocytes. J Virol 60: 1125–1129

Reddehase MJ, Mutter W, Koszinowski UH (1987a) In vivo application of recombinant interleukin-2 in the immunotherapy of established cytomegalovirus infection. J Exp Med 165: 650–656

Reddehase MJ, Mutter W, Münch K, Bühring H-J, Koszinowski UH (1987b) CD8-positive T lymphocytes specific for murine cytomegalovirus immediate-early antigens mediate protective immunity. J Virol 61: 3102–3108

Reddehase MJ, Zawatzky R, Weiland F, Bühring H-J, Mutter W, Koszinowski UH (1987c) Stable expression of clonal specificity in murine cytomegalovirus-specific large granular lymphoblast lines propagated long-term in recombinant interleukin-2. Immunobiology 174: 420–431

Reddehase MJ, Jonjić S, Weiland F, Mutter W, Koszinowski UH (1988) Adoptive immunotherapy of murine cytomegalovirus adrenalitis in the immunocompromised host: CD4-helper-independent antiviral function of CD8-positive memory T lymphocytes derived from latently infected donors. J Virol 62: 1061–1065

Reddehase MJ, Rothbard JB, Koszinowski UH (1989) A pentapeptide as minimal antigenic determinant for MHC class I-restricted T lymphocytes. Nature 337: 651–653

Reed EC, Bowden RA, Dandliker PS, Lilleby KE, Meyers JD (1988) Treatment of cytomegalovirus pneumonia with ganciclovir and intravenous cytomegalovirus immunoglobulin in patients with bone marrow transplants. Ann Intern Med 109: 783–788

Reiser HC, Kühn J, Doerr HW, Kirchner H, Munk K, Braun RW (1986) Human cytomegalovirus replicates in primary human bone marrow cells. J Gen Virol 67: 2595–2604

Rice GPA, Schrier RD, Oldstone MBA (1984) Cytomegalovirus infects human lymphocytes and monocytes: virus expression is restricted to immediate-early gene products. Proc Natl Acad Sci USA 81: 6134–6138

Rodgers BC, Scott DM, Mundin J, Sissons JGP (1985) Monocyte-derived inhibitor of IL-1 induced by human CMV. J Virol 55: 527–532

Rothbard JB, Taylor RW (1988) A sequence pattern common to T cell epitopes. EMBO J 7: 93–100

Rothbard JB, Lechler RI, Howland K, Bal V, Eckels DD, Sekaly R, Long EO, et al. (1988) Structural model of HLA-DR1 restricted T cell antigen recognition. Cell 52: 515–523

Sattentau QJ, Weiss RA (1988) The CD4 antigen: physiological ligand and HIV receptor. Cell 52: 631–633

Schickedanz J, Philipson L, Ansorge W, Pepperkok R, Klein R, Koszinowski UH (1988) The 89,000-M_r murine cytomegalovirus immediate-early protein stimulates c-*fos* expression and cellular DNA synthesis. J Virol 62: 3341–3347

Schrier RD, Nelson JA, Oldstone MBA (1985) Detection of human cytomegalovirus in peripheral blood lymphocytes in a natural infection. Science 230: 1048–1051

Schrier RD, Rice GPA, Oldstone MBA (1986) Suppression of NK activity and T cell proliferation induced by fresh isolates of CMV. J Infect Dis 153: 1084–1091

Selgrade MK, Ahmed A, Sell KW, Gershwin ME, Steinberg AD (1976) Effect of murine cytomegalovirus on the in vitro responses of T and B cells to mitogens. J Immunol 116: 1459–1465

Selgrade MK, Nedrud JG, Collier AM, Gardner DE (1981) Effects of cell source, mouse strain, and immunosuppressive treatment on production of virulent and attenuated murine cytomegalovirus. Infect Immun 33: 840–847

Selgrade MK, Collier AM, Saxton L, Daniels MJ, Graham JA (1984) Comparison of the pathogenesis of murine cytomegalovirus in lung and liver following intraperitoneal or intratracheal infection. J Gen Virol 65: 515–523

Sethi KK, Brandis H (1979) Induction of virus specific and H-2 restricted cytotoxic T cells by UV inactivated murine cytomegalovirus. Arch Virol 60: 227–238

Shanley JD (1987) Modification of acute murine cytomegalovirus adrenal gland infection by adoptive spleen cell transfer. J Virol 61: 23–28

Shanley JD, Pesanti EL (1985) The relation of viral replication to interstitial pneumonitis in murine cytomegalovirus lung infection. J Infect Dis 151: 454–458

Shanley JD, Pesanti EL (1986) Murine cytomegalovirus adrenalitis in athymic nude mice. Arch Virol 88: 27–35

Shanley JD, Jordan MC, Cook ML, Stevens JG (1979) Pathogenesis of reactivated latent murine cytomegalovirus infection. Am J Pathol 95: 67–77

Shellam GR, Allan JE, Papadimitriou JM, Bancroft GJ (1981) Increased susceptibility to cytomegalovirus infection in beige mutant mice. Proc Natl Acad Sci USA 78: 5104–5108

Sinigaglia F, Guttinger M, Kilgus J, Doran DM, Matile H, Etlinger H, Trzeciak A et al. (1988) A malaria T-cell epitope recognized in association with most mouse and human MHC class II molecules. Nature 336: 778–780

Smith MG (1954) Propagation of salivary gland virus of the mouse in tissue cultures. Proc Soc Exp Biol Med 86: 435–440

Starr SE, Allison AC (1977) Role of T lymphocytes in recovery from murine cytomegalovirus infection. Infect Immun 17: 458–462

Stenberg RM, Thomsen DR, Stinski MF (1984) Structural analysis of the major immediate early gene of human cytomegalovirus. J Virol 49: 190–199

Stenberg RM, Witte PR, Stinski MF (1985) Multiple spliced and unspliced transcripts from human cytomegalovirus immediate early region 2 and evidence for a common initiation site within immediate early region 1. J Virol 56: 665–675

Sullivan KM (1987) Immunoglobulin therapy in bone marrow transplantation. Am J Med [Suppl 4A] 83: 34–45

Tegtmeyer PJ, Craighead JE (1968) Infection of adult mouse macrophages in vitro with cytomegalovirus. Proc Soc Exp Biol Med 129: 690–694

Townsend ARM, Rothbard J, Gotch FM, Bahadur G, Wraith D, McMichael AJ (1986) The epitopes of influenza nucleoprotein recognized by cytotoxic T lymphocytes can be defined with short synthetic peptides. Cell 44: 959–968

Townsend ARM, Bastin J, Gould K, Brownlee G, Andrew M, Coupar B, Boyle D, et al. (1988) Defective presentation to class I-restricted cytotoxic T lymphocytes in vaccinia-infected cells is overcome by enhanced degradation of antigen. J Exp Med 168: 1211–1224

Volkmer H, Bertholet C, Jonjić S, Wittek R, Koszinowski UH (1987) Cytolytic T lymphocyte recognition of the murine cytomegalovirus nonstructural immediate-early protein pp89 expressed by recombinant vaccinia virus. J Exp Med 166: 668–677

Wabuke-Bunoti MAN, Fan DP, Braciale TJ (1981) Stimulation of anti-influenza cytolytic T lymphocytes by CnBr cleavage fragments of the viral hemagglutinin. J Immunol 127: 1122–1125

Weiland F, Keil GM, Reddehase MJ, Koszinowski UH (1986) Studies on the morphogenesis of murine cytomegalovirus. Intervirology 26: 192–201

Weller TH, Hanshaw JB, Scott DE (1960) Serological differentiation of viruses responsible for cytomegalic inclusion disease. Virology 12: 130–132

Wise TG, Manischewitz JF, Quinnan GV, Aulakh GS, Ennis FA (1979) Latent cytomegalovirus infection of BALB/c mouse spleens detected by an explant culture technique. J Gen Virol 44: 551–556

Wofsy D, Mayes DC, Woodcock J, Seaman WE (1985) Inhibition of humoral immunity in vivo by monoclonal antibody to L3T4: studies with soluble antigens in intact mice. J Immunol 135: 1698–1701

Zinkernagel RM, Doherty PC (1979) MHC-restricted cytotoxic T cells: studies on the biological role of polymorphic major transplantation antigens determining T cell restriction specificity, function and responsiveness. Adv Immunol 27: 52–177

Immune Response to Human Cytomegalovirus Infection

L. RASMUSSEN

1 Introduction 222
2 Intracellular Viral Proteins 222
2.1 Immediate-Early (α) Proteins 223
2.2 Delayed Early (β) Proteins 223
2.2.1 DNA-Binding Protein 223
2.2.2 72-kDa Protein 224
2.2.3 Viral DNA Polymerase 224
2.3 Late (γ) Proteins 224
2.3.1 51-kDa DNA-Binding Protein 224
3 Structural Proteins 224
3.1 Intracellular Development of Virions 224
3.2 Proteins Associated with Extracellular Virion Forms 226
3.2.1 Viral Matrix Proteins 226
3.2.2 Major Nucleocapsid Protein 227
3.2.3 28-kDa Structural Protein 227
3.2.4 46-kDa DNAse 227
3.2.5 Protein Kinase 228
4 Envelope Glycoproteins 228
4.1 gB Homolog 229
4.2 gH Homolog 231
4.3 gcII 232
5 Proteins Identified by Sequence Analysis Only 233
5.1 MHC Class I Antigen Homolog 233
6 Patterns of CMV Infection 233
7 Antigenic Properties of Viral Proteins 234
7.1 Humoral Immune Responses 234
7.1.1 Antibodies Reactive with Specific Viral Proteins 235
7.1.2 Virus-Neutralizing Antibody 237
7.1.3 Cytolytic Antibody 238
7.1.4 Nonantiviral Consequences of the Humoral Immune Response 238
7.1.5 Mechanism of Interaction of CMV with B-Lymphocytes 239
7.2 Cellular Immune Response 239
7.2.1 T-Helper Cell Responses 239
7.2.2 Cytotoxic T-Cell Responses to Viral Antigens 241
7.2.3 Nonspecific Immune Responses 243
8 Conclusions 244
References 246

Division of Infectious Diseases, Stanford Medical School, Stanford, California 94305, USA

Current Topics in Microbiology and Immunology, Vol. 154
© Springer-Verlag Berlin · Heidelberg 1990

1 Introduction

The purpose of this article is to review immune responses to cytomegalovirus (CMV) which may be initiated or guided by specific gene products of the virus. In light of the clinical importance of CMV as a pathogen, increasing efforts are being made to understand the immune response to CMV and how it relates to protection from severe clinical disease. The genome of CMV is 230 kilobases and has the capacity to code for aproximately 200 proteins, each of which may be subject to posttranslational modification by cleavage, phosphorylation, glycosylation, or sulfation. The spectrum of proteins is therefore complex, but our understanding of the immunologic structure of CMV has improved greatly in the past few years, largely as a result of the application of monoclonal antibodies and recombinant DNA technology to the problems of gene and protein identification. The rational design of a subunit CMV vaccine is dependent upon progress in studies of both the virology and immunology of CMV. In this review, I will first summarize what is currently known about the protein structure of human CMV. In that section I will focus on those proteins and glycoproteins that have either been characterized according to function or have been localized to a specific area within the genome. The formidable task of grouping the CMV gene products that have been described to date has been accomplished in a recent review by LANDINI and MICHELSON (1988). Second I will describe the general patterns of immune responsivity to CMV. I will emphasize the human immune responses which have been associated with protection or are thought to be important for containment of virus infection. However, studies in animal models or with non-human CMV strains will be discussed where appropriate. Immune responses which can be stimulated with defined viral proteins will be described.

2 Intracellular Viral Proteins

The proteins described in this section will be those which can be detected in infected cells but are not necessarily destined to be incorporated into the virion structure or viral envelope. The replication cycle of CMV is complex and limited largely to human fibroblast cell cultures, although exceptions have been reported (SMITH 1986). The sequential order of gene expression that is common to other herpesviruses occurs (WALTHEN and STINSKI 1982). Viral genes are expressed at immediate-early (0–2 h), early (2–24 h), and late (after 24 h) times after infection and proteins are classified as α, β, or γ. The proteins that are synthesized during the immediate-early and early periods are generally associated with regulation of virus replication while the late or γ proteins are structural elements, although there are exceptions to this general rule. Most of the envelope glycoproteins of CMV are synthesized during the early and late times after cellular infection and they will be reviewed separately in Sect. 4.

2.1 Immediate-Early (α) Proteins

The immediate-early (IE) genes of CMV are those which are transcribed and translated prior to onset of de novo viral DNA and protein synthesis. This group of genes is being intensively investigated because their regulation may be important in latent CMV infection. The molecular biology of this genetic region has recently been summarized by STINSKI (1984). For CMV (Towne strain) there are three IE gene-coding regions between 0.709 and 0.751 map units within the HindIII region of the unique long sequence. Region one (0.739–0.751) has been designated the major IE gene or IE1. The product of this gene is a 491-amino-acid protein which is modified after translation to give a polypeptide of 75 kDa. It is known that one modification which occurs is phosphorylation and accounts for the size variation among different strains of CMV such as Towne, AD169 and Davis (GIBSON 1981a). The adjacent second region (IE2), from 0.732 to 0.739, codes for proteins which are found in low concentration. A third region between 0.709 and 0.728 codes for a 1.95-kb mRNA that translates into a 68-kDa protein. A second transcriptionally active area at IE times is in a different region of the genome entirely and is located at the junction between HindIII fragments Z and J of strain AD169 (WILKINSON et al. 1984). The sequence of this region has been determined and three mRNAs have been identified by transcription analysis (KOUZARIDES et al. 1988). The predicted translation product of one of the mRNAs has features characteristic of a membrane-bound glycoprotein. The reading frame has the potential to encode a 487-residue polypeptide with a molecular weight of 56 kDa. This finding is of interest because it represents the first example of a potential glycoprotein gene which is transcribed at IE times after infection. As will be discussed in some detail in Sect. 6.2.2, the gene products of both human and murine CMV may be important targets for the HLA-restricted cytotoxic response.

2.2 Delayed Early (β) Proteins

The early proteins of CMV are classified operationally as those that are synthesized before the onset of viral DNA synthesis, as determined using phosphonoacetic acid specifically to block viral DNA polymerase.

2.2.1 DNA-Binding Protein

A major early CMV DNA-binding protein of 129 kDa is present in strain Colburn CMV (GIBSON et al. 1981). The Towne equivalent protein is140 kDa. The protein appears to be the counterpart of the HSV DNA-binding protein ICP8 (ANDERS et al. 1987; KEMBLE et al. 1987). The gene is located within the region between the CMV (AD169) EcoR1 (P/V) and HindIII (F/D) site. The open reading frame within this region has predicted amino acid homology with BALF4 of EBV and to ICP8 of HSV. For Towne strain the gene has been mapped to the EcoRI V and Q fragments (ANDERS and GIBSON 1988). Immunologically the DB129 and DB140 are cross-reactive, suggesting that they are products of homologous genes (ANDERS et al. 1987). By indirect immunofluorescence, this DNA-binding protein was localized within the intranuclear inclusions characteristic of replicating CMV and similar to the nuclear localization of HSV-1 ICP8.

2.2.2 72-kDa Protein

A 72-kDa protein has been purified by immunoaffinity from virus-infected cells using monoclonal antibody that detects early, but not IE, antigens (RODGERS et al. 1987).

2.2.3 Viral DNA Polymerase

A DNA polymerase induced after CMV infection can be distinguished from host cell enzymes by chromatographic behavior, template primer specificity, and sediment-ation behavior. It binds preferentially to single-stranded DNA (MAR et al. 1981, 1985). The sequence and transcriptional analysis of the DNA polymerase gene has been reported by two groups (KOUZARIDES et al. 1987; HEILBRONN et al. 1987). The DNA polymerases of CMV, EBV, and HSV show considerable amino acid homology with a number of highly conserved regions. This close similarity of the herpes group virus-induced enzymes enabled a region to be identified on the CMV genome whose amino acid sequence showed a striking homology to the HSV DNA polymerase amino acid sequence. The CMV DNA polymerase gene is an 850-bp region within the EcoR1 M fragment of strain AD169 in the long unique region with one continuous open reading frame. There is a highly conserved domain of 133 amino acids shared with HSV and the putative EBV polymerase sequences. One 5.4-kb early transcript appears to code for the 140-kDa polymerase protein.

2.3 Late (γ) Proteins

2.3.1 51-kDa DNA-Binding Protein

The 51-kDa DNA-binding protein was first described by GIBSON (1983). The protein is phosphorylated but is not a structural constituent of virus particles. Expression occurs even when viral DNA replication is blocked, but the gene product, also referred to as ICP36, accumulates to abundant levels during the late phase of viral replication. The gene has been localized to a 2800-bp EcoR1 fragment (map coordinates 0.228–0.240) on both the CMV (Towne) and CMV (AD169) genome (MOCARSKI et al. 1985).

3 Structural Proteins

3.1 Intracellular Development of Virions

The generation of extracellular CMV begins in the nucleus of the host cell where nucleocapsids with icosahedral symmetry are formed. The nucleocapsid acquires an envelope during the maturation process. The envelope has been reported to be derived from both the internal nuclear membrane (SMITH and DE HARVEN 1973) and from the endoplasmic reticulum (SEVERI et al. 1979). There is some evidence that there may be two distinct lamellae in the lipid envelope (FARRAR and ORAM 1984), which may explain the differences in the earlier observations. There are in excess of 30 proteins that can be detected on the various forms of the extracellular virion (KIM et al. 1976; GUPTA et al. 1977; STINSKI 1977; GIBSON 1983). The capsid proteins are the most abundant but the membranes contain a discrete population of proteins and glycoproteins (FARRAR and ORAM 1984; STINSKI 1977; STINSKI et al. 1979).

GIBSON (1981b) used biochemical fractionation to identify and characterize virus particles as they were synthesized within the infected cell. Four types of virus particles were identified, based on intracellular compartmentalization, sedimentation properties in rate-velocity sucrose gradients, protein composition, and infectivity. By analogy with the particles of HSV, they were given alphabetical designations. A-capsids have the simplest structure with at least three protein species (145, 34, 28 kDa) and, along with B capsids, are present in the nuclear fraction of infected cells. C capsids are present in the cytoplasmic fraction and virions can be recovered either from cells or extracellular fluids. The 145- to 155-kDa protein constitutes 90% of A capsid mass, which is consistent with it being the major structural component of the icosahedral capsid. The A 28-kDa protein is important in maintaining structural integrity. The B capsid has a 36-kDa protein which may be involved in DNA packaging and/or nucleocapsid envelopment. It is closely related to a 45-kDa protein which is present in much lower molar amounts. Both are probably exposed on the capsid surface. The C capsid is more complex with a 205 and 66 K band. The 66-kDa protein is 70% of the non A capsid protein mass, is phosphorylated, and apparently serves as interface between the nucleocapsid and the outer envelope proteins. The infectious virions have at least seven proteins not found in A, B, or C capsids. Virions all contain approximately 20 protein species ranging in molecular weight from 20 to 200 kDa with a predominant 60- to 70-kDa band. The involvement of intracellular particles in the assembly pathway of herpesviruses is not yet established. Empty A capsids may be precursoral forms of DNA-containing B, C capsids and virions.

The 36-kDa protein detected on B capsids is probably involved in virus assembly (IRMIERE and GIBSON 1985). Noninfectious enveloped particles are enveloped B-capsids, and B capsids may be precursors of virions. The maturation of B capsids to virions involves the modification or elimination of the 36-kDa assembly protein from the particle.

In addition to the intracellular capsid forms, there are at least three distinct species of extracelluar enveloped particles. These are (a) complete infectious particles which contain DNA, capsid, matrix protein, and envelope, (b) particles that are structurally and compositionally similar to virions but contain no DNA and are referred to as noninfectious enveloped particles, and (c) large enveloped spherical aggregates, known as dense bodies, that are composed primarily of protein and contain neither DNA nor a capsid.

3.2 Proteins Associated with Extracellular Virion Forms

3.2.1 Viral Matrix Proteins

The viral matrix, as described by GIBSON (1981b), represents the area located in the virion between the nucleocapsid and the envelope. It is present in virions, dense bodies, and C capsids, pointing to a role in the assembly of CMV. Also it is present in large amounts in the nucleoplasm of infected cells but is not an integral part of the intranuclear inclusions which are pathognomonic of CMV infection (WEINER et al. 1986). The viral matrix protein has at least three components: (a) the lower matrix protein of 64–69 kDa, (b) the upper matrix protein of 69–71 kDa, and (c) the 150-kDa basic phosphoprotein.

The lower matrix protein is one of the most abundant proteins synthesized during the infectious cycle. The protein accumulates in both the nucleus and cytoplasm of infected cells and can be detected on the extracellular forms. It represents aproximately 95% of the protein mass in dense body particles (ROBY and GIBSON 1986). This polypeptide, which is phosphorylated, has been referred to in various reports as pp65 (NOWAK et al. 1984), 69-kDa matrix-like protein (IRMIERE and GIBSON 1983), HCMV gp 64 (CLARK et al. 1984), or ICP 27 (GEBALLE et al. 1986). There is now evidence, based upon data obtained after exchange of reagents among laboratories, that all of these sizes probably represent the same protein. The protein was first isolated in large quantity using high-pressure liquid chromatography purification and represents about 15% of the total viral protein. The gene coding for the lower matrix protein is located within with EcoR1 A fragment of CMV (Towne strain) (NOWAK et al. 1984; PANDE et al. 1984) and the sequence has been determined (RUEGER et al. 1987). The sequence of the lower matrix phosphoprotein is not the same as the protein of similar molecular weight sequenced by DAVIS and HUANG (1985) but was identical to that reported by PANDE et al. (1984). The phosphoprotein is also distinct from the approximately 65-kDa comigrating virion envelope protein described by BRITT and AUGER (1986). The lower matrix protein is a late gene product (GEBALLE et al. 1986) which is transcribed in the absence of viral DNA replication and may be controlled by posttranscriptional events. It is not clear how the protein is distributed on the different types of extracellular virus particles. Some have reported that the lower matrix protein is not detectable on virions (GIBSON and IRMIERE 1984; KIM et al. 1983; LANDINI et al. 1987b) but is only assembled into cytoplasmic dense bodies and not virions. However, others (BRITT and VUGLER 1987) have reported that the lower matrix protein is an internal, nonglycosylated virion phosphoprotein which was inaccessible to antibodies in virions or on the surface of infected cells.

The upper matrix protein of 71 kDa, sometimes referred to as the 74-kDa protein (ROBY and GIBSON 1986), is transcribed from the same region of the genome as the lower matrix protein. However, it is not as abundant in infected cells as the lower matrix protein (GIBSON 1983; IRMIERE and GIBSON 1983). The lower matrix phosphoprotein is coded by the 5'-terminal part of an abundant 4-kb mRNA. The upper matrix phosphoprotein corresponds to the single translational reading frame form of a rare nonspliced 1.9-kb mRNA that is coterminal with the 4-kb transcript.

There is no immunologic cross-reactivity between the upper and lower matrix proteins (GIBSON 1983).

The 150-kDa basic phosphoprotein probably represents one of the matrix components of the virion (GIBSON 1983; ROBY and GIBSON 1986). This protein appears to be particularly reactive with human sera in immunoblot analysis (LANDINI et al. 1986). For strain AD169 the gene has been mapped to the *Hind*III fragments J and N and the nucleotide sequence has been published (JAHN et al. 1987). Despite the fact that phosphoproteins of approximately the same molecular size occur in the matrix of other herpesviruses (LEMASTER and ROIZMAN 1980), no sequence homology is demonstrable with other herpesviruses.

3.2.2 Major Nucleocapsid Protein

A major nucleocapsid protein of approximately 150 kDa is the principal structural element of the icosahedral capsid and constitutes approximately 90% of the capsid protein (GIBSON 1983). The basic phosphoprotein, also about 150 kDa, comigrates with the major nucleocapsid protein. However, the proteins can be well resolved by charge-size separation or the use of high-percentage polyacrylamide gels.

3.2.3 28-kDa Structural Protein

A 28-kDa structural protein is present in both the cytoplasm of infected cells during the late phase of the viral replication cycle and in the extracellular virus particles (RE et al. 1985). Monoclonal antibody to this protein detects antigen by immunofluorescence 48 h after infection and antigen expression requires viral DNA synthesis. There are no disulfide linkages and the protein is not a target for virus-neutralizing antibody. The 28-kDa protein is recognized by human sera and appears to be present in a number of wild CMV strains. This protein may be related to the 25-kDa structural protein described by PEREIRA et al. (1983), the 29-kDa phosphoprotein detected by NOWAK et al. (1984), and a protein of similar size described by MARTINEZ and ST. JOER (1986). The gene, mapped to the *Hind*III R fragment, is transcribed into a late 1.3-kb RNA (MEYER et al. 1988). Parts of the 28-kDa polypeptide that were expressed in *Escherichia coli* as hybrid proteins are recognized by human sera. The protein is phosphorylated and is present only in the outline of the cytoplasmic capsids as studied by immunoelectron microscopy (LANDINI et al. 1987b). Therefore the 28-kDa protein is probably a structural component of virions which is acquired in the cytoplasm and localized on the surface of the viral capsid. It is not present in dense bodies. This 28-kDa protein is probably different from the 28-kDa protein described by GIBSON (1981b) that appears only on intracellular capsid forms.

3.2.4 46-kDa DNAse

A 46-kDa polypeptide, present in extensively purified CMV particles, has been shown to have DNAse activity (RIPALTI et al. 1988). Monospecific anti-p46 sera produced in mice recognize an enzymatically inactive 76-kDa polypeptide in both noninfected and HCMV-infected cells.

3.2.5 Protein Kinase

The presence of virion-associated protein kinases is common to most herpesviruses (STEVELY et al. 1985). Protein kinase activity is present in all three extracellular CMV particles which have a viral envelope; specifically noninfectious-enveloped particles, dense bodies, and virions (ROBY and GIBSON 1986). A 67-kDa molecular weight phosphoprotein from nuclei of infected cells and virion preparations has been precipitated by CMV-specific monoclonal antibodies and shows protein kinase activity (DAVIS and HUANG 1985; DAVIS et al. 1984). The gene for this protein has been mapped to an area between 0.37 and 0.39 map units on the CMV genome. Protein kinase activity has also been detected in virions and infected cells which have been immunoprecipitated using a monoclonal antibody directed against an abundant 68-kDa virion structural protein (BRITT and AUGER 1986).

4 Envelope Glycoproteins

Examination of purified virus particles by electron microscopy shows that the virions are enclosed by an outer envelope which is osmotically fragile. The glycoproteins on the viral envelope are of interest because of their potential importance as antigens in both the humoral and cellular response. They can be targets for virus-neutralizing antibody, mediate viral entry, and may play a role in the release of the virion from the host cell. The glycoproteins of human strains of CMV show a complex electrophoretic profile. The interrelationships between all of the observed species are not yet well clarified. However, it has been estimated that there are from three to eight glycoproteins present on the envelope of CMV (FIALA et al. 1976; KIM et al. 1976; STINSKI 1976; GIBSON 1983; NOWAK et al. 1984; FARRAR and GREENAWAY 1986).

FARRAR and ORAM (1984) purified the envelope from virions and identified five-glycosylated components of 52, 67, 95, 130, and 250 kDa after oxidation of purified virus with sodium metaperiodate and subsequent labeling with sodium [^{3}H]borohydride. The most consistently identified polypeptides were the 52-, 95-, and 130-kDa forms.

The development of monoclonal antibodies to human CMV has provided a new mechanism for identifying viral components (PEREIRA et al. 1982, 1984) and in particular viral glycoproteins which are targets for virus-neutralizing antibody. By selecting for monoclonal antibodies which have functional activities, for example virus-neutralizing activity, it is possible to identify a target protein and analyze its biosynthesis and physical characteristics as well as the gene coding for its synthesis. Using this approach, it has been possible to identify at least three glycoproteins that are targets for virus-neutralizing antibody and are components of the viral envelope.

4.1 gB Homolog

This major envelope glycoprotein has been shown to be a complex of several proteins which are linked by disulfide bonds (NOWAK et al. 1984; LAW et al. 1985). It has also been referred to as p130/55 (RASMUSSEN et al. 1985a), gA (PEREIRA et al. 1982, 1984), and gcI (GRETCH et al. 1988c). There is informal agreement among workers in the area of CMV glycoproteins to refer to this glycoprotein as gB at this time. The gene products are referred to as the gB complex because of its genetic homology with the gB gene of HSV. This complex of proteins is detected by murine monoclonal antibodies which neutralize virus infectivity in the presence of guinea pig complement (PEREIRA et al. 1982; BRITT 1984; RASMUSSEN et al. 1985a). It is of interest that one group has reported the development of human hybridoma cell lines which neutralize virus infectivity and detect this same complex of proteins, indicating that in humans it is immunogenic (MATSUMOTO et al. 1986).

The complex is derived from intracellular processing and cleavage of a high molecular weight precursor protein. By pulse-chase analysis of infected cells the first species that is labeled is a high molecular weight species form in the molecular weight range of 130–160 kDa which is cleaved into a product of approximately 55 kDa that appears on the extracellular virion envelope in the absence of the precursor forms (NOWAK et al. 1984; LAW et al. 1985; RASMUSSEN et al. 1985a; CRANAGE et al. 1986; BENKO and GIBSON 1986; MACH et al. 1986). There is also an intermediate form of the protein in the molecular weight range of 92–116 kDa, detectable on the viral envelope, that is derived from the precursor 130- to 160-kDa protein since, after peptide digestion, common fragments can be detected (BRITT and AUGER 1986; GRETCH et al. 1988a, c). The primary form of the precursor protein is 92 kDa and is rapidly glycosylated to give an intermediate form of approximately 160 kDa that is rapidly trimmed to form the stable precursor protein and can be demonstrated reproducibly only in the presence of the processing inhibitor castanospermine (GRETCH et al. 1988a). Amino acid sequence analysis of the N-terminus of the 55-kDa viral glycoprotein showed that the gp55 is derived from the gp130 precursor by proteolytic cleavage and represents the C-terminal region of gp130. The cleavage enzyme is probably cellular in origin since processing of gB takes place in CV-1, CHO, and COS cells which are normally nonpermissive for CMV replication (SPAETE et al. 1988). There may be alternate cleavage patterns of the precursor protein since the molecular weights of the deglycosylated forms, when added together, exceed that of the polypeptide precursor (GRETCH et al. 1988a). Since the open reading frame for the gB gene predicts as many as seven dibasic protease recognition sites (CRANAGE et al. 1986), alternative cleavage of the gp130 may explain the diversity of related products within this complex.

The sugars that occur on the gB homolog complex are predominantly of the high-mannose type (RASMUSSEN et al. 1988) and are added rapidly to the primary forms during translation on the endoplasmic reticulum. The 55-kDa product may also contain O-linked oligosaccharides (BENKO and GIBSON 1986).

The gene coding for the gB complex was originally mapped to the right terminal sequence of the HindIII-F fragment between map coordinates 0.344 and 0.380 of HCMV (AD169) virion DNA (MACH et al. 1986). A monospecific rabbit antiserum against the gB product was used to screen a cDNA library that was constructed from polyA + RNA of CMV-infected cells in prokaryotic expression vector λ gt11. The sequence of the gene was subsequently defined (CRANAGE et al. 1986) by cloning an open reading frame for a CMV gene which possessed glycoprotein characteristics as determined by nucleotide sequencing. The glycoprotein gene was then cloned and expressed in vaccinia virus. By this approach the gB gene was shown to have homology with the gB gene of HSV, EBV, and the gpII of varicella-zoster virus, revealing that this gene is highly conserved among herpesviruses. It is also closely related to pseudorabies virus gII gene (ROBBINS et al. 1987) as well as Epstein-Barr and varicella-zoster viruses (EMINI et al. 1987). The sequence of the Towne strain of CMV gB gene has a 94% nucleotide similarity and a 95% amino acid similarity to the CMV (AD169) gene (SPAETE et al. 1988). These same workers have also shown that abundant levels of the gB transcript can be detected as early as 4 h postinfection while the gene product is not detected until 48 h after infection. This suggests that the gB gene may be regulated at the posttranscriptional level. The gB glycoprotein is not expressed in the presence of phosphonoformic acid, thus establishing that gB has the characteristics of a late gene product.

The location of the gp 55, both in viral particles and in cell membrane, was studied with indirect immunofluorescence and immunoelectron microscopy using antiglycoprotein B guinea pig antisera (LANDINI et al. 1987a). The glycoprotein was first observed on the plasma membrane of unfixed cells at 72 h p.i. By immunoelectron microscopy the plasma membrane was positive only where the virus and dense bodies budded through the membrane to form their own envelope. Extracellular viral particles, both viruses and dense bodies, appeared very strongly labeled on the external surface.

The immunogenicity of the gB complex has been demonstrated in guinea pigs for the induction of complement-dependent virus-neutralizing antibody (RASMUSSEN et al. 1985b; GONCZOL et al. 1986). The antibody produced in guinea pigs requires complement for neutralization, suggesting that the majority of epitopes on the protein require complement for the effective reaction with neutralizing antibody. However, it has recently been reported that both complement-dependent and -independent virus-neutralizing antibodies can be produced in response to immunization with recombinant gB gene product (BRITT et al. 1988). Using recombinant gB from prokaryotic expression vectors, there was almost exclusive production of low levels of complement-dependent neutralizing activity after immunization of mice. In contrast, mice immunized with recombinant vaccinia virus-derived gB gene product produced complement-independent neutralizing antibodies.

One epitope that is a target for virus-neutralizing antibody has been localized to a 186-amino-acid fragment of the 55-kDa glycoprotein (SPAETE et al. 1988). The other antigenic epitopes on the gB protein appear to be clustered in three major domains designated I, II, and III as determined by epitope analysis with a simultaneous two antibody binding assay and a panel of ten monoclonal antibodies (LUSSENHOP et al. 1988). Antibodies within individual domains I and II showed strong mutual inhibition of each other's binding. However, there were multiple antibody interactions between domains I and II. For example, the binding of most antibodies in I was augmented to some extent by antibodies from domain II.

However, this augmentation was dependent upon the native structure of gB. Synergistic effects on virus neutralization were also observed between antibodies in domains I and II in virus neutralization assay. Nonneutralizing antibodies gave enhanced neutralizing response in the presence of neutralizing antibodies. Two nonneutralizing antibodies in combination gave virus neutralization.

The function of the gB homolog gene product on the viral envelope is completely unknown at this point. It is of interest that the gB glycoprotein of herpes simplex virus appears to be involved in viral entry and cell fusion. While temperature-sensitive mutants have been used to establish a role for HSV gB in viral fusion and viral entry, the interpretation of these types of experiments is complicated by the presence of inactive gB. However, recently HSV gB null mutants have been used to show that gB is required for viral infectivity in a stage after viral attachment but before the expression of the virus-specific proteins (CAI et al. 1988). In addition, the gB contains different functional regions responsible for fusion induction and its inhibition.

4.2 gH Homolog

The second major glycoprotein which has been described is an envelope glycoprotein of approximately 86 kDa (RASMUSSEN et al. 1984). The glycoprotein is called gH because of its genetic homology with the gH gene of HSV and has recently been referred to as gcIII (GRETCH et al. 1988c). This glycoprotein can be immunoprecipitated from radiolabeled infected cells with murine monoclonal antibodies which neutralize virus infectivity in the absence of complement. The gH glycoprotein is a single gene product and no precursors can be demonstrated. In addition, the neutralizing epitope is present on both laboratory and clinical strains of human CMV. Biosynthetically the 86-kDa protein is detected in the cytoplasm of infected cells at late times (24–48 h) after infection. The glycoprotein, when purified by immunoaffinity chromatography, will induce complement-independent virus-neutralizing antibody in guinea pigs (RASMUSSEN et al. 1985b). The gene for gH homolog is in the HindIII L region of the U_L segment and has been sequenced and expressed in a vaccinia virus vector (CRANAGE et al. 1988). This gene was identified by nucleotide sequencing of CMV genomic DNA and the identification of an open reading frame with the characteristics of a glycoprotein-coding sequence. The predicted amino acid sequence was homologous to gH of HSV I (GOMPELS and MINSON 1986), the BXLF2 gene product of Epstein-Barr virus (EBV) (HEINEMAN et al. 1988) and varicella-zoster gpIII (KELLER et al. 1987). The gH glycoprotein gene in Towne strain is virtually identical to the AD169 gene and is in the HindIII H region of the U_L region (PACHL et al. 1988).

In addition to being targets for virus-neutralizing antibody, the gH glycoprotein may be involved in either intracellular spread or initiation of virus infectivity. The incorporation of monoclonal antibody into semisolid overlays of CMV-infected monolayers results in a decrease in size of the microfoci initiated by infectious CMV (RASMUSSEN, unpublished results). This reduction in microfocus size is not seen with antibody to the gB glycoprotein. The effect on apparent plaque size is similar to that reported for both monoclonal antibody to the HSV gH gene product (GOMPELS and MINSON 1986) and the varicella-zoster gH homolog, called gp III (KELLER et al. 1987). For EBV, monoclonal antibodies to an 85-kDa glycoprotein, which is also a homolog of the gH gene of HSV, will inhibit the cell fusion reaction that is important for cell-to-cell spread of EBV, but not virus attachment (MILLER and HUTT-FLETCHER 1988). In addition, anti-idiotype antibodies which bear the internal image of a neutralizing epitope on the gH glycoprotein have been shown to inhibit spread of CMV throughout the monolayer, suggesting that this viral glycoprotein may be interacting with cellular receptors (KEAY et al. 1988).

The physical characteristics of the gH glycoprotein have been described by RASMUSSEN et al. (1988). The glycoprotein contains only high-mannose-linked oligosaccharides which are added rapidly to a primary gene product of approximately 80 kDa. The oligosaccharides do not appear to be essential for immunogenicity in guinea pigs, but rather may play a protective or stabilizing role for the glycoprotein.

4.3 gcII

A glycoprotein complex present in the viral envelope with components of 93 kDa and 450 kDa in the unreduced state has been studied by KARI et al. 1986). After reduction the two most abundant species have molecular weights of 50–52 kDa and greater than 200 kDa. Minor species with molecular weights of 90, 116, and 130 kDa could also be detected. The monoclonal antibody used to detect the species within the complex neutralized virus infectivity in the absence of complement but also cross-reacted with herpes simplex and adenovirus in immunofluorescent assays. The glycoprotein complex has been extracted from human CMV envelopes with a nonionic detergent and separated by anion exchange high-performance liquid chromatography (KARI and GEHRZ 1988). The peptide maps of the 50- to 52-, 93-, and 200-kDa species are identical, showing that they are structurally similar. The 52-kDa component of the complex also appears to have a unique phenotype characterized by a high amount of O-linked oligosaccharides in comparison to other glycoproteins in the complex. The glycoproteins in this complex also appear to be heavily sialated.

The HXLF (HindIII-X left reading frame) gene family has five genes that share one or two regions of homology and are arranged in tandem within the Us component of CMV genome (WESTON and BARRELL 1986). This multigene family encodes the gcII (GRETCH et al. 1988b). When the genes were cloned into an SP6 expression vector an abundant 1.62-kb bicistronic mRNA was detected. When these messages were translated in vitro, nonglycosylated and glycosylated gene products were immunoprecipitated by the monoclonal antibody 9E10 which is specific for a virion envelope glycoprotein complex. In addition, the amino acid composition of 42- to 52-kDa glycoproteins, purified from virion envelopes, has highest similarity to predicted amino acid composition of HXLF1 plus HXLF2 open reading frames, but is more similar to HXLF2 than to HXLF1. The glycoprotein could also be synthesized by the monocistronic 0.8-kb mRNA encoded by the HXLF2 gene as well as by the mRNAs predicted from the other HXLF genes. The 47- to 52-kDa glycoprotein has precursor proteins of 25–32 kDa. The origin and nature of the five homologous gene families within the short unique region may be important from an evolutionary standpoint because it is likely that these homologous ORFs represent gene duplications and expansions of the short unique component.

5 Proteins Identified by Sequence Analysis Only

5.1 MHC Class I Antigen Homolog

As the sequence of the entire CMV genome is being revealed, it becomes apparent that there are many open reading frames for glycoproteins that have yet to be detected immunologically. By RNA sequence analysis, it has been shown that CMV can code for a glycoprotein that appears to be homologous to the MHC class I antigens (BECK and BARRELL 1988). The CMV class I like protein gene is not spliced, in contrast to the cellular genes. Infectious CMV can bind $\beta 2$ microglobulin, a protein that is normally found in association with the class I major histocompatibility complex, and it has been proposed that CMV may use $\beta 2$ microglubulin binding as an infection mechanism (GRIFFITHS and GRUNDY 1988). Two CMV envelope proteins of 36 and 65 kDa have been identified which can bind to $\beta 2$ microglobulin. Interaction of these two proteins with cellular class I molecules via $\beta 2$ microglobulin displacement or exchange might be a pathway for CMV receptor-mediated infection. The gene for the class I HLA-like molecule can code for a 65-kDa protein, assuming that 7 or 8 of the 13 potential glycosylation sites are actually glycosylated in vivo.

6 Patterns of CMV Infection

The detailed aspects of the pathogenesis of CMV have been reviewed by several authors (OSBORN 1981; HO 1982; ONORATO et al. 1985; KINNEY et al. 1985). In normal individuals, an initial infection with CMV is usually asymptomatic but can produce a mononucleosis-like syndrome accompanied by fever, hepatitis, fatigue, and circulating atypical lymphocytes. Following the initial infection there is a prolonged, inapparent infection during which the virus remains latent in multiple cells and tissues throughout the body without causing detectable damage or clinical illness.

The consequences of CMV infection are most severe in immunocompromised patients; for example, allograft recipients and fetuses who are infected in utero (STAGNO and WHITLEY 1985). Maternal-fetal transmission of CMV to the fetus may result in symptomatic infection, known as cytomegalic inclusion disease, in a small percentage of mothers who are undergoing primary infection. The congenital infection is characterized by hepatosplenomegaly, jaundice, thrombocytopenic purpura, low birth weight, microcephaly, and, in the most severe form, irreversible damage to the CNS (HANSHAW 1983). However, the majority of infants who are born infected with CMV are asymptomatic. One N 1000 newborns in the United States are born with some evidence of CMV infection (PASS et al. 1986). The incidence equates to about 36,000 new cases each year. The long-term consequences of this type of early colonization are unknown; however, at least 10% of this group are at risk for symptomatic consequences such as hearing loss, impaired vision, or neuromuscular abnormalities. CMV is now the major known cause of infectious mental retardation in children. In immunocompromised patients; for example, allograft recipients and patients with AIDS, symptomatic disease is a frequent occurrence. The sequelae of either primary disease or reactivation of latent virus include interstitial pneumonitis, colitis, and hepatitis, to name a few. Virtually very major organ system is subject to CMV-induced pathology.

Evidence for latent CMV infection in blood and tissues has accumulated primarily from the transfer of organs and blood to either seronegative recipients or immunocompromised individuals. However, the site of latency in blood elements is unknown. Evidence for CMV in the blood of normal seropositive individuals has been reported (DIOSI et al. 1969; SHRIER et al. 1985) but this is an infrequent occurrence. Viral DNA has been detected in monocytes and granulocytes from immunocompromised individuals (SALTZMAN et al. 1988) but it is likely that much of the virus present is the result of phagocytosis.

7 Antigenic Properties of Viral Proteins

7.1 Humoral Immune Responses

The antibody response is normal individuals following primary CMV infection consists of an initial transient IgM response which is followed by persisting levels of IgG. Reactivation infections, studied chiefly in immunocompromised individuals, are not necessarily accompanied by an IgM response, pointing to the lack of reliability of this marker for infectivity in certain patient populations (RASMUSSEN et al. 1982; GRIFFITHS et al. 1982; PASS et al. 1983). A protective role for antibody is highly likely in some patient populations. A fetus is protected against the debilitating effects in utero of CMV if maternal antibody is present (STAGNO et al. 1982). Passively transferred CMV hyperimmune globulin may also confer a protective effect against symptomatic CMV-associated interstitial pneumonitis in bone marrow transplant recipients (WINSTON et al. 1987; HUART et al. 1987). However, other groups have found that hyperimmune globulin is only marginally effective (BORDGONI et al. 1987). In a recent retrospective analysis of a group of bone marrow transplant recipients there was no significant difference in the incidence of CMV infections between recipients of seropositive and seronegative marrow. However, the incidence of CMV pneumonitis and the mortality attributable to CMV infection were significantly greater in the group with seronegative than those with seropositive donors (GROB et al. 1987).

Because antibody appears to be an important protective factor in primary infections, it is likely that its major role is to prevent the generalized spread of virus which can ultimately produce a symptomatic infection. However, it is clear that circulating antibodies neither eliminate virus infectivity nor prevent infection with a second strain of CMV (CHOU 1986; GRUNDY et al. 1986).

7.1.1 Antibodies Reactive with Specific Viral Proteins

There have been many studies in which the reactivity of human sera to viral proteins from either infected cells or purified extracellular virions has been evaluated. In normal individuals, antibody to at least 15 CMV associated proteins can be detected by either immunoblot analysis (GOLD et al. 1988) or immunoprecipitation of radiolabeled CMV-infected cells (PEREIRA et al. 1982, 1984; ZAIA et al. 1986; HAYES et al. 1987). When radiolabeled CMV-infected cells are fractionated into cytoplasmic and nuclear preparations for immunoprecipitation with human sera from normal individuals with CMV mononucleosis, the most intense reactions were found to occur with the high molecular mass proteins of 50- to 214-kDa in the cytoplasmic fraction and the more rapidly migrating proteins of less than 50 kDa in the nuclear antigen preparation (HAYES et al. 1987). In addition, each individual serum exhibited different patterns of reactivity. The basis for the variability is not clear but could relate to strain differences in the host, varying antibody affinity, or loss of critical epitopes during preparation of the antigen. There may also be patterns of "early," "late," and "variable" responses to specific groups of CMV-associated proteins (GOLD et al. 1988). The "early" responses occurred most frequently to proteins of 80, 66, 50, 40, 35, and 30 kDa. The "late" responses were to species of 100, 60, and 22 kDa. "Variable" responses were noted to proteins of 115, 63, 58, and 42 kDa. In addition, there were observed differences between reactivity to laboratory strain AD169 and clinical isolates. In bone marrow transplant patients, the pattern of the polypeptide-specific humoral immune response to CMV-infected cells is similar to the normal immune response, but qualitatively variable (ZAIA et al. 1986). In the group of patient sera studied by these workers, the predominant sites of antibody reactivity were with the 64-kDa (probably the lower matrix), the 50-kDa (probably the major nonstructural DNA-binding protein), and a 36-kDa (undefined) polypeptide.

In a group of renal transplant patients, the p150 (the basic phosphoprotein which has been mapped to the HindIII J region of the CMV genome) is a useful marker for assessing the occurrences of previous CMV infection (LANDINI et al. 1986). However, early during the course of a primary infection, no antibody to the p150 can be detected (LANDINI, personal communication). This suggests that antibody to the p150 may be useful marker for primary infection in certain patient populations; for example, to help distinguish primary from recurrent infection in pregnant females with CMV infection. The 28-kDa protein, described in a previous section, can also be detected by sera with IgG, but not IgM, antibody to CMV.

The IE antigens can stimulate humoral immunity in humans. There are at least four immediate early polypeptids which can be immunoprecipitated from infected cell extracts (BLANTON and TEVETHIA 1981; THE et al 1974). Early antigens, which are thought to be important in regulating the synthesis of late polypeptides, consist of at least 16 proteins that can be immunoprecipitated from lytically infected cells. In a recent study indirect immunofluorescent staining of CMV cells which had been infected in the presence of 75 μg cytosine arabinoside/ml was used to evaluate human sera from 500 normal blood donors (SWEET et al. 1985). A positive test was evaluated by reaction of human sera with CMV-infected nuclei to give a characteristic nuclear staining pattern. Five hundred normal blood donors were studied; three were positive for viruria and antibody to early antigen. There is some confusion and disagreement in CMV serology due to the almost total lack of information concerning the numbers, relative amounts, and especially relationships of antigens in IE, early, and late CMV antigen preparation. Some IE and early antigens may still be synthesized at late times and multiplicity of infection can affect IE and early antigen expression and detection. Currently there is no consistent relationship that can be observed between donor virological status and numbers or types of antibodies to the various CMV antigens. Further studies are needed to determine whether any specific CMV antibody is associated with presence of CMV genome in donor blood cells or is a marker for infectivity.

Thus it is clear that while the studies described in the preceeding paragraphs represent important first steps in the analysis of the humoral immune response to CMV there are still major problems in interpretation of the data. It is apparent that we still do not have a clear picture of the biosynthetic relationships among the CMV proteins that can be visualized by these methods. Moreover, we know that some of the important viral epitopes involved in, for example, virus-neutralizing activity can be destroyed by the denaturing conditions necessary for immunoblotting (RASMUSSEN et al. 1988). We also know that some viral proteins can comigrate in SDS-gels and are indistinguishable on the basis of apparent molecular size. The best example of this is the major structural protein and the basic phosphoprotein of CMV which comigrate in SDS gels with an apparent molecular size of 150 kDa and require charged-gel analysis for separation (ROBY and GIBSON 1986). Therefore antibody responses to a protein band are subject to misinterpretation without proof that there is only a single protein present.

The antibody response to cytomegalovirus polypeptides captured by monoclonal antibodies in the solid phase has also been used to study the humoral antibody response to CMV (CREMER et al. 1985). In these studies it was shown that antibody to the glycoprotein that we now know to be the gB homolog (referred to in the cited study as gA) was present in serum samples at a higher concentration in primary and reactivated infection and persisted longer than antibody to the other tested antigens. In contrast, antibody to antigen captured by a monoclonal which detected a polypeptide with an apparent molecular weight of 150 kDa (probably the basic phosphoprotein described previously) was present at a lower concentration, rose more slowly in infection, and persisted for a shorter time than did antibody to the other antigens. Other antigens tested were a group designated gC (polypeptides from 66 to 46 kDa and gD) and four antigenically related polypeptides from 49 to 25 kDa, which probably represent the late intracellular DNA-binding protein (see

Sect. 2.3.1). It is of interest that in this study the antibodies with different specificities for the polypeptides were detected at different times after seroconversion. This could mean that detection of some antibodies may be useful in evaluating the course of infection, as has been shown with antigens of Epstein-Barr virus (HENIE et al. 1974) and hepatitis B (Dienstag 1982). However, further studies are necessary to determine whether equivalent concentrations of antigen are bound by each of the monoclonal antibodies to assure equivalent sensitivity for each antigen.

More recently the gcII and gB homolog glycoprotein complexes have been isolated from gradient-purified Towne strain of CMV by anion-exchange high-pressure liquid chromatography. Sera from a small group of seropositive individuals were studied and found to have antibody that immunoprecipitates both of the glycoprotein complexes (LIU et al. 1988).

The lower matrix protein has also shown to be immunogenic in both humans and rabbits by immunoprecipitation studies (FORMAN et al. 1985).

The human antibody response to six isolated DNA-binding proteins found in CMV-infected cells, probably similar to the 51-kDa intracellular DNA-binding protein (see Sect. 2.3.1), was studied by Western blot technique (GERGELY et al. 1988). In sera from patients with acute infection, reactions with all six proteins were detected. The strongest reactivity was wih the 52- and 35-kDa proteins. The sera from some healthy CMV-seropositive donors reacted only with the 52-kDa DNA-binding protein.

The use of purified viral proteins for immunologic studies provides a level of improvement over the use of mixtures of viral proteins. However these types of studies must also be interpreted with caution. For example, it is possible to have copurification of immunologically unrelated proteins even with the use of a highly specific monoclonal antibody. The 51-kDa CMV DNA-binding protein (ICP36) is a frequent contaminant of immunoaffinity-purified preparations of gp86 and gp130/55 and can be immunogenic in experimental animals in concentrations which cannot be detected immunologically or physically in inoculum (RASMUSSEN, unpublished data). Unequivocal analysis of the humoral immune response must await the availability of cloned gene products.

7.1.2 Virus Neutralizing Antibody

Virus-neutralizing antibodies are produced during CMV infection (STALDER and EHRENSBERGER 1980), but whether they are directly involved in protection is not yet clear. Infectious CMV antibody complexes have been described (RUNDELL and BETTS 1980) and infectious virus can be found in saliva (TAMURA et al. 1980) or cervical secretions (WANER et al. 1977) despite presence of antibody. The apparent inefficient neutralization of CMV in vivo may be the result of masking of viral determinants by binding of the host protein B2-microglobulin (McKEATING et al. 1987).

We know that there are three viral glycoproteins, the gB homolog, the gH homolog, and the gcII, that are targets for virus-neutralizing antibody. Both the gH homolog and the gB homolog are immunogenic for the production of virus-neutralizing antibody in experimental animals. It is of interest that the neutralizing antibody produced against the gB homolog in animals is complement dependent, as are most of the monoclonal antibodies that detect this glycoprotein. In contrast, polyvalent neutralizing antibody to the gH homolog is complement independent. The importance of these glycoproteins in the neutralizing antibody response in humans has yet to be determined. However, in view of the ability of some antibodies to the viral glycoproteins not only to neutralize virus infectivity but also to inhibit cell-cell spread, one must consider the possibility that virus-neutralizing activity may only reflect the activity of an antibody with a more fundamental role in containing the infection.

7.1.3 Cytolytic Antibody

Both IgM and IgG in CMV hyperimmune sera are capable of lysing CMV-infected cells in the presence of added guinea pig complement (BETTS and SCHMIDT 1981; MIDDELDORP et al. 1984). While the target antigens for the cytolytic antibody are not yet defined, there is some evidence to suggest that they are antigens present on the surface of CMV-infected cells rather than those which are present on the viral envelope (MIDDLERDOP et al. 1986). The cytolytic antibodies could be detected in both acute and convalescent-phase sera from renal allograft patients as well as nonimmunocompromised patients with community-acquired symptomatic disease. The antibody-mediated cytolytic response was absent in patients with the fatal CMV infection.

7.1.4 Nonantiviral Consequences of the Humoral Immune Response

It has recently been reported that the sequence of the variable regions of the heavy and light polypeptide chains of a human-neutralizing IgG1 monoclonal antibody have striking homology to IgM rheumatoid factors of the Wa idiotypic family (NEWKIRK et al. 1988). The serologic and structural similarity of the major idiotypic family of rheumatoid factor antibodies and the anti-CMV antibody may provide a link between the immune response to a common virus such as CMV and rheumatoid arthritis.

The importance of anti-idiotype antibodies, arising as a consequence of the production of antiviral antibodies, in either regulating immunity to CMV or altering pathogenesis, is unexplored. The potential importance of anti-idiotypic antibodies in control of infectious disease has been reviewed (DRESSMAN and KENNEDY 1985). It has been shown that anti-idiotype antibodies are generated during the couse of a virus infection, for example, measles in mice (KRAH and CHOPPIN 1988). Some anti-idiotype antibodies could be protective. For example, anti-idiotype antibodies which are both "internal image" and "antireceptor" may limit virus spread by blocking viral entry. Anti-idiotype antibodies developed against neutralizing monoclonal antibodies to the gH homolog glycoprotein do have the ability to reduce plaque size of CMV in fibroblast cultures, suggesting that they may be blocking viral entry (or exit) (KEAY et al. 1988). The detection and analysis of anti-idiotype antibodies to specific viral antibodies is a new and possibly fruitful pathway for exploration of immune parameters which affect the course of CMV disease.

7.1.5 Mechanism of Interaction of CMV with B-Lymphocytes

The effects of CMV on B-cell differentiation have not yet been extensively studied. However, there is some evidence that CMV can directly activate B cells in vitro (HUTT-FLETCHER et al. 1983). However, other studies have shown that CMV is a potent B-cell activator in the presence of T cells (YACHIE et al. 1985). The specific memory T cells were shown to be CD4 + phenotype and proliferation of the antigen-specific cells was necessary for B-cell activation. The activation was limited to cells from immune human donors. These studies suggest that CMV may be different from EBV where Ig production is stimulated in nonimmune donors and does not require accessory cells.

The importance of these studies relates to the clinical observations that (a) atypical lymphocytes appear in the peripheral blood of patients with acute infection, (b) occasionally the presence of autoantibodies can be detected in human sera, and (c) the increased serum immunoglobulin levels in AIDS patients have been attributed to accompanying CMV infection (KANTOR et al. 1970; LANE et al. 1983). Further studies of the potent activation of both B and T cells may provide explanations for some of the immune abnormalities observed in patients with acute CMV infection.

7.2 Cellular Immune Response

The cellular immune system carries out numerous functions that may be important in control of virus infection. The importance of cellular immunity in CMV infection is clear from clinical observations. In patients undergoing immunosuppressive therapy or with AIDS, who have profound defects in cell-mediated immunity but normal levels of circulating antibody, symptomatic CMV infections such as interstitial pneumonitis, retinitis, colitis, hepatitis and encephalitis are common.

The delayed hypersensitivity response and T-lymphocytes may be critical for maintenance of the latent or limited replication that is characteristic of latent infection. Aspects of cellular immunity include (a) antigen recognition, (b) lymphokine production, and (c) cytotoxic kill of infected cells. These reactions are mediated by T-helper (CD4 +), T-cytotoxic/suppressor (CD8 +), and natural killer lymphocytes. Much of our information about the functions of each of these cellular phenotypes has been obtained in various animal models of herpesvirus infection (ROUSE et al. 1988; DIX 1987). In the following section I will describe how CMV interacts with the various cellular components of the immune system to generate detectable immune responses which may be important for containment or resolution of the infection.

7.2.1 T-Helper Cell Responses

Antigen presentation to T cells requires some type of association with gene products of the major histocompatibility complex. It is also considered to be a general finding at this point that some antigens and/or viral peptides are more effective at stimulating T cells than reacting with B cells and vice versa. There is some evidence to suggest that antigen recognition by T-lymphocytes is somewhat dependent upon linear epitopes whereas B-lymphocytes will preferentially recognize conformational determinants. T-helper cells usually recognize the viral antigens that are present on intact viral particles. When peripheral blood mononuclear cells from seropositive subjects were stimulated in vitro with CMV antigen consisting of virus particles, the T-cell lines which were generated were of the helper phenotype and did not kill CMV-infected target cells (BORYSIEWICZ et al. 1983). The response of T-helper cells to viral antigens can be quantitated by measurement of the amount of incorporation of a radiolabeled nucleotide precursor into cells cultured in vitro with antigen.

Antigen-specific T-helper cells recognize processed antigen in association with class II MHC genes expressed on the surface of macrophages as well as on other cell types; for example activated B cells, dendritic cells, epidermal Langerhans cells, and human dermal fibroblasts. EBV-transformed lymphocyte cell lines are also capable of presenting CMV antigen to CMV-specific T-helper clones in MHC-restricted fashion (LIU et al. 1987). However, the efficiency of presentation was better by autologous mononuclear cells than the lymphoblastoid cell lines. Studies have been performed to determine whether certain products of the MHC region preferentially restrict recognition of CMV and whether there is variation among haplotypes in CMV recognition. Products of all three HLA class II families (DR, DQ, DP) can function to restrict CMV recognition (LINNER et al. 1986; GEHRZ et al. 1987a). The primary restricting determinants appear to be subtypic to the serologically determined antigen and that subtypic restriction is very closely associated with single Dw specificities. A defect in proliferation of T-helper cells, not related to defective antigen presentation, has been shown in infants who are congenitally infected with CMV (GEHRZ et al. 1987b). How this immunodeficiency relates to the pathogenesis of the infection has yet to be determined.

T-helper lymphocytes are also the primary source of lymphokines such as interferons and interleukins. There have been many demonstration of interferon production in vitro after stimulation of T-lymphocytes with CMV antigens. These have been summarized recently (GRIFFITHS and GRUNDY 1987). α-, β-, and γ-interferon can all be detected in vitro in lymphocytes stimulated with CMV antigens. γ-interferon is of particular interest in herpesvirus infections because of its positive association with containment of recurrent herpes labialis in humans (RASMUSSEN et al. 1974; CUNNINGHAM and MERIGAN 1984). Herpes labialis disease is focal and lends itself to both recovery of γ-interferon from sites of active virus replication as well as quantitation of virus at the site of replication. In this system it has been shown that the gD glycoprotein will stimulate γ-interferon in vitro; however, combinations of purified glycoproteins are required to elicit a maximum response, comparable to that obtained with whole virus (TORSETH et al. 1987b). Locally, all three species of interferon can be detected in lesions, and the γ-interferon titer correlates with the interval between lesions (TORSETH and MERIGAN 1987; TORSETH et al. 1987a). It is more difficult to establish a role for γ-interferon in pathogenesis of CMV infection than for herpes labialis. CMV is a generalized infection and it is not possible to recover γ-interferon from sites of virus replication and correlate virus at the infected tissue level with systemic γ-interferon. Defects in γ-interferon have been identified in

CMV infection (GEHRZ and LEONARD 1985) but they are usually in association with other immune defects in activation and/or proliferation of CMV-specific T-helper cells. The significance of γ-interferon, particularly in response to glycoproteins of CMV, is an area that is totally unexplored at this point.

The lower matrix protein of CMV has been shown to induce a proliferative response in seropositive humans that is associated with both IL-2 secretion and IL-2 receptor expression (FORMAN et al. 1985). In addition, the envelope glycoprotein, gB homolog, of CMV can also stimulate T-lymphocyte blastogenesis in hyperimmunized guinea pigs (GONCZOL et al. 1986) and in normal seropositive individuals (GONCZOL et al. 1987), indicating that the gB glycoprotein can stimulate T-helper cells in vivo and in vitro. A 72-kDa early (β) protein can also stimulate helper T-lymphocytes (RODGERS et al. 1987) as measured in assays for both humoral and cellular immunity. This protein is of interest because it can also stimulate cytotoxic class I restricted CD8$^+$ cytotoxic T-lymphocytes.

7.2.2 Cytotoxic T-Cell Responses to Viral Antigens

Cytotoxic T-lymphocytes (CTLs) probably play a pivotal role in CMV infections since the ability to develop a specific cytotoxic response is correlated with successful resolution of disease in patients (MEYERS 1984; QUINNAN et al. 1982). The idea that viral glycoproteins were exclusively involved in stimulation of protective host cell responses has been abandoned. Recent findings in viral immunology coverage to the conclusion that, in addition to the viral genes which code for classical cell membrane glycoproteins, there are also proteins located mainly in the nucleus of the infected cell, which specify immunodominant determinants recognized by CTL in conjunction with class I and class II major histocompatibility glycoproteins. This area has recently been reviewed (ROUSE et al. 1988). Examples of nonstructural antigens which are targets for cytotoxic T-lymphocytes include the nonstructural large T-antigen of the papovavirus group and the internal virion nucleoprotein of the orthomyxovirus influenza A . In these systems the predominant cytolytic cell is a class I restricted CD8 + phenotype. The phenotype of the cytotoxic response is dependent to a certain degree upon the state of the sensitizing antigen. For example, when infected cells are used as antigens there may be some cytotoxicity which is class II restricted for the same system and mediated by CD4 + lymphocytes.

The role of cytotoxic lymphocytes in CMV infection has been studied in detail in the murine CMV model infection. A substantial body of evidence points to the importance of the murine CMV IE gene products as major targets for MLC-restricted cytotoxic T-lymphocytes. A single gene gives rise to three abundant polypeptides of 89, 84, and 76 kDa transcribed from the major IE region of the murine CMV genome (KEIL et al. 1985). The 84- and 76-kDa forms are apparently posttranslational modifications of the 89-kDa protein. In vitro translation of IE infected cell RNA gives only the 89-kDa form. In the acutely infected mouse, there are murine CMV-specific cytotoxic T-lymphocytes present in the draining lymph nodes. There are apparently two population of H2-restricted cytotoxic T-lymphocytes demonstratable (REDDEHASE and KOSZINOWSKI 1984; REDDEHASE et al. 1984a, b). One population is specific for cell membrane-incorporated viral structural antigens whereas the second population detects an antigen whose appearance is correlated with the synthesis of viral IE proteins. Long-term cytolytic T-lymphocyte lines, specific for distinct antigens associated with the different phases of the replication cycle, were derived from the lymph nodes of latently infected BALB/c mice (REDDEHASE et al. 1986a). One clone was specific for a structural antigen of murine CMV and the other clone detected an IE antigen. Fortuitously, the clones were able to grow in the presence of interleukin-2 only and did not require continued stimulation with antigen. These cell lines were used to trace the expression of the IE antigen throughout the viral replication cycle (REDDEHASE et al. 1986b). The expression of the target antigen is mainly a late -phase event which is correlated with the reexpression of the major IE gene. In the presence of cycloheximide there is enhanced expression of the IE antigen on the cell surface. However, without enhancement, high numbers of cytolytic T-lymphocytes were required. Therefore the IE membrane antigen is expressed in an amount sufficient for cytotoxic T-lymphocyte effector function without inhibition of de novo viral DNA synthesis. A 10.8-kb fragment which is abundantly transcribed at immediate times, when transfected into L cells, gave rise to antigens which were recognized by specific cytolytic T-lymphocytes (KOSZINOWSKI et al. 1987a). Only cells that expressed the IE gene and the appropriate class I MHC gene (L^d) were recognized by the cytotoxic T-cell clones. Within the transfected region, only the transcription unit IE 1 is essential for the specific cytotoxic reaction (KOSZINOWSKI et al. 1987b). Because transcripts from IE region 1 are spliced and translated into proteins of different size, it was necessary to construct the continuous pp89 coding sequence without introns to prove the identity of the transfected product and pp89 (VOLKMER et al. 1987). When the continuous coding sequence, with introns removed by site-directed mutagenesis, was used to infect mice, HLA-restricted T-lymphocytes with specificity for the IE gene products were detected. A recombinant vaccinia virus which expressed the 89-kDa protein induced protective immunity in BALB/c mice. Mice were protected against challenge with a lethal dose of murine CMV but not from infection and morbidity (JONJIC et al. 1988).

Experimental infection of mice with murine CMV is an appropriate model for the study of pathogenesis of human CMV since the latent infection in the natural host can be reactivated by immunosuppression (BRODY and CRAIGHEAD 1974). As in humans, infection of very young animals or immunosuppression of older animals is required to produce symptomatic disease. The resulting interstitial pneumonitis observed in mice (REDDEHASE et al. 1985) may be a model for the interstitial pneumonitis which is a major cause of death in human bone marrow transplant recipients (NEUMAN et al. 1973). This system may also provide a useful model for the study of the adrenal necrosis with presumed herpesvirus etiology (TRAPPER et al. 1984) in patients with AIDS (SHANLEY and PESANTI 1986). The cytotoxic CD8 + lymphocytes have been shown to control virus infection in various tissues in the infected mouse. Using transfer of memory T-lymphocytes from latently infected BALB/c mice, which require specific antigenic restimulation to generate cytolytic effector (CD8 +) T cells, immunosuppressed mice were protected from symptomatic disease (REDDEHASE et al. 1987, 1988). The antiviral efficacy of the therapeutically transferred cells was lower in adrenal glands than in lungs and spleen but prophylactic transfer was effective in protecting against adrenal gland infection. The authors propose that the effector T-lymphocytes cannot infiltrate the adrenal gland in sufficient time in an acutely infected mouse, whereas prophylactic transfer prevents colonization of tissue by virus. The transfer of helper (CD4 +) lymphocytes has also been shown to restrict murine CMV replication in the adrenal gland during acute infection (SHANLEY 1987).

In humans the presence of cytotoxic T-lymphocytes has been correlated positively with protection from CMV disease (QUINNAN et al. 1982; ROOK et al. 1984). Both class I (BORYSIEWICZ et al. 1983, 1988a, b) and class II restricted (LINDSLEY et al. 1986) cytotoxic T-lymphocytes can be demonstrated in humans infected with CMV.

It is not yet clear whether the IE antigen gene products will have the same immunologic significance in humans as has been shown for murine CMV. CMV proteins appearing in any one of the three phases of CMV replication (IE, early, and late) can serve as target antigens for class I restricted cytotoxic T-lymphocytes (BORYSCIEWICZ et al. 1983; CHARPENTIER et al. 1986). The population of T-lymphocytes specific for a late structural glycoprotein (gB) is a minor fraction of the cytotoxic population. The human cytotoxic T-lymphocyte precursors recognizing infected cells prior to viral DNA replication are the predominate cell type (BORYSIEWICZ et al. 1988b). In acute herpes simplex virus infections of mice, a significant proportion of the class I HLA-restricted cytotoxic T cells obtained from draining lymph nodes of mice acutely infected with HSV 1 recognize IE gene products in expressing target cells (MARTIN et al. 1988). However, the cytotoxic T-lymphocytes that were reactive with the IE proteins did not, in this case, dominate the response and accounted for less than 30% of the total anti-HSV response. It is also clear that in both murine models and human HSV infection the envelope glycoproteins of HSV are also important targets for cytotoxic T lymphocytes. Thus, it appears that there will be differences in both the antigens needed for the stimulation of protective cytotoxic T-lymphocyte responses as well as the phenotypes of the primary effector cell among the herpesviruses.

7.2.3 Nonspecific Immune Responses

The natural cytotoxic effects of lymphocytes are of special interest because they may have a direct effect on the virus-infected cell. By lysing infected cells early in the course of infection, the amount of infectious virus which is produced could be severely restricted. Natural killer (NK) cells are a subset of leukocytes which are distinct from T or B cells or myelomonocytic cells. Morphologically they are identifiable as "large granular lymphocytes". They are able to kill virus-infected cells without showing conventional immunologic specificity or memory. Their cytotoxic activity is enhanced by biological response modifiers, such as interferon or interleukin-2. The cellular lineage is not yet clear. They do have T-cell markers which favors their being a part of the T-cell-derived immunologic repertoire. NK cells expresses a low-affinity Fc receptor for aggregated IgG or CD106 antigen which is recognized by a series of monoclonal antibodies (PERUSSIA et al. 1983a, b).

The target structure for NK cells is thought to be a cellular structure rather than a viral gene product.

NK cells probably have a very important role in limiting the severity of virus infection in the period preceding the development of T-cell-mediated immunity. Evidence for the protective role of NK cells in murine CMV is substantial and has been reviewed recently by GRIFFITHS and GRUNDY (1987). In healthy individuals who were seropositive for CMV, there were significantly higher numbers of cells bearing the phenotype of NK lymphocytes than in the blood of CMV-seronegative individuals (GRATAMA et al. 1987). An increase in numbers of NK and NK-activated cells was the only difference observed between children with congenital CMV infection and asymptomatic patients (CAUDA et al. 1987).

In bone marrow transplant patients at high risk for CMV infection, there is evidence that natural cytotoxicity of CMV targets is an important correlate of the acquisition and outcome of CMV infection after marrow transplant. Detection of NK activity prior to the onset of CMV infection, followed by the development of specific T-lymphocyte cytotoxicity, was associated with a good clinical outcome (QUINNAN et al. 1982). More recently it has been shown that survival from CMV infection was longer in patients whose peripheral blood mononuclear cells had the ability to lyse CMV-infected cell targets during the first 20–60 days after transplant (BOWDEN et al. 1987).

However, in one study, NK cells, identified in bronchoalveolar lavage cells from immunocompromised patients with CMV pneumonitis, were analyzed. In the group with fatal pneumonitis, cells identified morphologically as large granular lymphocytes were present in higher percentages than in patients who recovered from the pneumonitis. The basis for the apparent lack of association with positive clinical outcome is not clear (ESCUDIER et al. 1986).

It has also been shown that HLA DR + cells provide an important accessory function for NK activity against CMV-infected cells. The soluble factor that stimulates NK cytotoxic activity when HLA-DR + cells are cocultivated with CMV-infected targets has been identified as interferon-α (BANDYOPADHYAY et al. 1986). IL-2 can also enhance NK activity against CMV-infected targets an its action is usually independent of α-interferon production (BANDYOPADHYAY et al. 1987).

8 Conclusions

Within the past several years there has been remarkable progress in identifying the proteins and glycoproteins of human CMV. We know that there are distinct proteins that can be identified at all stages of the viral replication cycle. Some of these have been well characterized and have a known genetic locus. We also know now that the proteins which are present on the extracellular forms of the virus are not necessarily the same as those which are synthesized intracellularly. In addition there may be differences in the protein profile of intracellular and extracellular assembled virions. We do not know the relationship of the plasma mambrane proteins, probably an important aspect of the biogenesis of human CMV, to the proteins that are ultimately destined to become a part of the infectious virus particle. The interrelationships between many of the molecular species that are observed are being established. For example, we are beginning to understand the pattern of biosynthesis of some of the glycoprotein complexes that will ultimately appear on the viral envelope, specifically the gB homolog complex. We are still faced with the problem of determining whether single bands on protein gels represent one or multiple protein species. The best examples of this type of problem are the comigrating basic phosphoprotein and the major nucleocapsid protein, which are of the same molecular size but represent two distinct gene products.

The immunologic approach to the identification of viral gene products with monoclonal antibodies, especially those with functional activity, has been very useful for isolating and identifying viral gene products. It is clear that there are many more viral gene products possible than those that have been identified to this point. We do not know whether antibodies prepared in nonhuman species will recognize the same proteins that stimulate antibody production in humans. Moreover, we do not know whether functional epitopes are identical in human and nonhuman species. Some of these questions can be approached by the use of human monoclonal antibodis; however, the repertoire of these remains small.

We are only beginning to understand the importance of each of the antigens that are synthesized during the infectious cycle of the virus in the human immune response. The studies in murine and human CMV infections have shown very clearly that the targets for immune recognition for virus-infected cells are different from those for virions. Specifically, the IE antigens, present in infected cells but not virions, are the major targets for attack by HLA-restricted cytotoxic T-lymphocytes. Also at least three glycoproteins exist on the viral envelope that are targets for virus-neutralizing antibody. Finally the basic phosphoprotein appears to be a highly immunogenic component of the virion matrix and may be of considerable value diagnostically for recognition of early CMV infection.

The study of the CMV antigens which are important in immunity is being impeded by the lack of genetically pure preparations in sufficient quantitiy for study. Preparation of pure antigens from virus-infected cells is not a reasonable approach for obtaining sufficient material for immunologic studies of the magnitude necessary for evaluation of their importance. The yields, particularly of the envelope glycoproteins, are so low by methods such as immunoaffinity chromatography that this method is quite impractical for preparation of large quantities of CMV antigens. Viral antigens extracted from infected cells, even after immunoaffinity with highly specific antibody, may be contaminated with copurifying proteins that will interfere with their usefulness as immunologic reagents. Progress in the study of the importance of individual viral proteins will be greatly facilitated by the availability of recombinant gene products for use in serologic studies. The existence of different virus strains leads one to ask whether there are antigenic differences that are associated with pahtogenicity. There is little or no information about the protein composition of wild-type viral strains. The problems of propagating sufficient quantities of early passage virus for adequate analysis makes a study of this question difficult.

Despite the compelling evidence that HLA-restricted cytotoxic T-lymphocytes that are specific for IE viral proteins are important for protection of both human and mouse CMV infection, we still do not know how the effect is mediated in vivo. We do not know whether the cytotoxic T-cell killing is the mechanism by which immunity is expressed in vivo since cytotoxic clones have other immune functions such as γ-interferon production that may be indirectly involved in cellular cytotoxicity. We also do not know how the IE antigen presents to cytotoxic T-lymphocytes. There is no detectable reactivity on the cell surface, using monoclonal antibody to the major IE gene products in immunofluorescent assays (OTTO et al. 1988). It is not clear how cytotoxic T-lymphocytes recognize an antigen which is primarily intracellular. It is also high likely that a replicating viral entity is necessary to stimulate cytotoxic T-lymphocytes. For immunotherapy, particularly by vaccine, it will be important to understand both the mechanism by which cytotoxic T-lymphocytes are stimulated in vivo and as the methods for generating them in a way that will not be harmful to the host.

The paradox of the importance of antibody in CMV infection is not yet resolved. While antibody is protective in certain patient groups, we know that the intracellular spread of infectious virus occurs despite the presence of high titers of circulating (and virus-neutralizing) antibody. We do not know whether we are evaluating, by our currently available serologic methods, an appropriate parameter of humoral immunity for determining whether a host is protected from either CMV infection or reactivation. It is possible that additional assays for functional antibody; for example, cytolytic antibody or antibody that inhibits spread of virus from cell to cell, will be more significant correlates of protection from disease than virus-neutralizing antibody.

There is also the interesting question of biological significance of the nucleotide homologies among herpesvirus, particularly for the envelope glycoproteins. We do not know whether this is simply a reflection of the evolution of the different members of the herpesvirus group or whether these homologies manifest themselves in some type of immunologic cross-reactivity that may be fundamental for control of infection by the whole family of viruses.

Thus it is clear that, while progress is being made in the study of the interaction of human CMV with the cells of the human immune system, there are still critical questions to be answered about both the virus and the host response. CMV, as a human pathogen with multifaceted impact, remains a challenging target for scientific investigation.

References

Akrigg A, Wilkinson G, Oram J (1985) The structure of the major immediate early gene of human cytomegalovirus strain AD 169. Virus Res 2: 107–121

Anders D, Gibson W (1988) Location, transcript analysis and partial nucleotide sequence of the cytomegalovirus gene encoding for an early DNA-binding protein with similarities to ICP8 of herpes simplex virus type 1. J Virol 62: 1364–1372

Anders D, Irmiere A, Gibson W (1986) Identification and characterization of a major early cytomegalovirus DNA-binding protein. J Virol 58: 253–262

Anders D, Kidd J, Gibson W (1987) Immunological characterization of an early cytomegalovirus single-strand DNA-binding protein with similarities to the HSV major DNA-binding protein. Virology 161: 579–588

Bandyopadhyay S, Perussia B, Trinchieri G, Miller D, Starr S (1986) Requirement for HLA-DR + accessory cells in natural killing of cytomegalovirus-infected fibroblasts. J Exp Med 164: 180–195

Bandyopadhyay S, Miller D, Matsumoto-Kobayashi M, Clark S, Starr S (1987) Effects of interferons and interleukin 2 on natural killing of cytomegalovirus-infected fibroblasts. Clin Exp Immunol 67: 372–382

Beck S, Barrell BG (1988) Human cytomegalovirus encodes a glycoprotein homologous to MHC class-I antigens. Nature 331: 269–272

Benko D, Gibson W (1986) Primate cytomegalovirus glycoproteins: lectin-binding properties and sensitivities to glycosidases. J Virol 59: 703–713

Betts R, Schmidt S (1981) Cytolytic IgM antibody to cytomegalovirus in primary cytomegalovirus infection in humans. J Infect Dis 143: 821–826

Blanton R, Tevethia M (1981) Immunoprecipitation of virus-specific immediate-early and early polypeptides from cells lytically infected with human cytomegalovirus strain AD 169. Virology 112: 262–273

Bordigoni P, Janot C, Aymar J, Witz F, et al. (1987) Clinical and biological evaluation of the preventative role of anti-cytomegalovirus specific immunoglobulins in bone marrow grafts. Nouv Reg Fr Hematol 29: 289–293

Borysiewicz L, Morris S, Page J, Sissons J (1983) Human cytomegalovirus-specific cytotoxic T lymphocytes: requirements for in vitro generation and specificity. Eur J Immunol 13: 804–809

Borysiewicz L, Graham S, Hickling J, Mason P, Sissons J (1988a) Human cytomegalovirus-specific cytotoxic T cells: their precursor frequency and stage specificity. Eur J Immunol 18: 269–275

Borysiewicz L, Hickling J, Graham S, Sinclair J, Cranage M, Smith G, Sissons J (1988b) Human cytomegalovirus specific cytotoxic T cells-relative frequently of stage specific CTL recognizing the 72 kDa immediate early protein and glycoprotein B expressed by recombinant vaccinia viruses. J Exp Med 168: 919–931

Bowden R, Day L, Amos D, Meyers J (1987) Natural cytotoxic activity against cytomegalovirus-infected target cells following marrow transplantation. Transplantation 44: 504–508

Brady A, Craighead J (1974) Pathogenesis of pulmonary cytomegalovirus infection in immunosuppressed mice. J Infect Dis 129: 677–689

Britt W (1984) Neutralizing antibodies detect a disulfide-linked glycoprotein complex within the envelope of human cytomegalovirus. Virology 135: 369–378

Britt W, Auger D (1986) Synthesis and processing of the envelope gp55–116 complex of human cytomegalovirus. J Virol 58: 185–191

Britt W, Vulger L (1987) Structural and immunological characterization of the intracellular forms of an abundant 68,000 M$_r$ human cytomegalovirus protein. J Gen Virol 68: 1897–1907

Britt W, Vulger L, Stephens E (1988) Induction of complement-dependent and -independent neutralizing antibodies by recombinant-derviced human cytomegalovirus gp55–116 (gB). J Virol 62: 3309–3318

Cai W, Gu B, Person S (1988) Role of glycoprotein B of herpes simplex virus type 1 in viral entry and cell fusion. J Virol 62: 2596–2604

Cauda R, Prasthofer E, Grossi C, Whitley R, Pass R (1987) Congenital cytomegalovirus: immunological alterations. J Med Virol 23: 41–49

Charpentier B, Michelson S, Martin B (1986) Definition of human cytomegalovirus-specific target antigens recognized by cytotoxic T cells generated in vitro by using an autologous lymphocyte system. J Immunol 137: 330–336

Chou S (1986) Acquisition of donor strains of cytomegalovirus by renal-transplant patients. N Engl J Med 314: 1418–1423

Clark B, Zaia J, Balce-Directo L, Ting Y (1984) Isolation and partial chemical characterization of a 64,000-dalton glycoprotein of human cytomegalovirus. J Virol 49: 279–282

Cranage M, Kouzarides T, Bankier A, Satchwell S, Weston K, Tomlinson P, Barrell B, et al. (1986) Identification of the human cytomegalovirus glycoprotein B gene and induction of neutralizing antibodies via its expression in recombinant vaccinia virus. EMBO J 5: 3057–3063

Cranage M, Smith G, Bell S, Hart H, Brown C, Bankier A, Tomlinson P, et al. (1988) Identification and expression of a human cytomegalovirus glycoprotein with homology to the Epstein-Barr virus BXLF2 product, varicella-zoster virus gpIII, and herpes simplex virus type 1 glycoprotein H. J Virol 62: 1416–1422

Cremer N, Cossen C, Shell G, Pereira L (1985) Antibody response to cytomegalovirus polypeptides captured by monoclonal antibodies on the solid phase in enzyme immunoassays. J Clin Microbiol 21: 517–521

Cunningham A, Merigan T (1984) Leu-3 positive T cells produce gamma interferon in patients with recurrent herpes labialis. J Immunol 132: 197–202

Davis M, Huang E (1985) Nucleotide sequence of a human cytomegalovirus DNA fragment encoding a 67-kilodalton phosphorylated viral protein. J Virol 56: 7–11

Davis M, Mar E, Wu Y, Huang E (1984) Mapping and expression of a human cytomegalovirus major viral protein. J Virol 52: 129–135

Dienstag J (1982) Serologic testing for hepatitis. Lab Manage 22: 21–28

Diosi P, Moldovan E, Tomescu N (1969) Latent cytomegalovirus infection in blood donors. Br Med J 4: 660–662

Dix R (1987) Prospects for a vaccine against herpes simplex virus types 1 and 2. Prog Med Virol 34: 89–128

Dressman G, Kennedy R (1985) Anti-idiotypic antibodies: implications of internal image based vaccines for infectious diseases. J Infect Dis 151: 761–765

Emini E, Luka J, Armstrong M, Keller P, Ellis R, Pearson G (1987) Identification of an Epstein-Barr virus glycoprotein which is antigenically homologous to the varicella-zoster virus glycoprotein II and the herpes simplex virus glycoprotein B. Virology 157: 552–555

Escudier E, Fleury J, Cordonnier C, Vernant J, Bernaudin J (1986) Large granular lymphocytes in bronchoalveolar lavage fluids from immunocompromised patients with cytomegalovirus pneumonitis. Am J Clin Pathol 86: 641–645

Farrar G, Greenaway P (1986) Characterization of glycoprotein complexes present in human cytomegalovirus envelopes. J Gen Virol 67: 1469–1473

Farrar G, Oram J (1984) Characterization of the human cytomegalovirus envelope glycoproteins. J Gen Virol 65: 1991–2001

Fiala M, Honess R, Heiner D, Heine J, Murnane J, Wallace R, Guze L (1976) Cytomegalovirus proteins. I. Polypeptides of virions and dense bodies. J Virol 19: 243–254

Forman S, Zaia J, Clark B, Wright C, Mills B, Pottathil R, Racklin B, et al. (1985) A 64,000 dalton matrix protein of human cytomegalovirus induces in vitro immune response similar to those of whole viral antigen. J Immunol 134: 3391–3395

Geballe A, Leach F, Mocarski E (1986) Regulation of cytomegalovirus late gene expression; gamma genes are controlled by posttranscriptional events. K Virol 57: 864–874

Gehrz R, Leonard T (1985) Cytomegalovirus (CMV)-specific lymphokine production in congenital CMV infection. Clin Exp Immunol 62: 507–514

Gehrz R, Fuad S, Liu Y, Bach F (1987a) HLA class II restriction of the T helper cell response to cytomegalovirus (CMV). I. Immunogenetic control of restriction. J Immunol 138: 3145–3151

Gehrz R, Liu Y, Peterson E, Fuad S (1987b) Role of antigen-presenting cells in congenital cytomegalovirus-specific immunodeficiency. J Infect Dis 156: 198–202

Gergely L, Czedledy J, Vaczi L (1988) Human antibody response to human cytomegalovirus-specific DNA-binding proteins. Acta Virol (Praha) 32: 1–5

Gibson W (1981a) Immediate-early proteins of human cytomegalovirus strains AD 169, Davis, and Towne differ in electrophoretic mobility. Virology 112: 350–354

Gibson W (1981b) Structural and nonstructural proteins of strain Colburn cytomegalovirus. Virology 111: 516–537

Gibson W (1983) Protein counterparts of human and simian cytomegaloviruses. Virology 128: 391–406

Gibson W, Irmiere A (1984) Selection of particles and proteins for use as human cytomegalovirus subunit vaccines, Birth Defects 20: 305–324

Gibson W, Murphy T, Roby C (1981) Cytomegalovirus-infected cells contain a DNA-binding protein. Virology 111: 251–262

Gold D, Ashley R, Handsfield H, Verdon M, Leach L, Mills J, Drew L, Corey L (1988) Immunoblot analysis of the humoral immune response in primary cytomegalovirus infection. J Infect Dis 157: 319–326

Gompels U, Minson A (1986) The properties and sequence of glycoprotein H of herpes simplex virus type 1. Virology 153: 230–247

Gonczol E, Hudecz F, Ianocone J, Dietzschold B, Starr S (1986) Immune response to isolated human cytomegalovirus envelope proteins. J Virol 58: 661–664

Gonczol E, Ianacone J, Starr S, Plotkin S (1987) Immunization of seronegative and seropositive individuals with a protein complex of the HCMV envelope (Abstr). 12-th International Herpesvirus Workshop, 253

Gratama J, Kardol M, Naipal A, Slats J, Dan Ouden A, Stijnen T, d'Amaro J, et al. (1987) The influence of cytomegalovirus carrier status on lymphocyte subsets and natural immunity. Clin Exp Immunol 68: 16–24

Gretch D, Gehrz R, Stinski M (1988a) Characterization of a human cytomegalovirus glycoprotein complex (gcI). J Gen Virol 69: 1205–1215

Gretch D, Kari B, Gehrz R, Stinski M (1988b) A multigene family encodes the human cytomegalovirus glycoprotein complex gcII (gp47–52 complex). J Virol 62: 1956–1962

Gretch D, Kari B, Rasmussen L, Gehrz R, Stinski MF (1988c) Identification and characterization of three distinct families of glycoprotein complexes in the envelopes of human cytomegalovirus. Virology 62: 875–881

Griffiths P, Grundy J (1987) Molecular biology and immunology of cytomegalovirus. Biochem J 241: 313–324

Griffiths P, Grundy J (1988) The status of CMV as a human pathogen. Epidemiol Infect 100: 1–15

Griffiths P, Stagno S, Pass R, Smith R, Alford C (1982) Infection with cytomegalovirus during pregnancy: specific IgM antibodies as a marker of recent primary infection. J Infect Dis 145: 647–653

Groh J, Grundy J, Prentice H, Griffiths P, et al. (1987) Immune donors can protect marrow-transplant recipients from severe cytomegalovirus infections. Lancet 1: 774–776

Grundy J, Super M, Griffiths P (1986) Reinfection of a seropositive allograft recipient by cytomegalovirus from donor kidney. Lancet 1: 159–160

Gupta P, St Joer S, Rapp R (1977) Comparison of the polypeptides of several strains of human cytomegalovirus. J Gen Virol 34: 447–454

Hanshaw J (1983) Cytomegalovirus. In: Remington J, Klein J (eds) Infectious diseases of the fetus and newborn, 2nd edn. Saunders, Philadelphia, pp 104–142

Hayes K, Alford C, Britt W (1987) Antibody response to virus-encoded proteins after cytomegalovirus mononucleosis. J Infect Dis 156: 615–621

Heilbronn R, Jahn G, Burkle A, Freese U, Fleckenstein B, zur Hausen H (1987) Genomic localization, sequence analysis, and transcription of the putative human cytomegalovirus DNA polymerase gene. J Virol 61: 119–124

Heineman T, Gong M, Sample J, Kieff E (1988) Identification of the Epstein-Barr virus gp85 gene. J Virol 62: 1101–1107

Henle W, Henle G, Horwitz C (1974) Epstein-Barr virus specific diagnostic tests in infectious mononucleosis. Hum Pathol 5: 552–565

Ho M (1982) Cytomegalovirus biology and infection. Plenum, New York

Huart J, Baume D, Jouet J (1987) Specific anti-cytomegalovirus immunoglobulins in the prevention of cytomegalovirus infections in bone marrow allografts. Ann Med Interne (Paris) 138: 372–374

Hutt-Fletcher L, Balachandran N, Elkins M (1983) B cell activation by cytomegalovirus. J Exp Med 158: 2171–2176

Irmiere A, Gibson W (1983) Isolation and characterization of a non-infectious virion-like particle released from cells infected with human strains of cytomegalovirus. Virology 130: 118–133

Irmiere A, Gibson W (1985) Isolation of human cytomegalovirus intranuclear capsids, and demonstration that the B-capsid assembly protein is also abundant in noninfectious enveloped particles. J Virol 56: 277–283

Jahn G, Kouzarides T, Mach M, School B, Plachter B, Predy R, Satchwell S, et al. (1987) Map position and nucleotide sequence of the gene for the large structural phosphoprotein of human cytomegalovirus 1358–1367

Jonjic S, del Val M, Keil G, Reddehase M, Koszinowski U (1988) A nonstructural viral protein expressed by a recombinant vaccinia virus protects against lethal cytomegalovirus infection. J Virol 62: 1653–1658

Kantor G, Goldber L, Johnson B, Perechin M, Barnett E (1970) Immunologic abnormalities induced by post perfusion cytomegalovirus infection. Ann Intern Med 73: 553–558

Kari B, Gehrz R (1988) Isolation and characterization of a human cytomegalovirus glycoprotein containing a high content of O-lnked oligosaccharides. Arch Virol 98: 171–188

Kari B, Lussenhop N, Goertz Z, Wabuke-Bunoti M, Radeke R, Gehrz R (1986) Characterization of monoclonal antibodies reactive to several biochemically distinct human cytomegalovirus glycoprotein complexes. J Virol 60: 345–352

Keay S, Rasmussen L, Merigan T (1988) Syngeneic monoclonal anti-idiotype antibodies which bear the internal image of a human cytomegalovirus neutralization epitope. J Immunol 140: 944–948

Keil G, Fibi M, Koszinowski U (1985) Characterization of the major immediate-early polypeptides encoded by murine cytomegalovirus. J Virol 54: 422–428

Keller P, Davison A, Lower R, Rieman M, Ellis R (1987) Identification and sequence of the gene encoding gpIII, a major glycoprotein of varicella-zoster virus. Virology 157: 526–533

Kemble G, McCormick A, Pereira L, Mocarski E (1987) A cytomegalovirus protein with properties of herpes simplex virus ICP8: partial purification of the polypeptide and map position of the gene. J Virol 61: 3143–3151

Kim K, Sapienza V, Carp P, Moon H (1976) Analysis of structural polypeptides of purified human cytomegalovirus. J Virol 20: 614–611

Kim K, Sapienza V, Chen C, Wisniewski K (1983) Production of monoclonal antibodies specific for a glycosylated polypeptide of human cytomegalovirus. J Clin Microbiol 18: 331–343

Kinney J, Onorato I, Stewart J, Pass R, Stagno S, Chesseman S, Chin J, et al. (1985) Cytomegaloviral infection and disease. J Infect Dis 151: 772–774

Koszinowski U, Reddehase M, Keil G, Schickedanz J (1987a) Host immune response to cytomegalovirus: products of transfected viral immediate-early genes are recognized by cloned cytolytic T lymphocytes. J Virol 61: 2054–2058

Koszinowski U, Keil G, Schwarz H, Schickedanz J, Reddehase M (1987b) A nonstructural polypeptide encoded by immediate-early transcription unit 1 of murine cyomegalovirus is recognized by cytolytic T lymphocytes. J Exp Med 166: 289–299

Kouzarides T, Bankier A, Satchwell S, Weston K, Tomlinson P, Barrell B (1987) Sequence and transcription analysis of the human cytomegalovirus DNA polymerase gene. J Virol 61: 125–133

Kouzarides R, Bankier A, Satchwell S, Preddy E, Barrell B (1988) An immediate early gene of human cytomegalovirus encodes a potential membrane glycoprotein. Virology 165: 151–164

Krah D, Choppin P (1988) Mice immunized with measles virus develop antibodies to a cell surface receptor for binding virus. J Virol 62: 1565–1572

Landini M, Michelson S (1988) Human cytomegalovirus proteins. Prog Med Virol 35: 152–185

Landini M, Mirolo G, Coppolecchia P, Re M, LaPlaca M (1986) Serum antibodies to individual cytomegalovirus structural polypeptides in renal transplant recipients during viral infection. Microbiol Immunol 30: 683–695

Landini M, Severi B, Badiali L, Gonczol E, Morolo G (1987a) Structural components of human cytomegalovirus: in situ localization of the major glycoprotein. Intervirology 27: 154–160

Landini M, Severi B, Furlini G, DeGiorgi L (1987b) Human cytomegalovirus structural components: intracellular and intraviral localization of p28 and p65–69 by immunoelectron microscopy. Virus Res 8: 15–23

Lane H, Masur H, Edgar L, Whalen G, Rook A, Fauci A (1983) Abnormalities of B-cell activation and immunoregulation in patients with the acquired immunodeficiency syndrome. N Engl J Med 309: 453–458

Law K, Wilton-Smith P, Farrar G (1985) A murine monoclonal antibody recognizing a single glycoprotein within a human cytomegalovirus virion envelope glycoprotein complex. J Med Virol 17: 255–266

Lemaster S, Roizman B (1980) Herpes simplex virus phosphoproteins. II. Characterization of the virion protein kinase and of the polypeptides phosphorylated in the virion. J Virol 35: 798–811

Lindsley M, Torpley D, Rinaldo C (1986) HLA-DR-restricted cytotoxicity of cytomegalovirus-infected monocytes mediated by Leu-3-positive T cells. J Immunol 136: 3045–3056

Linner K, Monroy C, Bach F, Gehrz R (1986) Dw subtypes of serologically defined DR-DQ specificities restrict recognition of cytomegalovirus. Hum Immunol 17: 79–86

Liu Y, Fuad S, Gehrz R (1987) Epstein-Barr virus transformed lymphoblastoid cell lines as antigen-presenting cells and "augmenting" cells for human CMV-specific Th clones. Cell Immunol 108: 64–75

Liu Y, Kari B, Gehrz R (1988) Human immune responses to major human cytomegalovirus glycoprotein complexes. J Virol 62: 1066–1070

Lussenhop N, Goertz R, Wabuke-Bunoti M, Gehrz R, Kari B (1988) Epitope analysis of human cytomegalovirus glycoprotein complexes using murine monoclonal antibodies. Virology 164: 362–372

Mach M, Utz U, Fleckenstein B (1986) Mapping of the major glycoprotein gene of human cytomegalovirus. J Gen Virol 67: 1461–1467

Mar E, Patel P, Huang E (1981) Human cytomegalovirus-associated DNA polymerase and protein kinase activities. J Gen Virol 57: 149–156

Mar E, Chiou J, Cheng Y, Hang E (1985) Human cytomegalovirus-induced DNA polymerase and its interaction with the triphosphates of 1-(2'deoxy-2'fluoro-B-D-arabinofluaranosy)-5-methyluracil,-5-iodocytosine, and -5-methylcytosine. J Virol 56: 846–851

Martin S, Courtney R, Fowler G, Rouse B (1988) Herpes simplex virus type-1 specific cytotoxic T lymphocytes recognize virus nonstructural proteins. J Virol 62: 2265–2273

Martinez J, St Joer S (1986) Molecular cloning and analysis of three cDNA clones homologous to human cytomegalovirus RNAs present during late infection. J Virol 62: 531–538

Matsumoto Y, Sugano T, Miyamoto C, Masuho Y (1986) Generation of hybridomas producing human monoclonal antibodies against human cytomegalovirus. Biochem Biophys Res Commun 137: 273–280

McKeating J, Griffiths P, Grundy J (1987) Cytomegalovirus in urine specimens has host $\beta 2$ microglobulin bound to the viral envelope: a mechanism of evading the host immune response? J Gen Virol 68: 785–792

Meyer H, Bankier A, Landini M, Brown C, Barrell B, Ruger B, Mach M (1988) Identification and procaryotic expression of the gene coding for the highly immunogenic 28-kilodalton structural phosphoprotein (pp28) of human cytomegalovirus. J Virol 62: 2243–2250

Meyers J (1984) Cytomegalovirus infection following marrow transplantation: risk, treatment, and preventation. Birth Defects 20: 101–117

Middeldrop J, Tegzess A, Jongsma J, Roenhorst H, The T (1984) Immunity to human cytomegalovirus (HCMV). I. Humoral immune responses to HCMV-specific membrane antigens (CMV-MA) in normal and immunocompromised donors during acute and latent CMV infections. Birth Defects 20: 441–445

Middeldorp J, Jongsma J, The T (1986) Killing of human cytomegalovirus-infected fibroblasts by antiviral antibody and complement. J Infect Dis 153: 48–55

Miller N, Hutt-Fletcher L (1988) A monoclonal antibody to glycoprotein gp85 inhibits fusion but not attachment of Epstein-Barr virus. J Virol 62: 2366–2372

Mocarski E, Pereira L, Michael N (1985) Precise localization of genes on large animal virus genomes: use of lambda gt11 and monoclonal antibodies to map the gene for a cytomegalovirus protein family. Proc Natl Acad Sci USA 82: 1266–1270

Neuman P, Wasserman P, Wentworth B, Kao G, Lerner K, Storb R, Buckner C (1973) Interstitial pneumonia and cytomegalovirus infection as complications of human marrow transplantation. Transplantation 15: 478–485

Newkirk M, Gram H, Heinrich G, Ostberg L, Capra J, Wasserman R (1988) Complete protein sequences of the variable regions of the cloned heavy and light chains of a human anti-cytomegalovirus antibody reveal a striking similarity to human monoclonal rheumatoid factors of the Wa idiotypic family. J Clin Invest 81: 1511–1518

Nowak B, Sullivan C, Sarnow R, Thomas R, Bricout F, Nicolas J, Fleckenstein B, Levine A (1984) Characterization of monoclonal antibodies and polyclonal immune sera directed against human cytomegalovirus virion proteins. Virology 132: 325–338

Onorato I, Morens D, Martone W, Stansfield S (1985) Epidemiology of cytomegaloviral infections: recommendations for prevention and control. Rev Infect Dis 7: 479–497

Osborn J (1981) Cytomegalovirus: pathogenicity, immunology, and vaccine initiatives. J Infect Dis 143: 618–630

Otto S, Sullivan-Tailyour G, Malone C, Stinski M (1988) Subcellular localization of the major immediate early protein (IE1) of human cytomegalovirus at early times after infection. Virology 162: 478–482

Pachl C, Probert W, Hermsen K, Perot K, Masiarz F, Rasmussen L, Merigan T, Spaete R (1988) The human cytomegalovirus strain Towne glycoprotein-gene encodes glycoprotein p86. Virology 169: 418–426

Pande H, Baak S, Riggs A, Clark B, Shively J, Zaia J (1984) Cloning and physical mapping of a gene fragment coding for a 64-kilodalton major late antigen of human cytomegalovirus. Proc Natl Acad Sci USA 81: 4965–4969

Pass R, Griffiths P, August A (1983) Antibody response to cytomegalovirus after renal transplantation: comparison of patients with primary and recurrent infections. J Infect Dis 147: 40–46

Pass R, Hutto C, Ricks R, Cloud G (1986) Increased rate of cytomegalovirus infection among parents of children attending day-care centres. J Engl J Med 314: 1414–1418

Pereira L, Hoffman M, Gallo D, Cremer N (1982) Monoclonal antibodies to human cytomegalovirus: three surface membrane proteins with unique immunological and electrophoretic properties specify cross reactive determinants. Infect Immun 36: 924–932

Pereira L, Stagno S, Hoffman M, Volanakis J (1983) Cytomegalovirus-infected cell polypeptides immune-precipitated by sera from children with congenital and perinatal infections. Infect Immun 39: 100–108

Pereira L, Hoffman M, Tatsuno M, Dondero D (1984) Polymorphism of human cytomegalovirus glycoproteins characterized by monoclonal antibodies. Virology 139: 73–86

Perussia B, Starr S, Abraham S, Fanning V, Trinchieri G (1983a) Human natural killer cells analyzed by B73-1, a monoclonal antibody blocking Fc receptor functions. I. Characterization of the lymphocytes subset reactive with B73-1. J Immunol 130: 2133–2141

Perussia B, Acuto O, Terhorst C, Faust J, Lasurus R, Fanning V, Trinchieri G (1983b) Human natural killer cells analyzed by B73-1, a monoclonal antibody blocking Fc receptor functions. II. studies of B73-1-antibody-antigen interaction on the lymphocyte membrane. J Immunol 130: 2142–2148

Plotkin S, Michelson S, Pagno J, Rapp F (eds) (1984) Cytomegalovirus: pathogenesis and prevention of human infection. Birth Defects 20

Quinnan G, Kirmani N, Rook A, Manischewitz J, Jackson L, Moreschi G, Santos G, et al. (1982) HLA-restricted T-lymphocyte and non-T-lymphocyte cytotoxic responses correlate with recovery from cytomegalovirus infection in bone-marrow-transplant recipients. N Engl J Med 307: 7–13

Rasmussen L, Stevens D, Jordan G, Merigan T (1974) Interferon and transformation responses of human lymphocytes in recurrent herpesvirus hominis infections. J Immunol 112: 728–736

Rasmussen L, Kelsall D, Nelson R, Carney W, Hirsch M, Winston D, Preiksaitis J, Merigan T (1982) Virus specific IgG and IgM antibodies in normal and immunocompromised subjects infected with human cytomegalovirus. J Infect Dis 145: 191–199

Rasmussen L, Nelson R, Kelsall D, Merigan T (1984) Murine monoclonal antibody to a single protein neutralizes the infectivity of human cytomegalovirus. Proc Natl Acad Sci USA 81: 876–880

Rasmussen L, Mullenax J, Nelson R, Merigan T (1985a) Viral polypeptides detected by a complement dependent neutralizing murine monoclonal antibody to human cytomegalovirus. J Virol 55: 274–280

Rasmussen L, Mullenax J, Nelson M, Merigan T (1985b) Human cytomegalovirus polypeptides stimulate neutralizing antibody in vivo. J Virol 145: 186–190

Rasmussen L, Nelson M, Neff M, Merigan T (1988) Characterization of two different human cytomegalovirus glycoproteins which are targets for virus neutralizing antibody. Virology 163: 308–318

Re M, Landini M, Coppolecchia P, Furlini G, LaPlaca M (1985) A 28000 molecular weight human cytomegalovirus structural polypeptide studied by means of a specific monoclonal antibody. J Gen Virol 66: 2507–2511

Reddehase M, Koszinowski U (1984) Significance of herpesvirus immediate early gene expression in cellular immunity to cytomegalovirus infection. Nature 312: 369–371

Reddehase M, Keil G, Koszinowski U (1984a) The cytolytic T lymphocyte response to the murine cytomegalovirus II. Detection of virus replication stage-specific antigens by separate populations of in vivo active cytolytic T lymphocyte precursors. Eur J Immunol 14: 56–61

Reddehase M, Keil G, Koszinowski U (1984b) The cytolytic T lymphocyte response to the murine cytomegalovirus. I. Distinct maturation stages of cytolytic T lymphocytes constitute the cellular immune response during acute infection of mice with the murine cytomegalovirus. J Immunol 132: 482–489

Reddehase M, Weil F, Munch K, Jonjic S, Luske A, Koszinowski U (1985) Interstitial murine cytomegalovirus pneumonia after irradiation: characterization of cells that limit viral replication during established infection of the lungs. J Virol 55: 264–273

Reddehase M, Buhring H, Koszinowski U (1986a) Cloned long-term cytolytic T-lymphocyte line with specificity for an immediate-early membrane antigen of murine cytomegalovirus. J Virol 57: 408–412

Reddehase M, Fibi M, Keil G, Koszinowski U (1986b) Late-phase expression of a murine cytomegalovirus immediate-early antigen recognized by cytolytic T lymphocytes. J Virol 60: 1125–1129

Reddehase M, Mutter W, Munch K, Buhring H, Koszinowski U (1987) CD8-positive T lymphocytes specific for murine cytomegalovirus immediate-early antigens mediate protective immunity. J Virol 61: 3102–3108

Reddehase M, Jonjic S, Weiland F, Mutter W, Koszinowski U (1988) Adoptive immunotherapy of murine cytomegalovirus adrenalitis in the immunocompromised host: CD4-helper-independent antiviral function of CD8-positive memory T lymphocytes derived from latently infected donors. J Virol 62: 1061–1063

Ripalti A, Ladini M, LaPlaca M (1988) A 46 kD polypeptide, present in purified human cytomegalovirus, is provided with DNAse activity and is antigenically related to a higher molecular weight, enzymatically inactive, cellular protein. Microbiological 11: 69–76

Robbins A, Dorney D, Wathen M, Whealy M, Gold C, Watson R, Holland L, et al. (1987) The pseudorabies virus gII gene is closely related to the gb glycoprotein gene of herpes simplex virus. J Virol 61: 2691–2701

Roby C, Gibson W (1986) Characterization of phosphoproteins and protein kinase activity of virions, noninfectious enveloped particles, and dense bodies of human cytomegalovirus. J Virol 59: 714–727

Rodgers B, Borysiewicz L, Mondin J, Graham S, Sissons P (1987) Immunoaffinity purification of a 72 K early antigen of human cytomegalovirus: analysis of humoral and cell-mediated immunity to the purified polypeptide. J Gen Virol 68: 2371–2378

Rook A, Quinnan G, Fredrick J, Manichewitz J, Kirmani N, Dantzler T, Lee B, Currier C (1984) Importance of cytotoxic lymphocytes during cytomegalovirus infection in renal transplant recipients. Am J Med 76: 385–392

Rouse B, Norley S, Martin S (1988) Antiviral cytotoxic T lymphocyte induction and vaccination. Rev Infect Dis 10: 16–33

Rueger B, Klages S, Walla B, Albrecht J, Fleckenstein B, Tomlinson P, Barrell B (1987) Primary structure and transcription of the genes coding for the two virion phosphoproteins pp65 and pp71 of human cytomegalovirus. J Virol 61: 446–453

Rundell B, Betts R (1980) Physical properties of cytomegalovirus immune complexes prepared with IgG neutralizing antibody, anti-IgG, and complement. J Immunol 124: 337–342

Saltzman R, Quirk M, Jordan M (1988) Disseminated cytomegalovirus infection: molecular analysis of virus and leukocyte interactions in viremia. J Clin Invest 81: 75–81

Schrier R, Nelson J, Oldstone M (1985) Detection of human cytomegalovirus in peripheral blood lymphocytes in a natural infection. Science 230: 1048–1051

Severi B, Landini M, Musiahi M, Zerbini M (1979) A study of the passage of human cytomegalovirus from the nucleus to the cytoplasm. Microbiologica 2: 265–273

Shanley J (1987) Modification of acute murine cytomegalovirus adrenal gland infection by adoptive spleen cell transfer. J Virol 61: 23–28

Shanley J, Pesanti E (1986) Murine cytomegalovirus adrenalitis in athymic nude mice. Arch Virol 88: 27–35

Shrier R, Nelson J, Oldstone M (1985) Detection of human cytomegalovirus in peripheral blood lymphocytes in a natural infection. Science 230: 1048–1051

Smith J (1986) Human cytomegalovirus: demonstration of permissive epithelial cells and nonpermissive fibroblastic cells in a survey of human cell lines. J Virol 60: 582–588

Smith J, DeHarven E (1973) Herpes simplex virus and human cytomegalovirus replication in WI-38 cells. I. Sequence of viral replication . J Virol 12: 919–930

Spaete R, Thayer R, Probert W, Masiarz F, Chamberlian S, Rasmussen L, Merigan T, Pachl C (1988) Human cytomegalovirus strain Towne glycoprotein B is processed by proteolytic cleavage. Virology 167: 207–225.

Stagno S, Whitley R (1985) Herpesvirus infections of pregnancy. I. Cytomegalovirus and Epstein-Barr virus infections. N Engl J Med 313: 1270–1274

Stagno S, Pass R, Dworsky M, Henderson R, Moore E, Walton P, Alford C (1982) Congenital cytomegalovirus infection: the relative importance of primary and recurrent maternal infection. N Engl J Med 306: 945–949

Stalder H, Ehrensberger T (1980) Microneutralization of human cytomegalovirus. J Infect Dis 142: 102–105

Stevely W, Katan M, Stirling V, Smith G, Leader D (1985) Protein kinase activities associated with the virions of pseudorabies and herpes simplex virus. J Gen Virol 66: 661–673

Stinski M (1976) Human cytomegalovirus: glycoproteins associated with virions and dense bodies. J Virol 19: 594–609

Stinski M (1977) Synthesis of proteins and glycoproteins in cells infected with human cytomegalovirus. J Virol 23: 751–767

Stinski M (1984) The proteins of human cytomegalovirus. Birth Defects 20: 49–62

Stinski M, Mocarski E, Thomsen D, Urbanowski M (1979) Membrane glycoproteins and antigens induced by human cytomegalovirus. J Gen Virol 43: 119–129

Sweet G, Bryant S, Tegtmeier G, Beneke J, Bayer W (1985) Early and late antigens of human cytomegalovirus: electroimmunodiffusion assay of numbers, relationships, and reactivities with donor sera. J Med Virol 15: 137–148

Tamura T, Chiba S, Chiba Y, Nakao T (1980) Virus excretion and neutralizing antibody response in saliva in human cytomegalovirus infection. Infect Immun 29: 842–845

Tapper M, Rotterdam H, Lerner C, Al'Khafaji K, Seitzman P (1984) Adrenal cortical function in the acquired immunodeficiency syndrome. Ann Intern Med 100: 239–241

The T, Klein G, Langenhuysen M (1974) Antibody reactions to virus-specific early antigens (EA) in patients with cytomegalovirus (CMV) infection. Clin Exp Immunol 16: 1–12

Thomsen D, Stenberg R, Goins W, Stinski M (1984) Promoter-regulatory region of the major immediate early gene of human cytomegalovirus. Proc Natl Acad Sci USA 81: 659–663

Torseth J, Merigan T (1987) Significance of local gamma interferon in recurrent herpes simplex infection. J Infect Dis 153: 979–984

Torseth J, Nickoloff B, Basham T, Merigan T (1987a) Beta interferon produced by keratinocytes in human cutaneous infection with herpes simplex virus. J Infect Dis 155: 641–648

Torseth J, Cohen G, Eisenberg R, Berman P, Lasky L, Cerini C, Heilman C, et al. (1987b) Native and recombinant herpes simplex virus type 1 envelope proteins induce human immune T-lymphocyte responses. J Virol 61: 1532–1539

Volkmer H, Bertholet C, Jonjic S, Wittek R, Koszinowski U (1987) Cytolytic T lymphocyte recognition of the murine cytomegalovirus nonstructural immediate-early protein pp89 expressed by recombinant vaccinia virus. J Exp Med 166: 668–677

Walthen M, Stinski M (1982) Temporal patterns of human cytomegalovirus transcription: mapping the viral RNAs synthesized at immediate early, early, and late times after infection. J Virol 41: 462–477

Waner J, Hopkins D, Weller T, Allred E (1977) Cervical excretion of cytomegalovirus: correlation with secretory and humoral antibody. J Infect Dis 136: 805–809

Weiner D, Gibson W, Fields K (1986) Anti-complement immunofluorescence establishes nuclear localization of human cytomegalovirus matrix protein. Virology 147: 19–28

Weston K, Barrell B (1986) Sequence of the short unique region, short repeats, and part of the long repeats of human cytomegalovirus. J Mol Biol 192: 177–208

Wilkinson G, Akrigg A, Greenaway P (1984) Transcription of the immediate early genes of human cytomegalovirus strain AD 169. Virus Res 1: 101–116

Winston D, Ho W, Lin C, Bartoni K, Budinger M, Gale R, Champlin R (1987) Intravenous immune globulin for prevention of cytomegalovirus infection and interstitial pneumonia after bone marrow transplantation. Ann Intern Med 106: 12–18

Yachie A, Tosato G, Straus S, Blaese R (1985) Immunostimulation by cytomegalovirus (CMV): helper T-cell-dependent activation of immunoglobulin production in vitro by lymphocytes from CMV-immune donors. J Immunol 135: 1395–4000

Zaia J, Forman S, Ting Y, Vanderwal-Urbina E, Blume K (1986) Polypeptide-specific antibody response to human cytomegalovirus after infection in bone marrow transplant recipients. J Infect Dis 153: 780–787

Progress in Vaccine Development for Prevention of Human Cytomegalovirus Infection

E. Gönczöl and S. Plotkin

1   Introduction and Rationale for an HCMV Vaccine   255
2   Towne Live Virus Vaccine   256
2.1   Protective Effects of Towne Vaccine Against Low-Passage Toledo Strain
       Administered as a Challenge in Normal Vaccinated Volunteers   257
2.2   HCMV-Specific Lymphocyte Proliferation   259
2.3   Development of Virus-Neutralizing Antibodies   259
2.4   Recognition of Viral Proteins by Western Blot or Immunoprecipitation Assays   261
2.5   Implications for Functional Activity of Viral Proteins   264
3   Humoral and Cellular Immune Responses Induced in Human Volunteers by
       Immunoaffinity-Purified gA/gB protein   267
3.1   Preparation and Composition of the gA/gB Glycoprotein Complex   267
3.2   Immune Response to HCMV in Human Volunteers Immunized with the
       gA/gB Preparation   268
3.2.1   Immune Response of Seropositive Individuals   268
3.2.2   Immune Response of Seronegative Individuals   268
4   Conclusions and Prospects   271
References   272

1 Introduction and Rationale for an HCMV Vaccine

The infectious agent most frequently causing congenital malformations is the human cytomegalovirus (HCMV). HCMV infection is found in about 1% of newborns, and about 10%–15% of the infected children suffer either from immediate symptoms or late sequelae of the infection. Clinically apparent infections after birth are characterized by cytomegalic inclusion diseases (CIDs) in about 5% of the infected children. Another 5% have atypical involvement, usually with some damage of the CNS and 90% have no symptoms at birth. Among the most severely affected children mortality may be 30%. About 10%–15% of the children who are infected but asymptomatic at birth eventually develop mental retardation, chorioretinitis, microcephaly, and hearing loss (WELLER 1971; PASS et al. 1980; STAGNO et al. 1983, 1984).

HCMV infection in adults is usually symptomless or results in a self-limited infectious-mononucleosis-like syndrome. However, severe HCMV-caused diseases

The Wistar Institute, 36th Street at Spruce, Philadelphia, PA 19104, USA

Current Topics in Microbiology and Immunology, Vol. 154
© Springer-Verlag Berlin · Heidelberg 1990

develop in certain groups of the population, such as organ transplant patients and individuals with impaired immune functions (GLENN 1981).

Antibody seropositivity of a pregnant woman does not prevent the embryo or fetus from being infected by the reactivated virus. Moreover, seropositive individuals may become infected with a second or third HCMV strain, especially when immune functions are damaged. Although these observations would appear to discourage attempts to provide artificial immune protection, the analysis of the consequences of HCMV infections in previously seronegative individuals and of the reactivation or reinfection of seropositive individuals shows that immunity does make a difference. The congenitally infected children who are symptomatic at birth or who develop severe symptoms later are usually born to mothers who sustained primary HCMV infection during pregnancy. Congenitally infected children whose mothers underwent virus reactivation or reinfection during pregnancy are usually symptomless or have very mild symptoms. Likewise, although HCMV reinfection and reactivation does occur in seropositive organ transplant recipients, the symptoms are less severe and do not threaten the success of the transplantation (GLENN 1981). HCMV disease can be prevented in bone marrow transplant recipients if the transplant is accompanied by injection of HCMV antibody-containing γ-globulin preparation (MEYERS et al. 1983; WINSTON et al. 1984).

The clinical data mentioned above justify an effort to develop an HCMV vaccine. In our laboratory we have pursued two avenues of active immunization: live virus vaccine and subunit vaccine. These efforts will be described.

2 Towne Live Virus Vaccine

The first approach to vaccination against HCMV was that of an attenuated live vaccine. After early efforts (ELEK and STERN 1974), PLOTKIN et al. (1975) isolated and developed the Towne strain as a candidate vaccine. The strain was isolated from a congenitally infected infant, and then passaged 125 times in human fibroblasts before being prepared as a pool for clinical testing.

Human trials have been performed in normal, healthy volunteers, particularly pediatric nurses, and in renal transplant patients, who suffer a high morbidity due to primary HCMV infection. The properties of the strain and the results of tests thus far have been reported (FLEISHER et al. 1982; PLOTKIN et al. 1976, 1984, 1985; PLOTKIN and HUANG 1985) and are summarized in Table 1. The most noteworthy points are as follows.

1. Injection of the Towne virus is well tolerated aside from a local reaction which is due to the development of cellular immunity to HCMV.
2. The virus only replicates locally at the site of injection and is not excreted by vaccinees.
3. Extensive trials in renal transplant patients showed that the vaccine could not prevent HCMV superinfection, but did ameliorate the outcome of infection in a manner similar to natural immunity. The partial efficacy of both natural and vaccine-induced immunity was attributed to the suppression of the host's cellular immunity by the drugs used after transplantation.

Table 1. Comparison of infection due to natural virus and Towne live vaccine

	Natural infection	Live vaccine infection
Febrile illness	+	0
Lymphocytosis	+	0
Transaminase elevation	+	0
Local reaction	0	+
Reversed T-cell helper/suppressor ratio	+	0
Virus excretion	+	0
CF antibody	+	+ (1 year)
ACIF antibody	+	+
NEUT antibody	+	+
IgM antibody	+	+
Early antigens antibody	+	+
Lymphocyte proliferation[a] (HCMV specific)	±	+
T-cell cytotoxicity (HLA restricted)	+	+ (shorter duration)
Protection[b] in HCMV-exposed renal transplant recipients	83%	83%

[a] Becomes positive with recovery
[b] Against serious CMV disease

Challenge trials in normal vaccinated volunteers have been documented (PLOTKIN et al. 1989) and are described in the following section.

2.1 Protective Effects of Towne Vaccine Against Low-Passage Toledo Strain Administered as a Challenge in Normal Vaccinated Volunteers

The results of the challenge studies showed that the Towne vaccine induces both a full range of antibody responses and HCMV-specific cellular immune responses, and protects healthy volunteers against a certain dose [10–100 plaque-forming units (PFUs)] of low-passage Toledo strain.

The details of the study are as follows: A total of 25 volunteers with a normal immune-status were enlisted. After consent forms were received, 12 seronegative human volunteers were immunized with the Towne vaccine strain and challenged artificially with measured doses of a low-passage HCMV strain, the Toledo strain (PLOTKIN et al. 1985). As controls six seronegative and seven natural seropositive individuals were challenged with the Toledo strain.

The protective effect of the Towne vaccination is summarized in Table 2. Seronegatives developed infectious mononucleosis-type disease when injected with 10 or 100 PFUs Toledo strain, while natural seropositives showed the same symptoms when injected with 1000 PFUs. In contrast, the Towne strain vaccinees and the naturally seropositive individuals were protected against 10 PFUs Toledo strain with no signs of illness or infection. The 100-PFU dose of Toledo strain did not cause any illness in the seropositive control group while one of the seven Towne vaccinees complained of mild symptoms (headache, malaise) of the virus infection.

Table 2. Outcome of challenge with low-passage HCMV (Toledo strain) in seronegative, seropositive, and Towne vaccinated subjects

	Number positive/number observed								
	Seronegatives			Natural seropositives			Prior vaccinees		
Dose of Toledo	Illness[a]	Abnormal[b]	Infection[c]	Illness	Abnormal	Infection	Illness	Abnormal	Infection
1000 PFUs	—	—	—	2/5	5/5	3/5	—	—	—
100 PFUs	2/2	2/2	2/2	0/5	0/5	1/5	1/7	3/7	4/7
10 PFUs	4/4	4/4	4/4	0/2	0/2	1/2[d]	0/5	1/5[e]	0/5

[a]Clinical complaints
[b]Laboratory evidence of lymphocytosis, thrombocytopenia, or hepatitis
[c]Virus excretion or antibody rise
[d]Single positive specimen
[e]Single blood smear showing 10% atypical lymphocytosis

Virus infection was observed after the 100-PFU dose in one of the five natural seropositives and four of the seven Towne vaccinees as detected by virus excretion and seroconversion. These data clearly show that the outcome of HCMV infection is determined by the immune status of the individual and the dose of the infecting virus. A large dose can overwhelm even fully competent immunity. Smaller doses of HCMV may, however, result in symptomatic infection, asymptomatic infection, or no infection, depending on the host's immune status.

The immune status of the individuals in this trial was evaluated by an in vitro HCMV-specific lymphocyte-proliferation assay (PLOTKIN et al. 1989) and by neutralization, Western blot, and immunoprecipitation assays for HCMV antibodies (GÖNCZÖL et al. 1989a).

2.2 HCMV-Specific Lymphocyte Proliferation

The lymphocyte proliferation assay was carried out as described (STARR et al. 1980, 1981). Table 3 shows that the T-lymphocytes obtained as early as 2 weeks after the Towne strain immunization responded by HCMV-specific proliferation in an in vitro assay; two peak values were obtained at 2–4 weeks and at 12–16 weeks after the immunization. The significance and explanation for the two peaks are not clear.

2.3 Development of Virus-Neutralizing Antibodies

Virus-neutralizing antibodies were measured against the Towne and Toledo strain in microneutralization assays (GÖNCZÖL et al. 1986a).

Table 3. HCMV-specific lymphocyte proliferation of 12 seronegative volunteers immunized with Towne strain

	Weeks after immunization							
	0	2	4	6	8	12	16	52
Mean of stimulation indices[a]	1.0	16.5	18.8	3.9	6.5	22.2	11.2	8.6

[a] Stimulation index is defined as counts per minute (cpm) in HCMV antigen-stimulated cultures/cpm in control antigen-stimulated culture

Table 4. Neutralization titer[a] of 12 seronegative volunteers immunized with Towne strain and tested against Towne or Toledo strains

	Weeks after immunization					
Tested against	0	2	4	8	16	52
Towne	<4	<4	12	42.6	43.3	29.6
Toledo	<4	<4	5.6	19.0	32.0	17.2

[a] Neutralization titers as measured in the presence of C' are expressed as geometric means. Within each group a maximum four-fold difference was observed between the highest and lowest neutralization titer

Table 4 shows that the seronegative volunteers responded with the development of neutralizing antibodies to the Towne vaccine. The geometric mean titer of neutralizing antibodies was slightly higher against the Towne strain than against the Toledo strain at all times after the Towne strain injection. Table 5 summarizes the neutralizing antibody responses in individuals challenged with the Toledo strain. In seronegative individuals challenged with 10 PFUs (four individuals) or 100 PFUs (two individuals) of Toledo strain (group I) geometric mean neutralizing titers up to 1:724 were observed. There was no significant difference between the neutralization titers of individuals injected with 10 PFUs or 100 PFUs Toledo strain. However, strain-specific difference in the neutralization titer was clear, i.e., titers were two- to six-fold higher to the Toledo than to the Towne strain. In Towne vaccinees (group II) at 8 weeks after challenge there was a clear difference in the neutralization titer of individuals challenged with 10 or 100 PFUs Toledo strain. In five individuals who were challenged with 10 PFUs Toledo strain no increase in neutralization titer was observed against either strain; however, four individuals challenged with 100 PFUs Toledo strain responded with about a 20-fold increase in neutralizing antibody titer to both strains.

The neutralization titers of naturally seropositive individuals injected with 10 PFUs (two individuals) or 100 PFUs (three individuals were tested out of the five) (group III) did not change significantly after the challenge. The serum of one of three natural seropositive individuals who received 100 PFUs Toledo strain developed a fourfold increase in the neutralization titer to the Toledo strain and a twofold increase to the Towne strain at 16 weeks after challenge, resulting in a slight increase in the geometric mean titer of sera from all five individuals.

Table 5. Neutralization titer[a] of three groups of individuals challenged with the Toledo strain

Groups	Tested against	Weeks after challenge					
		0	6	7	8	12	16
I. Seronegatives challenged							
with 10 PFUs	Towne	<4	<4	11	69	152	181
($N = 4$)	Toledo	<4	4	76	152	430	724
with 100 PFUs	Towne	<4	<4	32	32	90	128
($N = 2$)	Toledo	<4	<4	64	128	512	724
II. Towne vaccinees challenged							
with 10 PFUs	Towne	32			32		32
($N = 5$)	Toledo	18			18		18
with 100 PFUs	Towne	26			512		512
($N = 4$)	Toledo	22			512		512
III. Natural seropositives challenged							
with 10 PFUs	Towne	72			72		72
($N = 2$)	Toledo	32			32		32
with 100 PFUs	Towne	51			64		64
($N = 3$)	Toledo	51			80		80

[a] Neutralization titers as measured in the presence of C′ are expressed as geometric means. Within each group a maximum fourfold difference was observed between the highest and lowest neutralization titer

All of the sera obtained from each of the individuals in the course of the experiment were also tested in virus neutralization assays in the absence of C'. The neutralization titers were significantly lower in the absence of C' than when tested in its presence, and strain-specific differences were clearly seen (data not shown). Our results confirm the earlier results showing strain-specific differences in virus neutralization activity of naturally HCMV-positive human sera (ANDERSEN 1970) and of animal sera after immunization with different HCMV strains (ANDERSEN 1971; GÖNCZÖL and ANDERSEN 1974). The differences in neutralization titers were not reflected in differential detection of any proteins of the Towne and Toledo strains in the immunoblot or immunoprecipitation assays (see results presented below), and possibly are due to differences in neutralizing epitopes.

2.4 Recognition of Viral Proteins by Western Blot or Immunoprecipitation Assays

The studies identifying viral protein(s) of importance in protective immunity showed that the gA/gB glycoprotein complex was recognized in the virus envelope by each of the sera with neutralizing activity.

The details of these studies are the following: The glycoprotein complexes of the virus envelope considered in this study were: (a) the 58- to 130-kDa glycoprotein complex, variously called gA (PEREIRA et al. 1982, 1984; GÖNCZÖL et al. 1986b), gp 55–116 (BRITT 1984; BRITT and AUGER 1986; BRITT et al. 1988), p130/55 (RASMUSSEN et al. 1985a, b, 1988), gB (CRANAGE et al. 1986; SPAETE et al. 1988), gcI (GRETCH et al. 1988a), and referred to as gA/gB in this publication; (b) the 86-kDa glycoprotein complex (RASMUSSEN et al. 1984, 1985b, 1988), also called gH (CRANAGE et al. 1988); and (c) the 47- to 52-kDa glycoprotein complex (KARI et al. 1986; FURLINI et al. 1987), also called gcII (GRETCH et al. 1988c).

Western blot assays were carried out using Towne strain or Toledo strain virions, purified from the culture medium of infected human fibroblast cells by sucrose gradient centrifugation (FURUKAWA et al. 1984; GÖNCZÖL et al. 1986b), as antigens. The sera of Towne vaccinees or Toledo-strain-injected individuals identified similar Western blot patterns with both virus strains. Similarly, immunoprecipitation assays using human fibroblast cells infected with the Towne and Toledo strains (MOI = 0.3 − 0.5 for both strains) labeled with $10\,\mu$Ci [^{35}S]methionine, prepared and used as 1×10^6 cpm/sample, showed no difference in the electrophoretic patterns of proteins of the two strains when immunoprecipitated by the antibodies of the Towne strain or Toledo-strain-injected individuals. Therefore, only the Western blots and immunoprecipitation patterns of the Towne strain antigens are presented.

Sera, drawn 4–8 weeks after immunization, from Towne vaccinees with low levels of neutralizing antibody (Table 4) reacted poorly when purified virions were used as antigen in Western blot assay. However, using a virus envelope preparation as antigen and the same sera in Western blot assay, a single band at the 58K position was seen (Fig. 1a). Immunoprecipitating antibodies to infected cell-specific antigens also developed in the Towne vaccinees. As shown in Fig. 2a, sera obtained at 4–16

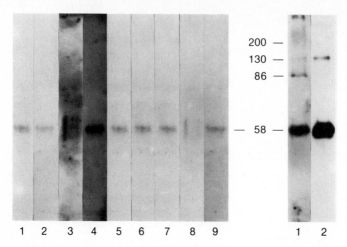

Fig. 1a, b. Autoradiograph of an immunoblot assay for detection of individual proteins in an envelope preparation by antibodies of seronegative volunteers (9 individuals tested of the 12) injected with Towne strain. Envelope antigen (10 μg protein/lane) was prepared, electrophoresed, and transferred to nitrocellulose. The strips were then incubated with serum samples (diluted 1:100) taken 4–8 weeks after injection. **a**, *lanes 1–9*, volunteers 1–9; **b**, *lane 1*, serum sample from one of the volunteers taken at 8 weeks after challenge with 100 PFUs Toledo strain; *lane 2*, anti-58 K–135 K glycoprotein complex guinea pig serum (GÖNCZÖL et al. 1986b). *Numbers* between **a** and **b** are kilodaltons

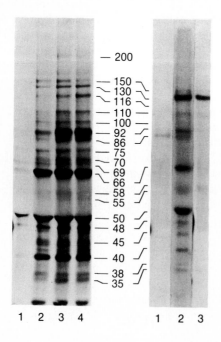

Fig. 2a, b. Immunoprecipitation assay for detection of individual proteins in infected cell lysates by antibodies of a seronegative volunteer injected with Towne strain. [^{35}S]methionine-labeled cell lysates were prepared and immunoprecipitated, and the precipitates were electrophoresed in 7.5% SDS-polyacrylamide gels, which were then fluorographed, dried, and exposed to X-Omat film (Eastman Kodak, Rochester, NY). **a**, *lane 1*, 0 week; *lane 2*, 4 weeks; *lane 3*, 8 weeks; *lane 4*, 16 weeks. **b** *lane 1*, 1G6 monoclonal antibody to the 86 **K** protein (RASMUSSEN et al. 1984); *lane 2*, 16 weeks serum of the Towne vaccinee shown in **a**; *lane 3*, 15D8 monoclonal antibody (RASMUSSEN et al. 1985a) to the 130- to 58-kDa protein complex. Both the 1G6 and the 15D8 monoclonal antibodies were kindly provided by Dr. L. Rasmussen, Stanford University School of Medicine, Stanford, CA

weeks after immunization revealed 35-, 38-, 40-, 42-, 45-, 48-, and 50-kDa species, two weak diffuse bands at the 55- to 58-kDa position, one strong band at the 66-kDa position, a triplet at 69–75 kDa, and bands at 86, 92,100, 110, 116, 130, 150, and 200 kDa. Figure 2b shows that the 86- and 130/55- to 58-kDa bands, immunoprecipitated by the 16-week serum of a Towne vaccinee, comigrated with proteins of similar molecular weight recognized by monoclonal antibodies 1G6 directed to the 86-kDa glycoprotein (lane 1) and 15D8 directed to the 130-kDa/55-kDa (gA/gB) glycoprotein complex (lane 3) in the envelope. The monoclonal antibodies 1G6 and 15D8 were kindly provided by Dr. L. Rasmussen, Stanford University, School of Medicine, Stanford, CA.

Figure 3 shows a typical Western blot pattern of seronegative individuals injected with 10 PFUs Toledo strain. The serum first reacted with a 66-kDa protein in a virion preparation at 6 weeks after challenge (lane 3). Sera obtained at 7 and 8 weeks after the Toledo injection detected (in order of intensity and time of appearance) the 66-, 150-, and 200-kDa proteins, a smear above the 150-kDa and 200-kDa proteins and 50-, 58-, 38-, 40-, 86-, and 28-kDa proteins in the virion preparation (lanes 4 and 5). Sera analyzed at 12 and 16 weeks after Toledo injection detected the same proteins (lanes 6 and 7) but on the blots of 7- and 8-week sera the 66-, 150-, and 200-kDa proteins appeared more intense than on the blots of the 12- and 16-week sera, whereas for the 28-, 40-, 58-, and 86-kDa proteins the reverse was true. Note that the neutralizing activity of the 16-week sera was significantly higher than that of the 7- or 8-week sera (Table 5, group I). In Western blot assays the sera

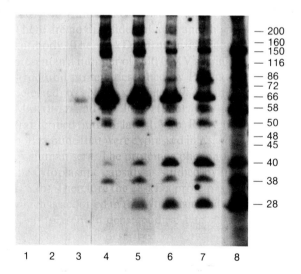

Fig. 3. Autoradiogram of an immunoblot assay for detection of individual proteins in purified virions by antibodies of a seronegative volunteer injected with 10 PFUs Toledo strain. Purified virions (10 µg protein/lane) were lysed, electrophoresed, and transferred to a nitrocellulose sheet. The strips were then incubated with serum samples (dilution 1:100) taken at different times (weeks) after injection. *Lanes: 1,* 0 week; *2,* 4 weeks; *3,* 6 weeks; *4,* 7 weeks; *5,* 8 weeks; *6,* 12 weeks; *7,* 16 weeks; *8,* mixture of four high-titer sera from naturally seropositive individuals. *Numbers* on the right are kilodaltons

of the Toledo-strain-injected individuals, obtained at 6 weeks after injection, which detected only the 66-kDa protein in the antigen prepared from virions (lane 3) recognized no proteins in the antigen prepared from virus envelope (data not shown). These sera also had no neutralizing activity (Table 5, group I).

The higher neutralizing titer of the sera of Towne vaccinees after challenge with 100 PFUs Toledo strain was correlated with a strong detection of the 58-kDa glycoprotein and the recognition of the 86-, 130-, and > 200-kDa glycoproteins in the envelope preparation (Fig. 1b, lane 1). The positive control guinea pig serum raised by immunization with an immunoaffinity-purified gA/gB glycoprotein complex (GÖNCZÖL et al. 1986b), detected a broad band at the 58-kDa molecular weight position and a weaker band at the 130-kDa position (Fig. 1B, lane 2), suggesting that the 58-kDa protein detected by human sera with low neutralizing activity (Table 4, Fig. 1a) is indeed the same component of the gA/gB major glycoprotein complex of the envelope.

The immunoblot pattern of seropositive, Toledo-strain-challenged individuals using either virion or envelope preparations was the same before and after the challenge except for some changes in the intensity of the reactivity of certain viral proteins in two of the five individuals tested. Thus, the 66-kDa protein blot was more intense after reaction with the 12- and 16-week sera than that obtained with earlier serum from one of the individuals (data not shown). The neutralizing activity of the sera from this individual, like that of the sera from four other individuals in that group, did not change after the injection. As mentioned, one of the naturally seropositive Toledo-injected individuals, who received 100 PFUs, responded with a slight increase in neutralizing titer, serum from the same individual recognized a 86-kDa and a 58-kDa viral protein with slightly greater intensity at 12 and 16 weeks after the injection in an immunoblot assay (data not shown).

2.5 Implications for Functional Activity of Viral Proteins

Our results show that antibodies recognizing the gA/gB glycoprotein complex in Westen blot or immunoprecipitation assays were detected with each of the neutralizing sera, but with none of the sera without neutralizing activity. These results are in correlation with previous observations. For example, virus-neutralizing and nonneutralizing murine and human monoclonal antibodies directed to this complex have been developed in several laboratories (CRANAGE et al. 1986; FURLINI et al. 1987; KARL et al. 1986; MASUHO et al. 1987; NOWAK et al. 1984; PEREIRA et al. 1982; RASMUSSEN et al. 1985a), indicating the high immunogenicity of this complex and its possible involvement in the protective immunity. The gA/gB complex in virion preparations or infected cell lysate is readily detectable by Western blot or immunoprecipitation assays using HCMV-positive human sera (GÖNCZÖL et al. 1986b; RASMUSSEN et al. 1985a). The immunoaffinity-purified gA/gB complex induces neutralizing antibodies (GÖNCZÖL et al. 1986b; RASMUSSEN et al. 1985b) and a cell-mediated immune response in experimental animals, as detected by a lymphocytic proliferation assay in vitro (GÖNCZÖL et al. 1986b). Table 6 shows that the titer of neutralizing antibodies and the HCMV-specific

Table 6. Immune response of guinea pigs to HCMV gA/gB preparation

No. of guinea pigs	Immunizing antigen	Neutralization titer[a]	Lymphocyte stimulation index[b]
20	gA/gB	512	10.2
20	viral envelope	362	10.5

[a] Neutralization titers as measured in the presence of C' are expressed as geometric means. Within each group a maximum fourfold difference was observed between the highest and lowest neutralization titer
[b] Stimulation index is defined as counts per minute (cpm) in HCMV antigen-stimulated cultures/cpm in control antigen-stimulated culture

lymphocyte proliferation of the gA/gB-immunized guinea pigs were comparable with those of animals immunized with the whole envelope.

The structure of the gA/gB protein has been the subject of several studies. Briefly, the unglycosylated polypeptide precursor in the infected cells is a 92- to 105-kDa protein (BRITT et al. 1988; CRANAGE et al. 1986; PEREIRA et al. 1984; RASMUSSEN et al. 1985a) encoded by a gene located in the HindIII F fragment of the Ad-169 strain (map units 0.344–0.380) (MACH et al. 1986; CRANAGE et al. 1986). The unglycosylated polypeptide precursor is glycosylated to form a 138-kDa glycoprotein which has been characterized by endoglycosidase treatment as an N-linked high mannose carbohydrate which is present in disulfide-linked complexes in the infected cells (GRETCH et al. 1988a; RASMUSSEN et al. 1988). After cleavage of the glycoprotein in the cells, the mature virions contain the cleavage products of the complex, a 55-kDa and a 93- to 130-kDa glycoprotein which form disulfide-linked complexes in the virion (BRITT and AUGER 1986; GÖNCZÖL et al. 1986b; RASMUSSEN et al. 1985a, 1988). The 93- to 130-kDa glycoproteins can be separated into two electrophoretic forms, 93 and 130 kDa (FARRAR and GREENAWAY 1986; GRETCH et al. 1988a). The peptide profiles of a 46-kDa polypeptide (a deglycosylated form of the 55-kDa polypeptide) and a 46- to 56-kDa and a 60- to 70-kDa polypeptide (the deglycosylated forms of the 93-kDa and 130-kDa glycoproteins, respectively) show that the peptide profile of the 93- and 130-kDa glycoproteins are very similar but the peptide profile of the 55-kDa glycoprotein shows only partial similarity with the peptide profiles of the 93-kDa and 130-kDa glycoproteins in electrophoretic behavior (GRETCH et al. 1988a). The 55-kDa and 93- to 130-kDa glycoproteins are, however, antigenically related; antisera raised to the 55-kDa component recognized the 93- to 130-kDa glycoprotein in the virion in Western blot or immunoprecipitation assays (MACH et al. 1986; our unpublished observation).

The coding gene of the gA/gB glycoprotein of the Ad-169 strain (BORYSIEWICZ et al. 1988; BRITT et al. 1988; CRANAGE et al. 1986) as well as the gA/gB gene of the Towne strain (our unpublished data) have been cloned into vaccinia expression vector. The gA/gB vaccinia recombinants expressed the precursor and mature forms of the gA/gB complex in tissue culture cells (BRITT et al. 1988; BORYSIEWICZ et al. 1988; CRANAGE et al. 1986; our unpublished data) as detected by Western blot, immunoprecipitation, and immunofluorescence assays. Experimental animals immunized with the gA/gB vaccinia recombinants developed neutralizing antibodies (BRITT et al. 1988; CRANAGE et al. 1986; our unpublished data).

One of the purposes of the neutralization assays carried out in the absence of C′ was to make some correlation between the neutralizing activity of the sera without C′ and the recognition of an 86-kDa protein in immunoprecipitation or Western blot assays. The 86-kDa protein bears an antigenic determinant which is recognized by a monoclonal antibody which neutralizes in the absence of C′ (CRANAGE et al. 1988; RASMUSSEN et al. 1984) and both the immunoaffinity-purified and the endoglycosidase-treated purified 86-kDa protein induce C′-independent neutralizing antibodies in animals (RASMUSSEN et al. 1985b, 1988). We were unable to make such a correlation; for example, sera taken at 4 weeks after Towne injection did not neutralize the Towne and Toledo strains in the absence of C′ (data not shown), but did detect a 86-kDa protein in the infected cell lysate by immunoprecipitation assays (Fig. 2A, lane 2). It is possible that the 86-kDa protein also bears a C′-dependent neutralization epitope. Examples of the presence of both C′-dependent (BRITT et al. 1988; RASMUSSEN et al. 1985a) and C′-independent (BRITT et al. 1988; MASUHO et al. 1987) neutralization epitopes are known for the gA/gB glycoprotein complex. The 86-kDa protein is easily labeled by [^{35}S]methionine and easily detected in immunoprecipitation assays. It seems that the relative abundance of this protein in the mature virion or envelope preparation is less than in the infected cell lysate, since it is detectable only by sera with high neutralization titer in immunoblot assays using virion or envelope preparations as antigen.

Sera of Towne vaccinees, taken either before or after Toledo strain challenge, did not recognize or recognized poorly (Fig. 1b, lane 1) the 47- to 52-kDa glycoprotein complex, called gCII (FURLINI et al. 1987; GRETCH et al. 1988b, c; KARI et al. 1986; LIU et al. 1988). This observation is in accordance with previous results, namely that human convalescent sera do not recognize this complex readily (GRETCH et al. 1988b). The reasons for limited recognition are not yet clear. The immunogenicity of the isolated 47- to 52-kDa glycoprotein complex has not been tested, although it seems to be highly immunogenic, at least in mice. Monoclonal antibodies to this complex with high neutralizing titer have been developed in several laboratories (FURLINI et al. 1987; KARI et al. 1986; PEREIRA et al. 1982).

Concerning the immune response to proteins other than the envelope glycoproteins of the virion, our results, in accordance with previous observations (LANDINI and MICHELSON 1988), show the following:

A 66-kDa protein was detected first in the virion preparation after injection of seronegative individuals with the Toledo strain (Fig. 3, lane 3), when the sera had no neutralizing activity (Table 5, group I). The Towne vaccinees (Table 5, group II) challenged with 100 PFUs Toledo strain develop an increased neutralization titer but the intensity of the 66-kDa band in Western blot assays did not increase after the challenge (data not shown). Serum from one naturally seropositive individual taken after the Toledo challenge gave a stronger signal at the 66-kDa position than before challenge; however, the neutralization titer did not increase (data not shown). Thus the 66-kDa protein, which is probably the major tegument phosphoprotein (GIBSON 1983; GIBSON and IRMIERE 1984), is a strong immunogenic antigen in the course of infection, but is not involved in virus neutralization.

During the immune response to the Towne and Toledo strains, antibodies also appeared that were directed to a 150-kDa protein (probably the 150-kDa major capsid protein) (GIBSON 1983; GIBSON and IRMIERE 1984). The role of this 150-kDa protein and of the other proteins (< 50, 69–75, 200, > 200 kDa) recognized by antibodies developed after injection with the Towne or Toledo strains is not clear.

3 Humoral and Cellular Immune Responses Induced in Human Volunteers by Immunoaffinity-Purified gA/gB Protein

Our other effort in the direction of active immunizations focused on viral subunits. A subunit HCMV vaccine would provide the immunogen protein(s) to the immune system without introducing the virus genome into the cells of the host. Although the attenuation of the Towne virus seems to preclude establishing virus. latency in immunized individuals (PLOTKIN and HUANG 1985), concerns still remain about using a complete live HCMV for vaccination.

Direct evidence for the importance of gA/gB glycoprotein complex in induction of immunity has been shown by immunization of seronegative and seropositive volunteers with the isolated gA/gB preparation (GÖNCZÖL et al. 1989b).

3.1 Preparation and Composition of the gAgB Glycoprotein Complex

The gA/gB protein was prepared as described (GÖNCZÖL et al. 1986b, 1989b). Briefly, all steps of the preparation were carried out under aseptic conditions. Monoclonal antibody CH-380 (PEREIRA et al. 1982) was purified and coupled to CNB-activated Sepharose 4B. Extracellular HCMV was purified by sucrose gradient centrifugation (FURUKAWA et al. 1984) and after 2 h treatment with the dialyzable, nonionic detergent, n-octyl-glycoside (Sigma), the virus envelope was separated from the nucleocapsid by centrifugation as described (FURUKAWA et al. 1984).

Virus envelope proteins were incubated with CNBr-activated Sepharose 4B beads (precolumn), then with immune adsorbent beads and loaded onto a column. The column was washed with PBS containing n-octyl-glycoside and a proteinase inhibitor, phenylmethylsulfonylfluoride (PMSF, Sigma). Bound protein was eluted with 3.0 M KSCN (Sigma) in PBS (pH 7.0) containing n-octyl-glycoside. Samples were dialyzed and concentrated. Sterility tests established the absence of any bacterial or yeast contamination. The absence of contamination with mouse, bovine, or human proteins was also determined.

The isolated gA/gB preparation was electrophoretically separated on polyacrylamide gel in reducing conditions and stained with silver. The gA/gB preparation contained a mixture of 52-, 58-, 92-, and 130-kDa proteins. A 66-kDa protein, a possible additional component of the complex (BRITT and AUGER 1986; CRANAGE et al. 1986; GÖNCZÖL et al. 1986b; GRETCH et al. 1988a; RASMUSSEN et al. 1985b, 1988), was also present in the mixture. The presence of multiple bands is consistent with the heterogeneity of the gA/gB complex. As described earlier in this chapter and in Chaps. 6 and 8, the 130-, 93-, 58-, and 52-kDa proteins are cleavage products of a higher molecular weight glycosylated precursor, present in disulfide-linked complexes in the infected cells and in the virus envelope (BRITT 1984; BRITT and AUGER 1986; BRITT et al. 1988; CRANAGE et al. 1986; FARRAR and GREENAWAY 1986; FARRAR and ORAM 1984; GÖNCZÖL et al. 1986b; GRETCH et al. 1988a; PEREIRA et al. 1982, 1984; RASMUSSEN et al. 1985a, 1988). In Western blot assays a natural HCMV-positive human serum strongly recognized the 52-kDa and 58-kDa proteins, some additional bands at the position of 45- to 52-kDa, and recognized weakly the 93-kDa and 130-kDa proteins. The bands at the 45- to 52-kDa positions could be the differentially glycosylated polypeptides of the 58-kDa and 93- to 130-kDa proteins (GRETCH et al. 1988; RASMUSSEN et al. 1988).

3.2 Immune Response to HCMV in Human Volunteers Immunized with the gA/gB Preparation

After consent forms were signed, two seropositive and three seronegative individuals were immunized with the gA/gB preparation mixed in equal volume with $Al(OH)_3$. The immune response of the volunteers was evaluated by a lymphocyte proliferation assay in vitro and by neutralization, Western blot, immunoprecipitation, ELISA, and immunofluorescence assays. Sera from the gA/gB-immunized individuals showed no difference in neutralization titers, Western blot, and immunoprecipitation assays when Ad-169, Towne, or Toledo strains of HCMV were used as antigens, so only results with the Towne strain antigen are presented.

3.2.1 Immune Response of Seropositive Individuals

The immune responses of seropositive individuals after a single injection with the gA/gB preparation are summarized in Table 7. The lymphocyte stimulation index was increased in the 1st and 2nd week after injection, as shown most clearly by volunteer H. The virus neutralization activity was also increased soon after injection, reaching a four- to eightfold increase in titer by the 4th week after injection. One year after the injection the virus neutralization titer was still twofold higher than before the injection. A 58-kDa protein of the purified virion preparation was detected by higher dilutions of the postimmunization sera than by the sera obtained before the immunization (data not shown).

3.2.2 Immune Response of Seronegative Individuals

The immune response of seronegative individuals injected repeatedly with the gA/gB preparation is shown in Table 8 and Fig. 4. HCMV-specific lymphocyte proliferation was increased after the second or third injection of the gA/gB preparation and remained positive during the 1-year observation period, with a slight increase 5 months after the fourth injection. Neutralization antibodies were detectable in low titers and only transiently after the third injection, but a significant and rapid increase was observed after the fourth injection. The neutralization titer,

Table 7. Immune response to HCMV in seropositive volunteers immunized with purified gA/gB protein

Time (weeks)	Neutralization titer[a] of volunteers		Lymphocyte stimulation index[b] of volunteers	
	H	G	H	G
→ 0	32	64	9.6	ND
1	ND	ND	20.2	11.4
2	128	128	19.2	9.1
4	256	256	4.7	8.2
8	128	256	5.3	ND
12	128	256	6.0	5.0
28	ND	256	ND	ND
36	ND	128	ND	ND
44	128	128	8.6	ND
52	64	128	6.9	3.9

Arrow indicates the time of injection with gA/gB protein
[a] Neutralization titers, as measured in the presence of C', are expressed as geometric means. Within each group, a maximum fourfold difference was observed between the highest and lowest neutralization titer
[b] Stimulation index is defined as counts per minute (cpm) in HCMV antigen-stimulated cultures/cpm in control antigen-stimulated culture

Table 8. Immune response to HCMV in seronegative volunteers immunized with purified gA/gB protein

Time (weeks)	Neutralization titer[a] of volunteers			Lymphocyte stimulation index[b] of volunteers		
	T	W	S[c]	T	W	S[c]
→ 0	<4	<4	<4	0.9	1.2	0.8
→ 2	<4	<4	<4	3.0	1.4	1.6
3	<4	<4	<4	1.8	1.2	2.2
→ 4	16	<4	<4	1.8	8.6	1.4
8	64	16	16	6.7	3.6	5.1
16	4	4	<4	3.3	1.2	1.3
24	4	<4	<4	3.4	3.9	ND
→32	<4	<4	ND	3.9	4.3	ND
33	64	32	ND	1.9	3.7	ND
34	256	64	ND	4.7	3.5	ND
35	256	128	ND	5.3	ND	ND
40	256	128	ND	4.1	3.7	ND
44	64	64	<4	9.6	8.3	6.4
52	64	64	ND	9.6	5.4	ND

Arrows indicate the time of injection with gA/gB protein
[a] Neutralization titers, as measured in the presence of C', are expressed as geometric means. Within each group, a maximum fourfold difference was observed between the highest and lowest neutralization titer
[b] Stimulation index is defined as counts per minute (cpm) in HCMV antigen-stimulated cultures/cpm in control antigen-stimulated culture
[c] Volunteer S did not receive a fourth injection

even at 1 year after the first injection of the two individuals who received a fourth injection, was comparable with those of natural seropositives (see Table 7). The 52-kDa and 58-kDa proteins were detected in an envelope preparation by the sera obtained at 4 or 16 weeks (after the second or third injection) of the gA/gB-immunized seronegative individuals when tested in a Western blot assay (Fig. 5,

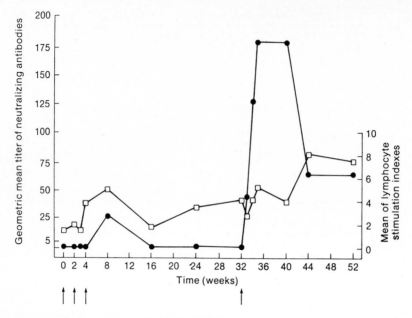

Fig. 4. Neutralizing antibody and lymphocyte proliferation responses to the Towne strain of HCMV in initially seronegative gA/gB vaccinees. Geometric mean (*GM*) titer of neutralizing antibodies and mean of stimulation indexes (*SI*) were calculated from data in Table 8. ●————●, GM titers of neutralizing titers; □————□, mean of LSI-S

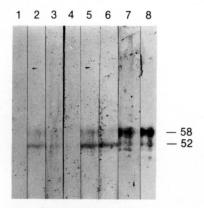

Fig. 5. Antibody response to HCMV envelope proteins of initially seronegative individuals after injection with three doses of gA/gB preparation. Viral envelope (Towne strain) was prepared, electrophoretically separated, and transferred to nitrocellulose sheets. Strips were then incubated with serum samples (dilution 1:50) of gA/gB vaccinee T (*lanes 1–3*), vaccinee W (*lanes 4–6*). *Lanes 1, 4*, serum samples obtained at week 0, before the first injection; *lanes 2, 5*, serum samples taken at 4 weeks; *lanes 3, 6*, serum samples taken at 16 weeks after the first injection and as controls; *lanes 7 and 8* were incubated with serum samples (dilution 1:50) from naturally seropositive volunteers G and H, respectively, taken 2 weeks after the gA/gB injection

lanes 2, 3, 5, 6). The intensity of the 52-kDa and 58-kDa bands was stronger and additional weak bands of the position of 93 kDa and 130 kDa were seen when sera obtained after fourth inoculaton in the 34th week of the study were used in the Western blot assay (data not shown).

In the initially seronegative individuals the observed priming effect on antibody production after the fourth injection indicated the generation and activation of immune memory cells. This could be useful in immunization of organ transplant recipients or other high-risk groups with the gA/gB preparation, since the subsequent natural HCMV infection might induce a very rapid increase in the neutralization titer in the individuals and provide some protection. Such a priming effect was observed in patients receiving HSV-type 2 glycoprotein subunit vaccine (ASHLEY et al. 1985).

Neutralization antibodies that developed after repeated injection with the gA/gB preparation similarly neutralized the Ad-169, Towne, and Toledo strains of HCMV. This is in agreement with previous studies when monoclonal antibodies directed to the gA/gB complex did not show any strain specificity to the Ad-169, Towne, Toledo strains in neutralization assays (KARI et al. 1986; RASMUSSEN et al. 1985a). However, as shown in Tables 4 and 5, strain-specific differences were observed in neutralization assays using sera of seronegative individuals injected with the Toledo strain and Towne strain. It seems that the differences in the neutralization activity of sera when whole, replicating viruses are used for immunization are dependent not upon the neutralizing epitopes of the gA/gB complex, but upon neutralizing epitopes carried by other proteins.

In this study we did not elaborate the optimal conditions (dose, schedule, etc.) for immunization with the gA/gB preparation. Large-scale immunization with this gA/gB preparation of individuals in high-risk groups is not feasible because of the time-consuming and expensive preparation of the protein. Because the gene of the gA/gB protein has been identified in the Ad-169 strain (CRANAGE et al. 1986; MACH et al. 1986) and in the Towne strain (SPAETE et al. 1988; our unpublished data), the availability of a subunit HCMV vaccine depends on finding a suitable expression vector, as in the case of subunit vaccines of several other viruses.

4 Conclusions and Future Prospects

A live attenuated vaccine virus protected vaccinees against infection and disease caused by a CMV challenge when the vaccinee's cellular immune responses were intact and the challenge dose was not too high. Immunosuppressed subjects given the vaccine were protected against disease but not infection when transplanted with a CMV-bearing kidney. In these successes, the live vaccine simulated natural immunity.

Subunit immunogens based on the viral envelope, or a single protein contained within the envelope (the gA/gB glycoprotein), can also induce neutralizing antibodies and CMV-specific cellular sensitization in humans. We have described indirect evidence for the importance of gA/gB in protective immunity, but direct challenge studies have not yet been performed.

Several possibilities must be considered before designing an HCMV-subunit vaccine. Other envelope glycoproteins, such as the 86-kDa and 47- to 52-kDa complexes, could also be important in the development of the protective immunity. Furthermore, recent results indicate that the major immediate early protein of HCMV might play a major role in cell-mediated immunity: immunoaffinity-purified immediate early protein elicited proliferative T-cell responses in seropositive individuals (RODGERS et al. 1987) and high frequency of immediate-early protein-specific cytotoxic lymphocytes was observed in asymptomatic, persistently infected individuals (BORYSIEWICZ et al. 1988).

The protection effect by challenge studies of the products of HCMV glyco-protein or immediate early genes is difficult to test.

In the murine CMV system it was shown that the major immediate-early protein of MCMV, expressed by a recombinant vaccinia virus, protected mice against mortality by a lethal MCMV infection and that the CD8$^+$ lymphocytes were involved in the protective effect (JONJIC et al. 1988). In natural MCMV infection, however, in addition to the CD8$^+$ lymphocytes, some other components, probably neutralizing antibodies, contribute to the protective effect, since mice first immunized with the vaccinia recombinant expressing the immediate early protein and then depleted of the CD8$^+$ lymphocytes lost protection against challenge virus. In contrast, mice immunized with MCMV and depleted of CD8$^+$ lymphocytes were still protected (JONJIC et al. 1988). If the mouse infection and immune system is comparable with the human CMV infection and human immune system, it is likely that a combination of the products of one or more glycoprotein gene(s) and the immediate early gene of HCMV is necessary for the protection of humans. However, before applying the results of the murine CMV system to humans, careful comparative studies on the biological properties of the murine and human CMV as well as on the relative importance of the components of mouse and human immune system must be carried out.

Active research on cytomegaloviruses and on the relevant subjects, for example on the identification of a viral expression vector acceptable for human use, certainly will provide the results necessary for the development of an HCMV subunit vaccine.

Acknowledgments. This work was supported by grant HD-18957 from the National Institute for Child Health and Development and by the Institut Merieux, France.

References

Andersen HK (1970) Complement-fixing and virus-neutralizing antibodies in cytomegalovirus infection as measured against homologous and heterologous antigen. Acta Pathol Microbiol Immunol Scand 78: 504–508

Andersen HK (1971) Serologic differentiation of human cytomegalovirus strains using rabbit hyperimmune sera. Arch Gesamte Virusforsch 33: 187–191

Ashley R, Mertz G, Clark H, Schick M, Salter D, Corey L (1985) Humoral immune response to herpes simplex virus type 2 glycoprotein in patients receiving a glycoprotein in subunit vaccine. J Virol 56: 475–481

Borysiewicz LK, Hickling JK, Graham S, Sinclair J, Cranage MP, Smith GL, Sissons JGP (1988) Human cytomegalovirus-specific cytotoxic T cells. Relative frequency of stage-specifc CTL recognizing the 72 kD immediate early protein and glycoprotein B-expressed by recombinant vaccinia viruses. J Exp Med 168: 919–931

Britt WJ (1984) Neutralizing antibodies detect a disulfide-linked glycoprotein complex within the envelope of human cytomegalovirus. Virology 135: 369–378

Britt WJ, Auger D (1986) Synthesis and processing of the envelope gp 55–116 complex of human cytomegalovirus. J Virol 58: 185–191

Britt WJ, Vugler L, Stephens EB (1988) Induction of complement dependent and independent neutralizing antibodies by recombinant-derived human cytomegalovirus gp 55–116 (gB). J Virol 62: 3309–3318

Cranage MP, Kouzarides T, Bankier A, Satchwell S, Weston K, Tomlinson P, Barrell B, et al. (1986) Identification of the human cytomegalovirus glycoprotein B gene and induction of neutralizing antibodies via its expression in recombinant vaccinia virus. EMBO J 5: 3057–3063

Cranage MP, Smith GL, Bell SE, Hart H, Brown C, Bankier AT, Tomlinson P, et al. (1988) Identification and expression of a human cytomegalovirus glycoprotein with homology to the Epstein-Barr virus BXLF2 product, Varicella-Zoster virus gpIII, and herpes simplex virus Type-1 glycoprotein H. J Virol 62: 1416–1422

Elek SD, Stern H (1974) Development of a vaccine against mental retardation caused by cytomegalovirus infection in utero. Lancet 1: 1–5

Farrar GH, Greenaway PJ (1986) Characterization of glycoprotein complexes present in human cytomegalovirus envelopes. J Gen Virol 67: 1469–1473

Farrar GH, Oram JD (1984) Characterization of the human cytomegalovirus envelope glycoprotein. J Gen Virol 65: 1991–2001

Fleisher GR, Starr SE, Friedman HM, Plotkin SA (1982) Vaccination of pediatric nurses with live attenuated cytomegalovirus. Am J Dis Child 136: 294–296

Furlini G, Gönczöl E, Szokan G, Ianacone J, Plotkin SA (1987) Monoclonal antibodies directed to two groups of viral proteins neutralize human cytomegalovirus in vitro. Hybridoma 6: 321–326

Furukawa T, Gönczöl E, Starr S, Tolpin MD, Arbeter A, Plotkin SA (1984) HCMV envelope antigens induce both humoral and cellular immunity in guinea pigs. Proc Soc Exp Biol Med 175: 243–250

Gibson W (1983) Protein counterparts of human and simian cytomegaloviruses. Virology 128: 391–406

Gibson W, Irmiere A (1984) Selection of particles and proteins for use as human cytomegalovirus subunit vaccines. Birth Defects 20: 305–324

Glenn J (1981) Cytomegalovirus infections following renal transplantation. Rev Infect Dis 3: 1151–1178

Gönczöl E, Andersen HK (1974) Studies on human cytomegalovirus strain variations by membrane-fluorescence. Arch Gesamte Virusforsch 44: 147–149

Gönczöl E, Furlini G, Ianacone J, Plotkin SA (1986a) A rapid microneutralization assay for cytomegalovirus. J Virol Methods 14: 37–41

Gönczöl E, Hudecz F, Ianacone J, Dietzschold B, Starr S, Plotkin SA (1986b) Immune responses to isolated human cytomegalovirus envelope proteins. J Virol 58: 661–664

Gönczöl E, Ianacone J, Furlini G, Ho W, Plotkin SA (1989a) Humoral immune response to cytomegalovirus Towne vaccine strain and to Toledo low passage strain. J Infect Dis (in press)

Gönczöl E, Ianacone J, Ho W, Starr S, Meignier B, Plotkin SA (1989b) Subunit human cytomegalovirus (HCMV) vaccine induces humoral and cellular immune-responses in human volunteers. Vaccine (in press)

Gretch DR, Gehrz RC, Stinski MF (1988a) Characterization of a human cytomegalovirus glycoprotein complex (gcI). J Gen Virol 69: 1205–1215

Gretch DR, Kari B, Rasmussen L, Gehrz R, Stinski MF (1988b) Identification and characterization of three distinct families of glycoprotein complexes in the envelopes of human cytomegalovirus. J Virol 62: 875–881

Gretch DR, Kari B, Gehrz RC, Stinski MF (1988c) A multigene family encodes the human cytomegalovirus glycoprotein complex gcII (gp 47–52 complex). J Virol 62: 1956–1962

Jonjic S, del Val M, Keil GM, Reddehase MJ, Koszinowski UH (1988) A nonstructural viral protein expressed by a recombinant vaccinia virus protects against lethal cytomegalovirus infection. J Virol 62: 1653–1658

Kari B, Lussenhop N, Goertz R, Wabuke-Burot M, Radeke M, Gehrz R (1986) Characterization of monoclonal antibodies reactive to several biochemically distinct human cytomegalovirus glycoprotein complexes. J Virol 60: 345–352

Landini MP, Michelson S (1988) Commented catalogue of human cytomegalovirus proteins. Prog Med Virol 35: 152–185

Liu Y-NC, Kari B, Gehrz RC (1988) Human immune responses to major human cytomegalovirus glycoprotein complexes. J Virol 62: 1066–1070

Mach M, Utz U, Fleckenstein B (1986) Mapping of the major glycoprotein gene of human cytomegalovirus. J Gen Virol 67: 1461–1467

Masuho Y, Matsumoto Y, Sugano T, Fujinaga S, Minamishima Y (1987) Human monoclonal antibodies neutralizing human cytomegalovirus. J Gen Virol 68: 1457–1461

Meyers JD, Leszczynski J, Zaia JA, Fluornoy N, Newton B, Snydman DR, Wright GG, et al. (1983) Prevention of cytomegalovirus infection by cytomegalovirus immune globulin after marrow transplantation. Ann Intern Med 98: 442–446

Nowak B, Sullivan C, Sarnow P, Thomas R, Bricout JC, Nicolas JC, Fleckenstein B, Levine AZ (1984) Characterization of monoclonal antibodies and polyclonal immune sera directed against human cytomegalovirus virion proteins. Virology 132: 325–338

Pass RF, Stagno S, Myers GJ, Alford CA (1980) Outcome of symptomatic congenital cytomegalovirus infection: Results of long-term longitudinal follow-up. Pediatrics 66: 758–762

Pereira L, Hoffman M, Gallo D, Cremer N (1982) Monoclonal antibodies to human cytomegalovirus: three surface membrane proteins with unique immunological and electrophoretic properties specify cross-reactive determinants. Infect Immun 36: 924–932

Pereira L, Hoffman M, Tatsuno M, Dondero D (1984) Polymorphism of human cytomegalovirus glycoproteins characterized by monoclonal antibodies. Virology 139: 73–86

Plotkin SA, Huang ES (1985) Cytomegalovirus vaccine virus (Towne strain) does not induce latency. J Infect Dis 152: 395–397

Plotkin SA, Furukawa T, Zygraich N, Huygelen C (1975) Candidate cytomegalovirus strain for human vaccination. Infect Immun 12: 521–527

Plotkin SA, Farquhar J, Hornberger E (1976) Clinical trials of immunization with the Towne 125 strain of human cytomegalovirus. J Infect Dis 134: 470–475

Plotkin SA, Friedman HM, Fleisher GR, Dafoe DC, Grossman RA, Smiley ML, Starr SE, et al. (1984) Towne vaccine induced prevention of cytomegalovirus disease after renal transplants. Lancet 1: 528–530

Plotkin SA, Weibel RE, Alpert G, Starr SE, Friedman HM, Preblub SR, Hoxie J (1985) Resistance of seropositive volunteers to subcutaneous challenge with low passage human cytomegalovirus. J Infect Dis 151: 737–739

Plotkin SA, Starr SE, Friedman HM, Gönczöl E (1989) Protective effects of Towne CMV vaccine against low passage CMV administered as a challenge. J Infect Dis (in press)

Rasmussen L, Nelson R, Kelsall D, Merigan T (1984) Murine monoclonal antibody to a single protein neutralizes the infectivity of human cytomegalovirus. Proc Natl Acad Sci USA 81: 876–880

Rasmussen L, Mullenax J, Nelson M, Merigan TC (1985a) Viral polypeptides detected by a complement-dependent neutralizing murine monoclonal antibody to human cytomegalovirus. J Virol 55: 274–280

Rasmussen L, Mullenax J, Nelson M, Merigan TC (1985b) Human cytomegalovirus polypeptides stimulate neutralizing antibody in vivo. Virology 145: 186–190

Rasmussen L, Nelson M, Neff M, Merigan TC Jr (1988) Characterization of two different human cytomegalovirus glycoproteins which are targets for virus neutralizing antibody. Virology 163: 308–318

Rodgers B, Borysiewicz L, Mundin J, Graham S, Sissons P (1987) Immunoaffinity purification of a 72 K early antigen of human cytomegalovirus: analysis of humoral and cell-mediated immunity to the purified polypeptide. J Gen Virol 68: 2371–2378

Spaete RS, Thayer RM, Probert WS, Masiarz FR, Chamberlain SH, Rasmussen L, Merigan TC, Pachl C (1988) Virology 167: 207–225

Stagno S, Pass RF, Dworsky ME, Alford CA (1983) Congenital and perinatal cytomegalovirus infections. Semin Perinatol 7: 31–42

Stagno S, Pass RF, Dworsky ME, Britt WJ, Alford CA (1984) Congenital and perinatal cytomegalovirus infections: clinical characteristics and pathogenic factors. Birth Defects 20: 65–85

Starr SE, Dalton B, Garrabrant T, Paucker K, Plotkin SA (1980) Lymphocyte blastogenesis and interferon production in adult leukocyte cultures stimulated with cytomegalovirus antigens. Infect Immun 30: 17–22

Starr SE, Glazer LP, Friedman HM, Farquhar JD, Plotkin SA (1981) Specific cellular and humoral immunity after immunization with live Towne strain cytomegalovirus vaccine. J Infect Dis 143: 585–589

Weller TH (1971) The cytomegalovirus: ubiquitous agents with protean clinical manifestations. N Engl J Med 285: 203–214

Winston DJ, Ho WG, Lin C-H, Budinger MD, Champlin RE, Gale RP (1984) Intravenous immunoglobulin for modification of cytomegalovirus infections associated with bone marrow transplantation: preliminary results of a controlled trial. Am J Med 76: 128–133

Subject Index

acute infection
– immunocompromised   50
– salivary gland   50
– tissue distribution   51
adoptive lymphocyte transfer
– prophylactic and therapeutic
    regimen   194–195
antibodies, to MCMV
– protective capacity   207
antigenic peptides, of MCMV IE protein pp89
– association with the MHC glycoprotein
    L^d 211
– inhibition of presentation   212–213
– recognition by CTL clone 1E1   211–212
– temporal regulation of expression   212–213
antigenic properties of viral proteins
– aplasia, of bone marrow   198–200
– cellular immune response   239–243
– cytolytic antibody   238
– cytotoxic T-cell   241–243
– humoral immune responses   234–239
– interferon   240–241
– lymphokines   240
– MHC class II
– non-specific immune response   243–244
– T-helper cell   240–241
– virus neutralizing antibody   237–238

bone marrow
– aplasia caused by MCMV   197–200
– stem cells, inhibition of generation   200

capsid proteins
– assembly protein gene   150
– DNA packaging   150
– major capsid protein   150
CD3, CD4   156
cis-acting sequences   34
consensus binding site   35
cytoimmunotherapy (see adoptive
    lymphocyte transfer)   194
cytolytic T lymphocytes (CTL)
– antigen-specificity, MCMV   202–204,
    206–212

– clonal expansion   203
– clone 1E1   206, 211–212
– frequency of precursors   203, 207
– interleukin-2-receptive precursors   203
– memory CTL in latency,
    MCMV   195, 196, 206

differential phosphorylation   32
DNA repair
– deoxyribonuclease gene   149
– diagnosis of HCMV   171
– DNase 1 hypersensitive sites   83, 90
– uracil-DNA glycosylase   148
DNA replication
– dUTPase gene   149
– helicase-primase   148
– major DNA-binding protein   39, 148
– origin binding protein   148

early genes (β)   37, 78
– DNA binding protein   39
– DNA polymerase   38
– EcoRI fragment I transcript   39
– EcoRI fragments R and d   26–33
– gB   38
– HWLF1   39
– HXLF   39–40
– ICP36   37–38
– nuclear phosphoprotein (76-kDa)   39
– transcription   26–40
– transcription-long repeat   33–37
early phase, MCMV
– inhibition of pp89 expression in   213
early phosphoproteins
– spliced early transcripts   149
early transcription   3, 33
enhancer   85
envelope glycoproteins
– gB homolog   229–231
– gCII   232–233
– gH homolog   231–232
enzymes of nucleotide metabolism
– deoxyribonucleoside kinases   147
– DHPG   147

– ribonucleotide reductase   147
– thymidine kinase   147

c-fos   12

β-galactosidase   63, 182
gB homolog   38, 155
GCN4 protein   10
gene expression   47
gene families   157
– gene function   62
gene layouts   160
gH homolog   155
G-protein coupled receptor family
– β-adrenergic receptors   160
– opsin family homology   159
glycoprotein complexes   172
glycoprotein genes
– anchor sequences   152
– glycoprotein exons   152
– N-linked glycosylation sites   152
– signal sequences   152
glycoproteins   171
– gA   267
– gB   268
glycosylated envelope proteins   172
guinea pig cytomegalovirus   101
– brain   104
– DNA sequence homology   111
– hematopoietic and lymphoid tissues   108
– IE protein synthesis   117
– IE transcription   116
– labyrinthitis   106
– placenta   107
– restriction endonuclease maps   110
– salivary gland   102

HCMV gene superfamily   162
hemopoiesis
– bone marrow aplasia   198–200
– effect of MCMV on stem cell
    generation   200
herpes simplex virus type 1   62
– β-herpesviruses   48
histopathology, prevention of   193, 196, 197
host range
– human CMV   48–49
– human fibroblast   49
host versus graft response   80
HQLF1 open reading frame   25
human glycoprotein hormone gene   10
human immunodeficiency viruses   14, 78

Immediate early genes (α)
– enhancer region   8–16, 85–90
– functional organization   6–16, 55–62
– genomic localization   3–4, 24–26, 55–58

– IE gene expression   24, 78, 83–96
– IE murine CMV   204
– IE1   24, 143
– IE2a   144
– IE2b   144
– 5.0 kb RNA   24
– Kozak consensus ATG   144
– major IE promoter (MIEP)   84–92
– NF-1/CTF binding domain   90–91
– spliced transcripts   144
– transcription   4–6, 26–39, 55–62, 84–85
immediate-early (IE), MCMV
– genes and proteins   204–205
– immunodominant antigens for
    CTL   202–204, 207
– phase in replication   203–204, 213
IEI enhancer region
– 18 bp repeat element   8
– cAMP-response element (CRE)   12
– DNAse 1 footprinting   8
– dyad symmetry   10
– heat shock   15
– modular organization   15
– 19 bp palindrome   9
– nucleoprotein complex   9
– protein kinase C   13
– repeat elements   8
– 17 bp repeat   15
– 21 bp repeat   15
– TPA   13
– transcription factors   9
– transcription factor AP-1   13
– transient expression   12
immediate early-1-upstream region
– DNAse 1 hypersensitive sites   8
– enhancer   7, 25
– enhancer trap   7
– IE promoter   7
– modulator region   8
– nuclear factor 1 (NF-1)   7
– trans-regulation factors   8
IE-2   24, 63
IE-3   24
immediate early gene expression
– NF-kβ   58–61
– protein-DNA complexes   58
– transactivation   55, 60
immediate early proteins
– transactivation   6
immediate early (α) gene regulation
    and function   55
immediate early transcription
– anisomycin   3
– cycloheximide   3
– immediate early (IE)   3
– IE-1 region   4, 55, 91
– IE-2 region   5, 91
– major IE protein   5
– nuclease mapping   5
– promoter   5
– polyadenylation signal   6

– splicing 5
IE protein pp89, MCMV
– antigenic peptides of 211–212
– as antigen for CTL 206–207
– deletion mutants of 205–210
– interaction with histones and DNA 205–206
– mapping of antigenic site 208–212
– regulatory function 205
immune response
– cell mediated immunity 52
– cytoxic T-cell response 52
– neutralizing antibodies 51
– subunit vaccine gA/gB 269–271
– Towne live virus vaccine 256–267
immunity
– human CMV 51–52
– murine CMV 51–52
– natural killer (NK) cell 52
immunity, protective
– CD8$^+$CD4$^-$T lymphocytes, role
   in 193–197, 201–202
– CD8$^-$CD4$^+$T lymphocytes, role
   in 195–196
– CD8$^-$CD4$^-$T lymphocytes, role
   in 201
– natural killer cells, role in 193
immunoaffinity-purified gA/gB 267
interleukin-2
– application in vivo 195
– in estimation of CTL precursor
   frequencies 203
– phenotype of responsive T lymphocytes 194
interstitital pneumonia 191, 196
intracellular viral proteins
– capsid proteins 225
– delayed early (β) proteins 223–224
– DNA-binding proteins 223–224
– immediate early (α) proteins 26, 29, 223
– late (γ) proteins 224
– viral DNA polymerase 224

c-jun 13

Kozak ATG 144, 145, 151, 158

late DNA-binding proteins
– ICP 36 family 37, 150
late genes 76
late transcription 3
latency
– human CMV 47, 50–51, 53–54
– mechanism 48
– murine CMV 62
– spleen 53
latent infection
– culture models 53
latent infection, MCMV
– control by CD8$^+$T lymphcytes 202

– escape from immune response 213
leucine zipper 95
live vaccines 256–267
L-S junction fragments 25

major early transcripts
– long repeats 145
– β2-microglobulin-binding 155
– strain differences 146–147
MHC antigens
– homolog 155
– T-cell receptor 156
MHC class I 233
modulator 90
morphogenesis, of MCMV virions 191
– implication of persistent infection 202
– relation to pathogenicity and
   attenuation 191, 192–193
murine cytomegalovirus 7, 51, 62, 87, 242
– cause of death 197, 200
– α gene expression 66
– immunocompetent host 191
– immunocompromised host 192
– persistence 64
– salivary gland 64, 66
mutagenesis
– murine CMV 61

neutralizing antibodies 182
NF-K-β-binding site 14, 57, 89
NF-1/CTF 90
NK cells 244
non-specific immune response 243
nonstructural viral proteins (MCMV)
– recognition by CTL 203, 207
– significance in protective
   immunity 203, 207–208, 214
nucleotide sequence homology 49

O-linked glycosylation 151

pathogenesis of CMV 48–51
peptides, antigenic 211–212
peripheral blood mononuclear cells 76
persistent infection 47
persistent infection, MCMV
– acinar glandular epithelial cells,
   of 191, 202
– CD4-T-lymphocyte deficiency,
   during 201–202
– cytoimmunotherapy, after 197
– salivary glands, in 191, 194–195, 202
phosphoenolpyruvate carboxykinase 12
phosphoproteins 29, 37, 171
phosphotransferase 149
postranscriptional 30, 54
prevention of infection 255

promoter 84
protein kinase 89, 149
proteolytic cleavage 155
pseudorabies 13

rat somatostatin gene 10
reading frames
– class 1 HLA (homologous) 129
– codon bias 136
– conserved spliced gene 131
– DNA replication 130
– dUTPase 130
– gB 130
– G + C content 136
– GCR family 129, 134
– helicase 132
– ICP 36 protein family 129
– IEI 132
– IE2A 132
– major capsid protein 131
– major DNA-binding protein 130
– major early transcript 128
– nucleotide composition 137
– phosphoproteins 91, 132
– phosphotransferase 131
– pp28 131
– pp65 131
– pp71 131
– pp150 129
– ribonucleotide reductase 129
– RL11 family 128, 133
– spliced IE glycoprotein 133
– UL 25 family 129
– UL 82 family 131
– uracil-DNA glycosylase 132
– US 1 family 133, 134
– US 2 family 133
– US 6 family 133, 134
– US 12 family 134
– US 22 family 129, 134
regulation of gene expression 54
renal transplants 79
resistance, to MCMV 191
RL11 family 128, 133
– immunoglobulin superfamily 157
– glycosylation 157
RNA polymerase III transcript 150

salivary glands, infection
    of 50, 190–196, 206
sequence analysis
– "a" sequence 126
– restriction maps 127
simian cytomegalovirus 7, 85, 89
SV40 T-antigen 9
SV40 enhancer 14
structural phosphoprotein genes
– matrix phosphoproteins 151

– 67-kDa nonglycosylated phosphoprotein
    154
– pp65 151
– pp71 151
– virion tegument 151
structural proteins
– complement-dependent neutralizing
    antibodies 182
– cross reactivity 176, 179
– dense body fraction 177, 178
– disulfide-linked glycoproteins 179
– extracellular virion forms 226
– β-galactosidase fusion proteins 174
– intracellular development of virions 225
– lambda gt11 cDNA 174
– lower matrix protein 177
– major capsid protein 131, 173, 227
– matrix protein 177
– phosphorylated structural
    polypeptides 177
– recombinant peptides 177
– viral matrix proteins 226
subunit vaccine 267–271

T-cell receptor homolog
– TCRγ 156
T-lymphocytes (see CD8-positive,
    see cytolytic, see
    immunity) 59, 259
T-lymphocytes (CD8-positive)
– antigen specificity,
    MCMV 202–204, 207–208
– antiviral efficacy in acute infection 194–199
– CD4-helper independent generation 201
– control of persistent and latent
    infection 201–202
– prevention of bone marrow aplasia 202
– prevention of viral histopathology 193,
    196–197
– protection by 208
– relation to CTL 202–203
temporal classes 22
teratocarcinoma cells 82
– HCMV replication 82–84
tissue specificity 75–96
trans-acting factors 29
transcriptional enhancers 54
transcription factors 35, 55
transmission of CMV 48

UL 37 IE gene
– glycoprotein 145
– spliced 145
– third position G + C 145
upstream regulatory elements 28, 35
US 3 IE gene
– 11 bp repeats 144
– enhancer 144

– glycosylation   144
– spliced transcripts   144
US 6 family
– glycoproteins   158
US 22 family
– spliced transcripts   158

vaccinia recombinant viruses
vaccine, experimental in
     MCMV   207–208
–antigenicity and immunogenicity of
     MCMV-ieI-VAC   207, 272

– deletion mutants of MCMV-ie1-VAC
     209–210
– experimental vaccine, as   207–208, 272
vasoactive intestinal polypeptide
     of proenkephalin   12
virus-host interactions   48
virus-neutralizing antibodies   259

zinc fingers   95